Comprehensive
Coronary
Care

Comprehensive Coronary Care

Nigel I Jowett

MD, MRCP, MB BS, MRCS, LRCP

Senior Medical Registrar
Coronary Care Unit
Leicester General Hospital

and

David R Thompson

PhD, BSc, SRN, RMN, ONC

Lecturer in Nursing
University of Liverpool

SCUTARI PRESS

© Scutari Press 1989

A division of Scutari Projects, the publishing company of
the Royal College of Nursing

First published 1989

British Library Cataloguing-in-Publication Data

Jowett, Nigel I.
  Comprehensive Coronary Care.
  1. Man. Heart. Coronary diseases
  I. Title   II. Thompson, David R
  616.1′23

  ISBN 1-871364-05-1

Typeset by Blackpool Typesetting Services Ltd, Blackpool
Printed in Great Britain at the Alden Press Oxford London and Northampton

Contents

*'One man is as good as another until he has
written a book'*

*From: The Letters of Benjamin Jowett (1899)
Volume 1, Abbott and Campbell.*

Dedicated to our wives who endured long absences whilst we were
bettering ourselves

Preface

The role of coronary care has changed markedly since its inception in the early 1960s, and it now has an extended importance for patients with other manifestations of coronary artery disease, and for those with critical cardiac dysfunction who require intensive care and cardiovascular monitoring. This book is intended as an up-to-date guide to this current practice of 'cardiac intensive care', and to provide a basis for further exploration of the subject. Because we believe that such practice is not the sole domain of either nursing or medical staff we have tried to utilise an integrated approach, suitable for all those concerned in patient management on the coronary care unit. Some of our material extends outside the traditional boundaries of coronary care, but we think it important that it is appreciated how the patients come to be there, and what may happen to them after they leave.

Whilst we hope that nurses never lose sight of their primary caring role, in reality much of their work in the area of coronary care involves a high degree of medical and technical expertise, and our book reflects this. We have assumed that nurse-readers have a basic understanding of primary nursing, the nursing process, nursing theories and conceptual models, and only salient features are mentioned in the text.

Nigel I Jowett
David R Thompson

1

Introduction to Coronary Care

Cardiovascular disease has become the major cause of morbidity and mortality in all Western industrialised countries (table 1.1). It is responsible for the deaths of 41 per cent of men aged 35 to 44 years, and of 52 per cent of men aged 45 to 54 years. In women, it is the second biggest killer (cancer being the first). Roughly half these cardiovascular deaths are due to coronary heart disease and one in five men will have a heart attack before retirement. Although the rising mortality rate has slowed over the last few years, coronary heart disease is still depriving the economy of people in their most productive years, and many young families of their parents. Coronary heart disease may present as congestive cardiac failure, conduction defects, dysrhythmias, angina pectoris or myocardial infarction. Most cases of unexpected death are also attributable to coronary heart disease. The detection of coronary atherosclerosis is often delayed because the degree of coronary artery disease may be masked by coronary reserve; coronary insufficiency only becomes obvious when there is disequilibrium between the demand for oxygen by the myocardium and the coronary blood supply. As a result, by the time clinical signs and symptoms of coronary heart disease have developed, atherosclerosis is usually in an advanced stage, with stenosed arteries lined by calcified and necrotic atheromatous plaques. Therapy would at this stage seem nothing more than palliative, and management should ideally concentrate on preventative measures.

In a recent World Health Organisation report (World Health Organisation, 1979), the concept of 'comprehensive cardiac care' was outlined as a systematic approach to the control of heart disease throughout the whole of its natural history. In the context of acute myocardial infarction, this comprises:

● Primary and secondary prevention of coronary heart disease
● Pre-hospital care of acute myocardial infarction (including 'bystander' resuscitation and coronary ambulances)
● The role of the coronary care unit
● Rehabilitation of the post-coronary patient

PRIMARY AND SECONDARY PREVENTION OF MYOCARDIAL INFARCTION

Primary prevention of coronary heart disease aims at either preventing the first heart attack, or delaying the appearance of other symptoms related to myocardial

Table 1.1. Age-standardised mortality from ischaemic heart disease in 1980. Rates per 100 000 population aged 40–69 years.

Males		Females	
Northern Ireland	630	Scotland	208
Finland	599	Northern Ireland	191
Scotland	592	New Zealand	178
Eire	499	Eire	160
England and Wales	482	England and Wales	136
New Zealand	468	Hungary	134
Czechoslovakia	438	Australia	133
Australia	421	Czechoslovakia	132
Hungary	410	United States of America	130
United States of America	398	Israel	128
Denmark	392	Finland	121
Canada	390	Canada	118
Norway	390	Denmark	112
Sweden	386	Bulgaria	100
Netherlands	323	Romania	93
West Germany	314	Sweden	90
Israel	314	Norway	86
Austria	293	Austria	80
Poland	282	Netherlands	78
Bulgaria	268	West Germany	75
Belgium	264	Belgium	72
Switzerland	219	Yugoslavia	71
Italy	212	Poland	66
Romania	202	Italy	53
Yugoslavia	197	Switzerland	47
France	137	France	30
Japan	65	Japan	24

(From Wells, 1987. Reproduced by permission of the Office of Health Economics)

ischaemia (such as dysrhythmias, heart failure and angina). Secondary prevention includes any treatment that reduces the risk of sudden death or a second heart attack in a patient who has already suffered one myocardial infarction. The two modes of prevention will not necessarily be the same since the underlying pathological processes and relative risks are not the same. The benefits of therapy will not necessarily be the same either.

Many different factors may lead to damage of the coronary vasculature to produce the same final result: accumulation of atheroma and coronary artery disease. Attention is usually focused on certain risk factors which have been implicated in the accelerated development of ischaemic heart disease (Joint Working Party of the Royal College of Physicians and the British Cardiac Society, 1976). These include hypertension, hyperlipidaemia, diabetes mellitus, cigarette smoking, obesity, physical inactivity and stress. However, these disorders alone are not implicated in all cases of coronary heart disease, and there may additionally be an inherited risk. The presence of early coronary heart disease in a first-degree relative is very common in young patients who present with myocardial infarction, and as such represents a strong risk factor. This, of course, may simply reflect the similarity of a shared environment and life-style, but it is likely that there is a significant genetic predisposition (Jowett, 1984).

The incidence of ischaemic heart disease is higher in certain populations. Even within individual countries there may be great variation in its incidence. There is also marked variation between the different social classes: higher rates are found in those with manual or unskilled jobs than in professional men. All these variations are strongly associated with 'life-style', which usually means the type of occupation, amount of daily exercise, and dietary, alcohol and smoking habits.

Population strategies such as that carried out in North Karelia, Finland, aimed at both primary and secondary prevention, and arose directly out of community concern over the high mortality from coronary heart disease. Major risk factor intervention took place with the help of environmental services to bring about a change in life-style. Follow-up studies have shown that the reduction in risk factors has persisted now that a healthier way of life has been established, and probably as a result there has been a reduction in mortality of about 20 per cent in men and 50 per cent in women. 'High-risk' intervention', as recently seen in the USA, involves the identification and treatment of those found to be at greatest risk of heart attacks. The Lipid Research Clinic study (1984) has clearly shown, for example, that reducing very high levels of serum cholesterol decreases the risk of angina and myocardial infarction. It is, however, important to realise that about half of all patients with ischaemic heart disease are not usually considered to be high risk.

There has been a recent decline in the mortality from coronary heart disease in some countries, including the USA and Australia (figure 1.1), whilst there has been little change or even an increase in Britain and Sweden (Heller et al, 1983; Stamler, 1985; Pell and Fayerweather, 1985). It is not known whether the decline in death rate represents a reduced incidence or fatality rate. Explanations as to why the mortality rate is falling have pointed to a combination of factors rather than a single cause (Goldman and Cook, 1984; Gillum et al, 1984; Kannel and Thom, 1984). What has been seen in those countries with a falling coronary mortality rate is a general change in life-style with a reduction in the smoking rate and ingestion of saturated fats, and an increase in levels of physical activity (especially jogging). Most of these risk factors are over-represented in the UK, and it is likely that only health education and intervention strategies directed at the whole population will lead to a fall in coronary heart disease mortality in this country.

It has been suggested that improved medical management of coronary heart disease may be responsible for a 40 per cent reduction in coronary mortality (Beaglehole, 1986). The major advance has come from resuscitation before admission to hospital and the improved recognition and control of hypertension. A smaller contribution has come from the work of coronary care units. The detection and treatment of potentially fatal dysrhythmias following myocardial infarction is obviously of major importance here. The incidence of ventricular fibrillation is about 5 per cent of admissions to coronary care, of which 90 per cent are usually reversed. Mortality at one year, however, is about 30 per cent. The role that coronary care units have played in the falling mortality rate from coronary heart disease is therefore likely to extend beyond the treatment of dysrhythmias, and has probably resulted from the improved control of heart failure and limitation of infarct size. Early surgical intervention, including coronary artery surgery, repair of surgical defects caused by myocardial

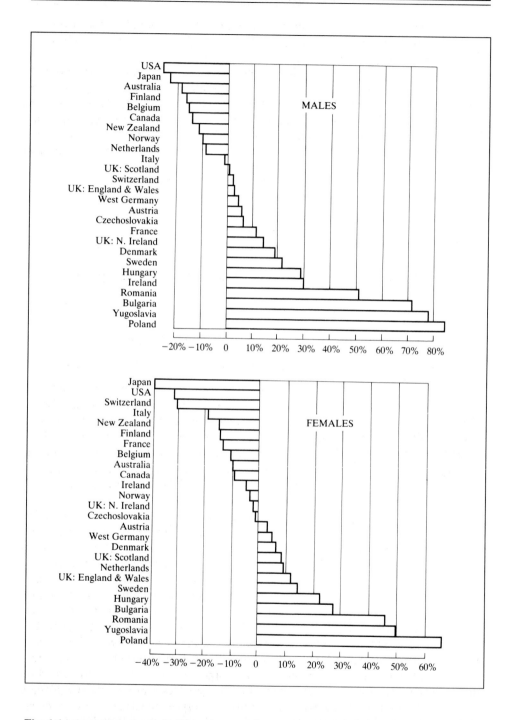

Fig. 1.1 Average percentage change in mortality from ischaemic heart disease at ages 40 to 69 years over 1968–1989 in (a) males and (b) females. (From Wells, 1987. Reproduced by kind permission of the Office of Health Economics)

infarction (such as left ventricular aneurysms and dysfunctional mitral valves) and coronary artery angioplasty are also having a major impact on the falling cardiovascular mortality (see chapter 15).

The control of coronary heart disease by secondary prevention has become more encouraging with recent reports on the use of beta-adrenergic blocking agents following myocardial infarction (Yusef et al, 1985). The evidence is that if these drugs are started within the first three weeks of myocardial infarction, the first-year mortality is reduced. There appears to be no major difference between the selected beta-blockers employed, but most work has focused on propranolol, timolol and metoprolol. Their value in acute administration (within hours of the infarct) is not so clear, but their use may reduce the incidence of dysrhythmias.

THE CORONARY CARE UNIT

Cardiac intensive care units have really been designed for three purposes.

1. To provide a separate area within the hospital for the care and monitoring of critically ill patients

2. To provide care by nurses and physicians with specialist training

3. To have personnel and equipment immediately available for resuscitation

Following the first description of cardiac resuscitation by Vesalius in the sixteenth century, there were many sporadic reports of success in restarting the arrested heart. However, it was not until 1933 that specific measures, including open heart massage and defibrillation, were suggested following work in animals (Hooker et al, 1933). Its application to humans had to wait until 1947, when Claude Beck used open heart massage and direct cardiac defibrillation to resuscitate a 14-year-old boy who developed ventricular fibrillation in the operating theatre following chest surgery (Beck et al, 1947).

It was only 30 years ago that it was first realised that these methods could be applied outside the operating theatre to those at greatest risk, i.e. patients who had sustained an acute myocardial infarction (Beck et al, 1956; Reagan et al, 1956). Later, the application of external defibrillation described by Zoll et al (1956) with Kouwenhoven's description of external cardiac massage (Kouwenhoven et al, 1960) formed the basis of cardiopulmonary resuscitation as we know it today. Julian (1961) suggested that all hospital staff should be trained in these new methods of resuscitation and, although frequently successful in practice, the primary problem of effective resuscitation then became the delay in reaching the patient following cardiac arrest. Hence, it was reasoned that for such methods to be effective a unit would be required where trained staff would be immediately available, and where patients at risk could be under constant supervision. It was in this way that the concept of coronary care units emerged. Before these units existed, treatment of acute myocardial infarction was exclusively directed towards the healing of the infarct and the prevention of cardiac rupture. However, the recognition of the importance of rhythm monitoring and prompt defibrillation revolutionised the management of coronary patients.

The first purpose-built coronary care unit was opened on 20 May 1962 by Hughes Day in Kansas City, and others quickly followed in Toronto and Philadelphia (Day, 1972). From then on, medical and public demand led to a rapid appearance of similar units, so that by the early 1970s most large hospitals had facilities for monitoring the acute coronary patient, either as part of a general ward or as a separate intensive care unit. Since the inception of these units, relatively few studies have been carried out to test their efficacy. No adequate long-term randomised trial has been carried out, and it seems unlikely now that one ever will be. There is little doubt that patient mortality has fallen for those initially cared for on coronary care (Chapman, 1979), but their value in uncomplicated myocardial infarction is questionable. There is evidence to suggest that some patients might fare better at home, or on ordinary medical wards (Hill et al, 1977). With the rising costs of medical health care, these issues should still be considered. It should not be forgotten that there are many patients who do not need to be rushed into hospital following a myocardial infarction, let alone into an intensive care unit. These include those living at a great distance from the hospital, the elderly and some others with coexisting illnesses.

THE ORGANISATION OF THE CORONARY CARE UNIT

The design, staffing and organisation of such cardiac intensive care units is of great importance. The style of management will vary from unit to unit, but it is important that decisions are democratic rather than autocratic. Failure to adopt this style is likely to interfere with overall patient management. Stress levels in staff members on the unit (which in turn will be transmitted to the patient) are likely to be high, and such an atmosphere is less likely to encourage individual initiative (Henderson, 1980). A unit providing intensive care for the acute coronary will need to be under the direction of a physician responsible for administration. However, it is desirable that selection and training of staff, unit policy and therapy is subject to discussion by all staff on the unit.

The design and layout of coronary care has to be a compromise between desirability and practicality. For psychological reasons, the patients may be better accommodated in individual rooms, so that they are unaware of other patients' problems, and are protected from the high drama of cardiac arrests. However, although this design may allow privacy and promote rest, it makes no allowance for direct vision of the patient by the staff. This factor is obviously a prime consideration in coronary care and, apart from its main role of spotting early signs of distress, may lead to a feeling of isolation by the patients, and fear about not being discovered if they were to collapse.

It should also be possible to move patients around without transfer between beds or trollies. This causes a great deal of physical effort, especially if the patient is overweight or arthritic. It may also involve involuntary use of the Valsalva manoeuvre producing potentially adverse vagal overstimulation. Doors should therefore be wide enough to permit the passage of beds in and out of the unit. Patient bed areas must be large enough to accommodate staff and equipment, and probably no smaller than $10\,\mathrm{m}^2$. Each bed should have piped oxygen and suction, and must be of suitable design for manoeuvring in case of resuscitation. The bedhead must be easily removable, and the base must be rigid (or easily made so with an 'arrest board'). Equipment should if possible be located on the walls and securely fixed. There should additionally be sufficient natural (and artificial) light, with window views to the outside world, so that the patient does not become unduly disorientated. Noise insulation and air-conditioning is important for comfort and to promote rest.

A separate procedure room is desirable for elective cardioversion and temporary pacing away from the main unit. Provision should be made for interviewing relatives in private, and this should be additional to a normal visitors' waiting room. Staff coffee and rest rooms are useful for periods of relaxation. A lecture room should perhaps also be included in the design of a cardiac intensive care unit, equipped with projection facilities and audiovisual aids, for continuing medical education and rehabilitation discussion group meetings.

STAFFING

Intensive care units have now been in existence for more than 30 years. In the United Kingdom and Scandinavia, they have principally become part of the department of anaesthesia. Elsewhere in Europe, the anaesthetists are in charge of surgical intensive care, and the department of internal medicine runs the medical intensive care units. Coronary care units have become entirely separate areas usually managed by physicians and/or cardiologists. Despite all the advances with machinery, recording equipment and other useful technology on intensive care units, the most important resource remains its staff. Both the equipment and the staff must work smoothly, reliably and efficiently all the time. There is usually a high work load, with many responsibilities and emotional demands, and although many people relish this atmosphere, others may find it overpowering. Ashworth (1986) has made reference to the classification of staff (and patients) as 'drains or radiators'. The former group leave you drained and exhausted after an encounter, whilst the 'radiators' radiate warmth and other good qualities, leaving you feeling better. Intensive care units need to develop a functional maturity, where each member is a radiator of professional competence and support. Although there will be times when, under pressure, we all become drains, inter-professional teamwork requires everybody involved to make a valued contribution from their personal resources towards efficient patient care. It is essential that the staff providing coronary care have been thoroughly trained, since the risks from apathy, over-enthusiasm or ignorance may be critical. They must be adept at the psychological handling of patients who may be easily upset by thoughtless words and deeds. Patients are usually investigated and treated by two groups of doctors: the junior house physicians and the supervising consultants. Whilst the consultant staff direct the management of the patients, it is the junior medical staff who are responsible for the day-to-day care of the patients on the unit. Since patients on these units require constant supervision, it is not possible for this to be undertaken on a 24-hour basis by medical staff. Accordingly, the responsibility has fallen to the nursing staff, and this has caused a major change in the role of nursing. The intensive care unit has provided a breakthrough for the nursing profession in elevating the nurse's participation in patient care far beyond anything in the past. The nursing staff have a vital role in the smooth running of coronary care, and in some units are almost entirely responsible for the care of patients. Because of the increased duties and responsibility assumed by intensive care nurses, the traditional doctor/nurse relationship has been altered, and often proves awkward to the uninitiated (Jowett, 1986). As part of the team approach, the nurse has emerged as the key to successful patient management.

PRE-HOSPITAL CARE AND BYSTANDER RESUSCITATION

'Sudden death' is a term used to describe an event which affects a group of people who at one moment appear fit and well, and then suddenly collapse to die in less than an hour (often immediately). Some of these will have experienced chest pain or dyspnoea in the preceding few days, and most will have a previous history of cardiovascular disease. The chance of survival is directly related to the speed with which resuscitative measures can be instituted. The event is presumably caused by a ventricular dysrhythmia (ventricular tachycardia or fibrillation), but whether this is triggered by coronary emboli, coronary thrombosis or biochemical abnormalities is unknown. As time passes actual myocardial necrosis will take place, with risk of heart failure or cardiogenic shock. The prognosis of the survivor of a heart attack is mainly dependent on the quantity of myocardium destroyed, although the age of the patient's heart is another important determinant. Infarcted tissue cannot be repaired, and damage will affect the heart's action as an efficient pump. The resultant cardiac failure and dysrhythmias caused by areas of necrosis and regional anoxia are the main treatable areas that will influence prognosis. In addition, other potentially fatal complications related to the infarction, such as peripheral embolisation and deep vein thromboses, will need to be considered. Primary ventricular fibrillation is the commonest cause of sudden death, and hence the urgency of rapid resuscitative measures. Approximately 30 to 50 per cent of deaths following myocardial infarction occur as sudden deaths. Studies is Seattle, USA, have shown that bystander initiated resuscitation results in a doubling of survival rates from 21 to 43 per cent; and, of those resuscitated, half leave hospital (Thompson et al, 1979). Pre-hospital care has in recent years taken on a more important role, often with specialist medical, nursing or paramedical staff employed as mobile emergency units in adapted 'coronary' ambulances (Pantridge and Geddes 1967). This has arisen because early-occurring ventricular fibrillation can be effectively treated if medical care is readily available and speedy resuscitation carries a good prognosis. The early correction of dysrhythmias and haemodynamic disturbances (such as autonomic imbalance) reduces the incidence of cardiogenic shock, and improved oxygenation of the myocardium in the early stages may help limit infarction size, and hence long-term prognosis too.

It is important to appreciate that intensive cardiac care facilities will not influence mortality rates in patients who delay a call for help (table 1.2). Success is likely if there has been a prompt call for help, efficient cardiopulmonary resuscitation and rapid admission to hospital.

Table 1.2. Time between onset of coronary symptoms and call for medical help in 200 patients admitted to coronary care* with and without previous myocardial infarction (MI).

Time (h)	Previous MI	No previous MI
<0.5	28	20
0.5–1	18	15
1–3	42	27
3–24	5	9
>24	7	29
Total	100	100

*Leicester General Hospital

IN-HOSPITAL CARE

Within hospital, rapid stabilisation, relief of pain and aggressive treatment of complications is indicated. Roughly half the patients admitted to coronary care have a complicated clinical course, and these complications mostly occur soon after admission. In general, the larger myocardial infarcts are more complicated and have a poorer prognosis; much depends upon how much functional myocardium is preserved. Intervention to salvage ischaemic myocardium has become a major target in the modern management of myocardial infarction (Hearse and Yellon, 1984), and pharmacological and mechanical therapies directed at improving myocardial oxygen supply and reducing myocardial work are the subject of current medical trials and research. In particular, the importance of relieving coronary obstruction and improving myocardial perfusion acutely by intracoronary thrombolysis or percutaneous coronary angioplasty will undoubtedly take on a more important role in the years to come.

The early success of coronary care units was probably due to better management of serious dysrhythmias, although the management of heart failure still remains a major problem. A better understanding of the pathophysiology of heart failure, with the introduction of improved haemodynamic monitoring methods and effective pharmaceutical agents, has now led to a further reduction in peri-infarction mortality. In fact, coronary care units have now extended their role to the management of cardiac problems not specifically due to acute myocardial infarction. These patients will include those with congestive cardiac failure, dysrhythmias and cardiogenic shock, and perhaps the term 'cardiac intensive care unit' (CICU) is more appropriate.

INTERMEDIATE CORONARY CARE

Since the risk of primary ventricular fibrillation is highest in the first 36 hours, there is little need for uncomplicated infarcts to remain on coronary care for longer than 24 to 48 hours. However, patients remain at increased risk of delayed complications such as ventricular fibrillation for 4 to 10 days, and late complications are responsible for up to a third of in-hospital deaths (Graboys, 1975). It is therefore perhaps justifiable to operate intermediate ('step-down') coronary care units. Such units might reduce this excess in-hospital mortality by the use of prolonged ambulatory monitoring and immediately available resuscitation facilities (Norris, 1982; Karliner and Gregoratos, 1981). An additional advantage may be that early rehabilitation and education can take place as a form of group therapy, perhaps with the patient's husband or wife being present.

REHABILITATION

Although no trial has shown the benefits of rehabilitation, there is no doubt that the quality of life may be improved by the relief of stress, anxiety and measures to prevent cardiac neurosis. Care for the cardiac patient should be directed not only towards physical problems, but also towards the patient's psychosocial well-being, and a realistic and optimistic approach by staff should be adopted. If the patient is going to die, death is likely to occur before discharge from hospital!

Early ambulation and early discharge are encouraged these days because prolonged bed rest and hospital therapy are usually not clinically necessary. This strategy will also prevent the complications caused by enforced bedrest (pressure sores, thromboembolic disorders, etc.), and additionally will reduce depression and physical weakness. Free discussion is to be encouraged at all times with advice on diet, smoking, exercise, work and sexual activity. The use of videotapes and pamphlets may be useful in this context.

CARDIAC INTENSIVE CARE AND THE NURSE

Cardiac intensive care by the nurse requires that she be skilled at:

1. Giving complete nursing care to the patient under her care

2. Collection and recording of clinical data, and taking appropriate action when necessary

3. Communication with her patient, his relatives, her colleagues and co-professionals

Expectations of the nursing staff by themselves and others is changing. Within the sphere of coronary care in particular, nurses are expected to take on greater responsibilities as well as learning new technical skills. This requires a willing approach, and for others to respect their expertise and authority. Nursing is not just keeping the patients fed, their beds made and bowels emptied. Unfortunately, in their attempts to throw off the submissive role of brainless handmaidens, some nurses have openly become 'anti-doctor', which is, of course, counter-productive. Both the medical and the nursing staff (and the allied professions) need to demonstrate interpersonal confidence and trust, with good communication and mutual support. The concept of intensive cardiac nursing is based on a team approach with the nurse and attending physician sharing the responsibility for patient care (Abdellah, 1972). Frequently their work overlaps, particularly in technical aspects, but it is perhaps more important for nurses to concentrate primarily on nursing matters rather than to become too engrossed in medical areas. Since the introduction of coronary care units, the role of the cardiac nurse has not been able to remain static. It has had to keep pace with advances in medicine and technology, which reflect the uniqueness of the nursing function within coronary care. Nurses have continually had to redefine their function in terms of the unit/patient needs rather than in the sphere of traditional nursing. Although this was not fully appreciated in the early days of coronary care units, as expectations of the function of the nurse have changed, so too has the attitude towards them. In former days, education programmes for nursing staff were virtually non-existent, and the few that did exist were not set up by the nursing profession, enabling it to determine its own particular educational needs. Programmes concentrated on pathophysiology, pharmacology and technology, with psychosocial, moral and spiritual issues being ignored. With this in mind, the Joint Board for Clinical Nursing Studies (JBCNS) was set up in 1970 to provide a post-basic course for the registered nurse. This was superseded by the four National Boards for Nursing, Midwifery and Health Visiting which are now responsible for the setting of the syllabus and approval of centres to run the courses (e.g. ENB course No. 124). Although this has certainly been a major advance in the United Kingdom, the JBCNS and to a lesser extent the ENB are still emphasising the technical and medical components, and have failed to provide sufficient emphasis on the theory and practice of nursing. Coronary care nursing means much more than the recording of vital signs and readings from machines. The nurse needs to be competent in assessing the various needs of the patient and his family to ensure the provision of physical comfort, safety and emotional support (Thompson, 1985). Although medical care has improved the physical well-being of the patient, successful recovery in terms of psychosocial outcome is still a problem (Wilson-Barnett, 1979). The illness itself, hospitalisation and therapy present their own problems, to say nothing of the effect of the alien and technical atmosphere of an intensive care unit, which frequently frightens trained medical and nursing staff on their first visit, let alone patients and their relatives.

Good coronary care nursing is based upon general nursing principles, to maintain as near normal life-styles as possible, and helping the patient perform daily activities. The nurse must be able to assess and interpret the patient's needs, set priorities, make judgements and take the necessary actions. It is only in addition to this that she need be skilled in technological advances, although experience in cardiopulmonary resuscitation (CPR) is obviously vital. Most cardiac patients are totally reliant on nursing support, whether being revived following cardiac arrest or in the physical and emotional support of themselves and their families. It is distressing to realise that many coronary care staff today are more skilled at invasive and technical manoeuvres than in recognising the need for them.

Until recently, nurses have tended to rely on others for guidance and direction rather than assuming the role of decision maker. The ability to make decisions quickly has become vital within coronary care (Thompson and Sutton, 1985), and can only come with expertise and knowledge. As professionals, nurses have a responsibility to themselves as well as to their patients and colleagues for continuing education. This includes frequent updating by reading relevant literature and keeping informed of professional issues and clinical practice. This should perhaps be seen as an obligatory and not an optional part of a professional approach to patient care. Clinical research and application by nurses is a relatively new concept in intensive care nursing, and should not be seen to be the domain of the medical staff.

The final contribution which nurses may make is in the role of the coronary care nurse in the community, and nurses should not perhaps view themselves as hospital based, in the isolation of the coronary care unit. They can perform a significant role in family education and physical rehabilitation of the patient (Hentinen, 1986). Their role is increasing in counselling sessions, exercise programmes and relaxation classes. Unfortunately, these rehabilitation services are as yet poorly developed in the United Kingdom, and rely heavily on community and voluntary services. There is now a role for the cardiac nurse as a community nurse specialist, as an expert nurse-practitioner in both the hospital and the community, and, as yet, the potential for this has not yet been seized (Thompson and Webster, 1986).

References

Abdellah F (1972) The nursing role in the coronary care system. In: *Textbook of Coronary Care,* eds. Meltzer L E and Dunning A J, pp. 35–51. Amsterdam: Excerpta Medica.

Ashworth P (1986) Doctors, nurses and others in ICU–'drains' or 'radiators'. *Intensive Care Nursing,* 1: 165–167.

Beaglehole R (1986) Medical management and the decline in mortality from coronary heart disease. *British Medical Journal,* 292: 33–35.

Beck C S, Pritchard W H and Feil H S (1947) Ventricular fibrillation of long duration abolished by electric shock. *Journal of the American Medical Association,* 135: 985–986.

Beck C S, Weckesser E C and Barry F M (1956) Fatal heart attack and successful defibrillation. *Journal of the American Medical Association,* 161: 434–436.

Chapman B L (1979) Effect of coronary care on myocardial infarction mortality. *British Heart Journal,* 42: 386–395.

Day H W (1972) History of coronary care units. *American Journal of Cardiology,* 30: 405–407.

Gillum R F, Folsom M R and Blackburn H (1984) Decline in coronary heart disease mortality. *American Journal of Medicine,* 76: 1055–1065.

Goldman L and Cook E E F (1984) The decline in ischaemic heart disease mortality rates. *Annals of Internal Medicine,* 101: 825–836.

Graboys T B (1975) In-hospital sudden death after coronary care unit discharge. *Archives of Internal Medicine,* 135: 512–514.

Hearse D J and Yellon D M (1984) *Therapeutic Approaches to Myocardial Infarct Size Limitation.* New York: Raven Press.

Heller R F, Hatward D and Hobbs M S T (1983) Decline in rate of death from ischaemic heart disease in the United Kingdom. *British Medical Journal,* 286: 260–262.

Henderson V (1980) Preserving the essence of nursing in a technological age. *Journal of Advanced Nursing,* 5: 245–260.

Hentinen M (1986) Teaching and adaption of patients with myocardial infarction. *International Journal of Nursing Studies,* 23: 125–138.

Hill J D, Holdstock G and Hampton J R (1977) Comparison of mortality of patients with heart attacks admitted to a CCU and an ordinary medical ward. *British Medical Journal,* ii: 81–83.

Hooker D R, Kouwenhoven W B and Langworthy A R (1933) Effects of alternating electrical currents on the heart. *American Journal of Physiology,* 103: 444–454.

Joint Working Party of the Royal College of Physicians and the British Cardiac Society (1976) Prevention of coronary heart disease. *Journal of the Royal College of Physicians of London,* 10: 213–275.

Jowett N I (1984) *Recombinant DNA gene-specific probes and the genetic analysis of diabetes, hyperlipidaemia and coronary heart disease.* MD Thesis, University of London.

Jowett N I (1986) The junior doctor on the intensive care unit. *Intensive Care Nursing,* **1:** 177–179.

Julian D G (1961) Treatment of cardiac arrest in acute myocardial ischaemia and infarction. *Lancet* **ii:** 840–844.

Kannel W B and Thom T J (1984) Declining cardiovascular mortality. *Circulation,* **70:** 331–336.

Karliner J S and Gregoratos G (1981) *Acute Coronary Care.* Edinburgh: Churchill Livingstone.

Kouwenhoven W B, Jude J R and Knickerbocker G G (1960) Closed chest cardiac massage. *Journal of the American Medical Association,* **178:** 1064–1067.

Lipid Research Clinics Coronary Primary Prevention Trial Results I and II (1984) *Journal of the American Medical Association,* **251:** 351–374.

Norris R M (1982) *Myocardial Infarction.* Edinburgh: Churchill Livingstone.

Pantridge J F and Geddes J S (1967) A mobile intensive care unit in the management of myocardial infarction. *Lancet,* **ii:** 271–273.

Pell S and Fayerweather W E (1985) Trends in the incidence of myocardial infarction and in associated mortality and morbidity in a large employed population 1957–1983. *New England Journal of Medicine,* **312:** 1005–1011.

Reagan L B, Young K R and Nicholson J W (1956) Ventricular fibrillation in a patient with probable acute coronary occlusion. *Surgery,* **39:** 482–486.

Stamler J (1985) The marked decline in CHD mortality rates in the United States 1968–1981. *Cardiology,* **72:** 11–22.

Thompson D R (1985) Intensive care nursing: neglected areas. *Nursing Mirror,* **160:** 38–42.

Thompson D R and Sutton T W (1985) Nursing decision-making in a coronary care unit. *International Journal of Nursing Studies,* **22:** 259–266.

Thompson D R and Webster R A (1986) The clinical nurse specialist in critical care. *Nursing Practice,* **1:** 136–142.

Thompson R G, Hallstrom A P and Cobb L A (1979) By-stander initiated cardiopulmonary resuscitation in the management of ventricular fibrillation. *Annals of Internal Medicine,* **90:** 737-740.

Wells N (1987) *Coronary Heart Disease: The Need for Action.* London: Office of Health Economics.

Wilson-Barnett J (1979) *Stress in Hospital: Patients' Psychological Reactions to Illness and Health Care.* Edinburgh: Churchill Livingstone.

World Health Organisation Working Group on the Development of Coronary Care in the Community (1979) *Review of Developments in Coronary Care in the Last 5 Years.* ICP/CVD 003(9).

Yusuf S, Peto R, Lewis J, Collins R and Sleight P (1985) Beta-blockade during and after myocardial infarction: an overview of randomised trials. *Progress in Cardiovascular Diseases,* **27:** 335-371.

Zoll P M, Linenthal A J, Gibson W, Paul M and Norman L (1956) Termination of ventricular fibrillation in man by externally applied countershock. *New England Journal of Medicine,* **254:** 727–732.

2

Anatomy and Physiology

THE ANATOMY OF THE HEART

The heart is a hollow muscular organ which is located behind the costal cartilages in the middle mediastinum. The size of the heart corresponds quite accurately with the size of the patient's clenched fist and weighs about 280–340 g. It lies obliquely in the chest, and resembles an inverted cone, with the base facing upwards, and the apex pointing downwards, forwards and to the left (figure 2.1). About two-thirds of the heart lies to the left, and one-third to the right of the median plane. The apex lies a little below and medial to the left nipple in the 5th intercostal space, and can usually be seen as the apex beat.

At the junction of the upper one-third and lower two-thirds of the heart, a deep oblique *atrioventricular groove* passes round the heart, separating the atria from the ventricles. From this, two other grooves extend towards the apex anteriorly (the *anterior interventricular groove*) and posteriorly (the *posterior interventricular groove*). These mark the position of the *interventricular septum* which separates the right and left ventricles internally. The junction of the posterior interventricular and posterior atrioventricular grooves is known as the *crux*. Internally, at this junction, the *interatrial septum* joins the interventricular septum.

The tough, fibrous pericardium encloses the heart and serves to limit any sudden cardiac distension. Within the fibrous pericardium and extending onto the surface

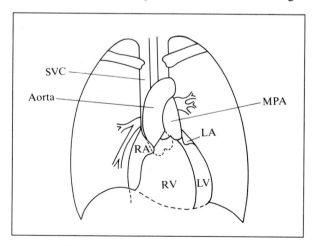

Fig. 2.1 Anterior view of the heart
RA = right atrium; LA = left atrium; RV = right ventricle; LV = left ventricle;
MPA = main pulmonary artery; SVC = superior vena cava.

of the heart is a thin, delicate membrane, the *serous pericardium*. This has been invaginated by the heart during development to form a two-layered structure. The outer parietal layer lines the inner surface of the fibrous pericardium, and the inner visceral layer (*epicardium*) covers the outer surface of the heart and the adjoining portions of the great vessels. Where the great vessels pass through the fibrous pericardium, the two layers of the serous pericardium are reflected back, and become continuous with one another. Between the two layers is a potential space, the *pericardial cavity*. This normally contains a small amount of fluid secreted by the serous pericardium, which acts as a lubricant to facilitate movement of the heart within the pericardial cavity.

The fibrous pericardium blends with the tunica adventitia of the great vessels and is firmly attached to the central tendon of the diaphragm below, and to the back of the sternum by the sternopericardial ligaments.

The chambers and valves of the heart

The heart consists of four chambers: two *atria* above and two *ventricles* below (figure 2.2). The right and left sides of the heart are separated by an interatrial septum and

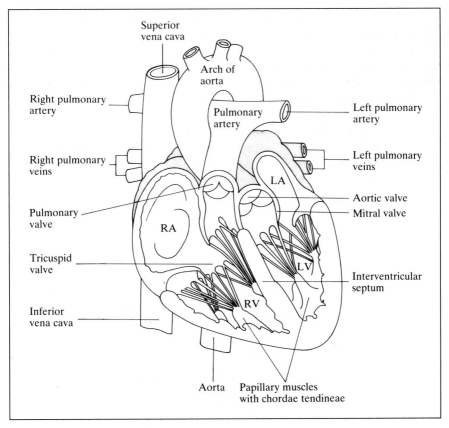

Fig. 2.2 The internal anatomy of the heart
RA = right atrium; LA = left atrium; RV = right ventricle; LV = left ventricle

an interventricular septum. The main valves of the heart are the *mitral* and *aortic* valves on the left side of the heart, and the *tricuspid* and *pulmonary* valves on the right side of the heart. They are complex avascular structures, and are very strong. During a normal lifetime they will open and close some 2700 million times.

The right atrium

The right atrium lies to the right and slightly behind the right ventricle, and anterior and to the right of the left atrium. It forms the lower right lateral heart border on the chest radiograph.

The right atrium is a thin-walled (2 mm) chamber which receives the venous return to the heart from the two largest veins in the body, the *superior and inferior venae cavae*. The right atrium also drains the coronary sinus and the anterior cardiac veins. The opening of the superior vena cava is valveless, but the inferior vena cava and the opening of the coronary sinus have rudimentary valves. The inner surfaces of the posterior and septal walls are smooth, whilst the surfaces of the lateral wall and the right atrial appendage are composed of parallel muscle fibres known as the *pectinate muscles*. Posteriorly, they end on a longitudinal elevation (the *crista terminalis*) which runs from the right side of the opening of the superior vena cava to the right side of the orifice of the inferior vena cava. This is marked externally on the surface of the right atrium by a shallow groove, the *sulcus terminalis*. On the interatrial septum is a depression known as the *fossa ovalis* which marks the site of the foetal foramen ovale. The floor of the right atrium is perforated by the right atrioventricular orifice and the tricuspid valve. This has three triangular cusps: septal, anterior and posterior.

The right ventricle

The right ventricle is located directly beneath the sternum. It is the most anteriorly located chamber, with its inferior border located beneath the xiphoid process. The crescent-shaped chamber has a relatively thin outer wall (5 mm), which is approximately one-third the thickness of the left ventricular wall. The pulmonary trunk rises from a cone-shaped area at the base of the ventricle called the *infundibulum*. Blood entering the infundibulum is ejected superiorly and to the right, through the pulmonary valve into the pulmonary artery. The pulmonary valve has three semilunar cusps: anterior, right and left. On the inner surface of the right ventricular wall are a number of irregular projections of raised muscle bundles (*trabeculae carneae*). The *papillary muscles* project into the ventricular cavity to become continuous with the *chordae tendineae,* which are attached to the free border of the cusps of the tricuspid valve. Contraction of the ventricle not only opposes the tricuspid valve cusps, but also prevents the valve being pushed back into the atrium by maintaining tension on the chordae tendineae. A large rounded muscle bundle, the *moderator band,* crosses the cavity of the right ventricle from the interventricular septum to the anterior wall. This conveys the right bundle branch of conducting tissue to the ventricular muscle. The right ventricle receives venous blood from the right atrium during ventricular diastole and expels it against low resistance (25–32 mmHg pressure) into the pulmonary circulation during ventricular systole.

The left atrium

The left atrium is the most posterior chamber and lies to the midline behind the right ventricle. It is the only cardiac chamber not normally visible on the chest radiograph. The left atrium receives blood from the pulmonary veins. It serves as a reservoir during left ventricular systole and as a conduit during left ventricular filling.

The chamber is irregularly cuboidal in shape, and somewhat smaller than the right atrium with slightly thicker walls (about 3 mm). A small conical pouch (the *auricle*) projects from the upper left corner. It receives the four pulmonary veins arranged in pairs on each side, and all four orifices are devoid of valves.

The interior of the left atrium is smooth, except in the auricle, where the ridges of the pectinate muscles occur. The left atrial aspect of the septum is roughened, being the flap valve of the fossa ovalis. In the floor is the circular left atrioventricular orifice, guarded by the mitral valve. This is so called because it possesses two unequal triangular cusps arranged like a Bishop's mitre.

The left ventricle

The left ventricle receives blood from the left atrium during ventricular diastole and ejects blood against high resistance into the systemic circulation during ventricular systole. It forms the lower left lateral cardiac border and lies posteriorly and to the left of the right ventricle, and below and to the left of the left atrium.

The chamber is conical, and its apex lies approximately in the 5th intercostal space within the midclavicular line. As it normally expels blood against a much higher resistance than the right ventricle, the walls of the left ventricle are much more muscular than the right ventricle (8–15 mm). The interventricular septum is also thick and muscular, except for a small membranous area. The septum separates the two ventricles and its upper portion additionally separates the right atrium from the left ventricle.

Below and posteriorly the left ventricle communicates with the left atrium through the left atrioventricular orifice and the mitral valve. The two papillary muscles are much larger than those of the right ventricle and, from these, chordae tendineae are attached to both cusps of the mitral valve. Above and anteriorly, the left ventricle opens into the aorta. The portion of the ventricular chamber immediately adjoining the aorta is known as the *vestibule*. The aortic valve is in continuity with the mitral valve by a fibrous double-looped band shaped like a figure 8. The aortic valve has three semilunar cusps (right, left and posterior) which are stronger than those of the pulmonary valve. At the origin of each cusp, the walls of the aorta show a slight dilatation or *sinus*. The right coronary artery arises from the right aortic sinus, and the left coronary artery from the left aortic sinus, the orifice of each artery arising above the level of the cusp. These three aortic sinuses are known collectively as the *sinuses of Valsalva*.

The atrioventricular junction

There is no muscular continuity between the atria and the ventricles except through the conducting tissue of the *atrioventricular (AV) node* and *AV bundle*. The aortic and mitral valves have strong fibrous rings which prevent the orifices from stretching and rendering the valves incompetent. These rings are continuous with a dense fibrocartilaginous mass, sometimes called the heart skeleton. This framework affords a firm anchorage for the attachment of the atrial and ventricular musculature as well as the valvular tissue. The pulmonary valve does not have a ring and that of the tricuspid valve is only partially formed.

The tissues of the heart

The main mass of the heart consists of muscular tissue (the *myocardium*), which is lined by the *endocardium,* and covered by the visceral layer of serous pericardium (the *epicardium*). Blood and lymphatic vessels, nerves, and specialised conducting tissues lie within the myocardial mass.

The epicardium

The epicardium consists of a single layer of mesothelial cells covering a thin layer of loose connective tissue which contains elastic fibres, small blood vessels and nerves. It is separated from the myocardium in places by a layer of adipose tissue which carries the coronary blood vessels.

The myocardium

The myocardium is composed of specialised involuntary cardiac muscle. Individual myocardial cells are grouped in bundles in a connective tissue framework which carries small blood and lymphatic vessels and autonomic nerve fibres. The density of capillaries in cardiac muscle cells is much greater than in skeletal muscle, because of its higher blood requirements. The myocardium is thickest towards the apex, and thins towards the base.

The myocardium consists of a network of muscle fibres which show transverse and longitudinal striation and which branch and connect with each other. The ends of the cells are in very close contact with adjacent cells, and the 'joints' can be seen as thick dark striations called *intercalated discs.* Because of the close relationship of one muscle fibre with the next, once contraction starts in any part, it cannot remain localised and spreads throughout the entire network of muscle cells.

The endocardium

The endocardium is in continuity with the lining of the blood vessels (*tunica intima*). It is much thinner than the epicardium, and consists of a lining of endothelial cells, a middle layer of dense connective tissue containing many elastic fibres, and an outer layer of loose connective tissue in which there are small blood vessels and specialised conducting tissue. The heart valves are formed by folds of endocardium, thickened by a core of fibrous tissue extending in from the tissue of the sulcus. The endocardium and myocardium are firmly bound together by connective tissue.

The conducting system

In addition to the purely contractile muscle fibres composing the atria and ventricles, the heart possesses certain specialised muscle cells which form the conducting system. These cells initiate and conduct electrical impulses within the heart to produce myocardial contraction. The conducting system comprises:

● The sino-atrial (SA) node
● The atrioventricular (AV) node
● The bundle of His
● The right and left bundle branches
● The peripheral ramifications of the bundle branches (Purkinje fibres)

The sino-atrial node

The sino-atrial node is the normal site of initiation of the heart beat. It is situated at the junction of the superior vena cava with the right atrium (figure 2.3). This junction is marked internally by the top end of the crista terminalis. The node is spindle-shaped, about 25 mm in length and about 3 mm in width. The framework of the node is collagenous, interlaced by bundles of small conduction fibres. There are numerous autonomic nerve endings in the node with parasympathetic fibres derived from the right vagus nerve. The blood supply is via the nodal artery, which in 60 per cent of people arises from the right coronary artery. In the remaining 40 per cent it arises from the left coronary artery.

Specialised pathways (*internodal tracts*) may exist in the atria, linking the SA and the AV nodes, but there is no histological evidence of this (Thompson, 1983). Conduction seems to occur preferentially along the thick muscle bundle of the right atrium.

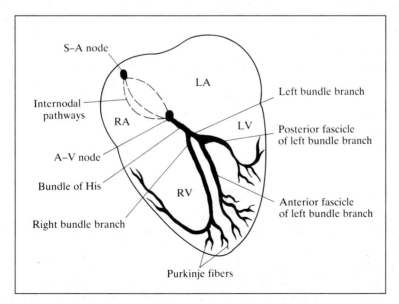

Fig. 2.3 The conducting tissues of the heart

The atrioventricular junction

The AV junction comprises the AV node and AV bundle (of His). The AV node lies between the opening of the coronary sinus and the posterior border of the membranous interventricular septum. The node is divided into a transitional zone and a compact portion. Its function is to cause a delay in transmission of the cardiac impulse from atria to ventricles so that the atria have time to expel their contents into the ventricles before systole.

The AV node has a similar structure to the SA node, but there is much less collagen in the framework, and the conduction fibres are thicker and shorter than those of the sinus node. There is a rich autonomic nerve supply, with the parasympathetic fibres being derived from the left vagus nerve. The blood supply is from a specific nodal artery (*ramus septi fibrosi*) which arises from the right coronary artery in 90 per cent of cases, and from the left circumflex artery in the remaining 10 per cent. The AV bundle extends from the AV node, along the posterior margin of the membranous portion of the interventricular septum, to the crest of the muscular septum. Here it bifurcates into the *right and left bundle branches*. The AV bundle is oval or triangular in cross-section. The fibres of the bundle run parallel to one another, unlike the fibres of the SA and AV nodes which interweave. The AV bundle and the proximal few millimetres of both bundle branches are supplied by the terminal branch of the AV nodal artery and from the septal branches of the left anterior descending artery.

The bundle branches

The right and left bundle branches extend subendocardially along both sides of the interventricular septum. The right bundle is a cord-like structure which passes down the right side of the interventricular septum towards the apex, lying more deeply beneath the endocardium than does the left main bundle. It then runs in the free edge of the moderator band to reach the base of the anterior papillary muscle, where it ramifies amongst the right ventricular musculature.

The left bundle branch is an extensive sheet of fibres which passes down the left side of the interventricular septum. The initial part of the left bundle is fan shaped, and breaks up into two interconnecting left and right hemifascicles (see figure 2.3). The terminal branches of the bundle branches are the *Purkinje fibres* which ramify within the ventricular myocardium.

The bundle branches are supplied by septal arteries from the left anterior descending artery.

The coronary circulation

The heart and proximal portion of the great vessels receive their blood supply from the two *coronary arteries* which originate from the sinuses of Valsalva (see figure 2.4).

The right coronary artery

The right coronary artery arises from the right coronary sinus of the aorta and runs forward to the atrioventricular groove, and gives off a small branch to the SA node.

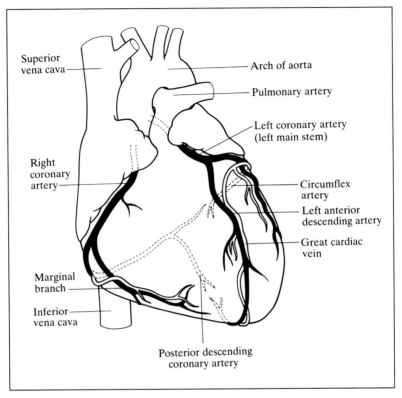

Fig. 2.4   The coronary circulation

It follows the sulcus downwards and round the inferior margin of the heart, giving off a marginal branch to supply the right ventricular wall. It then winds around the heart to the posterior aspect and passes down in the interventricular groove as the *posterior descending coronary artery* which supplies the ventricles and interventricular septum. Frequently a transverse branch continues in the posterior AV groove, supplying branches of the left atrium before anastomosing with the circumflex branch of the left coronary artery. Branches of the right coronary artery supply the conducting tissues, the right ventricle and the inferior (diaphragmatic) surface of the left ventricular wall.

The left coronary artery

The left coronary artery arises from the left posterior sinus of the aorta and runs to the left behind the pulmonary trunk, and then forwards between it and the left auricle to the AV groove. Here, it divides into two branches: an *anterior descending* branch and a *circumflex* branch.

The left anterior descending (LAD) artery descends in the anterior interventricular groove to the apex of the heart, where it turns round to ascend a short distance up the posterior interventricular groove, anastomosing with the posterior interventricular branch of the right coronary artery. Diagonal branches supply the anterior ventricular wall, and septal branches supply the interventricular septum.

The left circumflex branch passes round the left margin of the heart in the AV groove under the left atrial appendage, supplying branches to the left atrium and the left surface of the heart. In some individuals, the circumflex artery gives rise to the posterior descending artery, and this is called a left dominant coronary artery system. Other coronary artery variants include:

● Single coronary artery
● Circumflex branch arising from the right aortic sinus

The *left marginal* branch arises from the circumflex artery, and runs down the left margin of the left ventricle.

Within the myocardium, there are rich anastomoses between the right and left coronary arteries, but the vessels involved are small. These anastomoses are genetically determined, and can enlarge in the event of a gradual coronary artery occlusion, providing collateral circulation to the affected area of muscle. However, if the occlusion is sudden, necrosis of a segment of cardiac muscle will result, since these vessels cannot enlarge acutely.

The coronary veins

Most of the venous drainage of the heart is from veins which run with the coronary arteries, and drain directly into the right atrium. The *coronary sinus* occupies the posterior part of the AV groove, between the left atrium and left ventricle. It receives the great, middle and small *cardiac veins,* and opens directly into the right atrium. One or two large anterior cardiac veins also open directly into the right atrium, whilst smaller veins (*venae cordis minimae*) open directly into the heart chambers.

Lymphatic drainage

The heart is rich in lymphatic capillaries. Large vessels form the subendocardial and subepicardial lymphatic plexuses. The main collecting trunks accompany the larger blood vessels in the grooves of the heart. One large trunk ascends on each side of the heart to end in anterior mediastinal lymph nodes below the arch of the aorta and at the bifurcation of the trachea. The final drainage is to the thoracic duct, although there may be a connection with the bronchomediastinal trunk on the right side.

The nerve supply to the heart

Because of 'intrinsic rhythmicity', the heart can beat even if removed completely from the body. However, the heart is well supplied with both sympathetic and parasympathetic nerve fibres which can modify cardiac function by changing the heart rate and strength of myocardial contraction. Control of the autonomic nerves is via the cardiac centre in the medulla oblongata of the brain.

The sympathetic fibres derive from the cervical and upper thoracic sympathetic ganglia via the superficial and deep cardiac plexuses. The parasympathetic supply is from the vagus. Sympathetic nerve fibres supply the SA node, atrial muscle, AV node, specialised conduction tissue and the ventricular muscle. Parasympathetic nerve fibres supply mainly the SA node and AV node, and to a lesser extent the atrial and ventricular muscle.

Vagal stimulation to the heart is mediated by acetylcholine, which decreases heart rate and probably strength of ventricular contraction. The main action on the AV node is to slow conduction and lengthen the refractory period. In contrast, stimulation of the sympathetic fibres leads to the release of noradrenaline which acts specifically on beta-1 adrenergic receptors in cardiac muscle. Circulating adrenaline from the adrenal medulla may also elicit cardiac responses. Adrenergic stimulation increases both heart rate and force of contraction. Conduction velocity increases and there is shortening of the refractory period in the AV node.

The vagal and sympathetic nerves are distributed to the heart by the cardiac plexus which lies between the concavity of the aortic arch and the tracheal bifurcation. Pressure changes in the aorta and carotid arteries can affect cardiac performance. Sensory receptors (*baroreceptors*) can detect increased pressure in the aorta and carotid arteries. Sensory impulses travel via the vagus and glossopharyngeal nerves which pass to the vasomotor centre in the medulla causing slowing of the heart rate (Marey's reflex). These baroreceptors can be artificially stimulated by carotid sinus massage.

It is thought that most of the cardiac fibres of the right vagus terminate in the sinus node, while the majority of the fibres of the left vagus terminate in the AV node. Some vagal fibres probably terminate in the walls of the great veins near their entrance to the right atrium, and are responsible for the cardiac acceleration which accompanies increased venous return to the heart (Bainbridge reflex).

Chemoreceptors

Chemosensitive cells are located in two *carotid bodies* (at the carotid bifurcation) and several *aortic bodies* adjacent to the aortic arch. They detect changes in blood Po_2, Pco_2 and pH. The afferent impulses arising in these fibres alter respiration, heart rate and vasomotor tone. The efferent impulses from the chemoreceptors pass with the afferent fibres from the pressor-receptors via the glossopharyngeal and vagus nerves to the vasomotor centre in the medulla.

CARDIAC PHYSIOLOGY

The heart is a double pump which maintains two circulations: the pulmonary circulation and the systemic circulation. These serve to transport oxygen and other nutrients to the body cells, remove metabolic waste products from them, and convey substances (e.g. hormones) from one part of the body to another. At rest the heart beats at about 70 to 80 beats per minute, and pumps about 5 litres of blood. During exercise, the rate may approach 200 beats per minute, and the cardiac output may increase to as much as 20 litres.

Histology

The heart comprises two major types of cell:

- Myocardial cells specialised for contraction
- Automatic cells specialised for impulse formation

Myocardial cells

The myocardial cells provide the mechanical pumping action of the heart by shortening in response to electrical stimulation. Each cell is about 100 μm long and 15 μm wide, containing a central nucleus and numerous (about 150) myofibrils aligned along the cell's axis. Each fibril runs the length of the cell, and is made up of repeating functional subunits, or *sarcomeres,* containing actin and myosin arranged hexagonally. The thin *actin* filaments are attached to a limiting membrane (*Z-line*), and interdigitate with the thicker central *myosin* fibres. The sarcomeres of adjacent myofibrils are aligned at the Z-line. During contraction, the actin filaments slide together, bringing the Z-lines closer together. The forces that generate sliding (i.e. contraction)

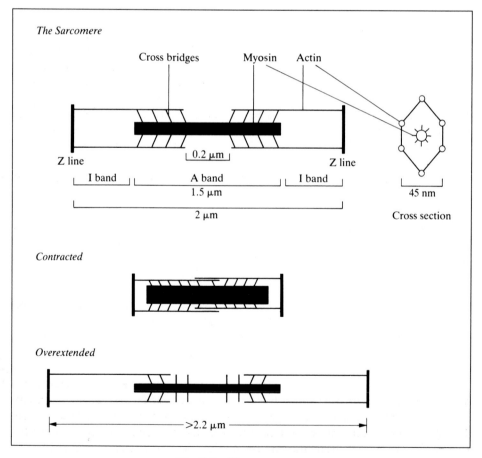

Fig. 2.5   The sarcomere

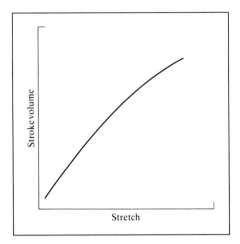

Fig. 2.6 Ventricular function (Starling's) curve

occur at bridges between the actin and myosin (figure 2.5). It is the heads of the myosin molecules that form these bridges and contain the enzyme ATPase responsible for breaking down ATP to provide the energy for contraction. It is likely that the greater the number of bridges, the more forceful the contraction. The thicker myosin filaments (seen as the *A band* on microscopy) are 1.5 μm in length, and have a central portion (0.2 μm) which is devoid of bridges. The thin actin filaments (seen as lateral *I bands*) are shorter (1 μm), so it can be seen that maximum bridging takes place when the overall sarcomere length is between 2.0 and 2.2 μm. If the sarcomere is stretched beyond these limits, some bridges become disengaged, which will limit the force of contraction. Starling's Law of the heart states that, within physiological limits, the greater the diastolic volume of the heart, the greater the energy of contraction. This is why the graphs demonstrating Starling's Law fall off at the upper limits of myocardial stretching (figure 2.6). However, this simplified concept is modified by the action of another contractile protein, *troponin.* This is attached to the actin filaments, and has an inhibitory effect which must be counteracted before actin and myosin can produce contraction. This is mediated by free calcium ions.

A large number of mitochondria are present (a third of the cell volume), which are responsible for generating the large amount of energy required to maintain cardiac contraction. Energy is produced by the process known as oxidative phosphorylation, in which substrates such as glucose, lactate and free fatty acids are oxidised to replenish the energy sources adenosine triphosphate (ATP) and creatine phosphate (CP).

The limiting cell membrane is known as the *sarcolemma,* and adjacent cells are held together by intercalated discs. Electrical resistance through these discs is about 1/400th of the resistance through the outside membrane of the myocardial fibre, allowing virtually free passage of electrical currents from one myocardial cell to the next without encountering significant resistance. The myocardial cells are so tightly bound together that stimulation of any single cell causes the action potential (AP) to spread to all adjacent cells, eventually spreading throughout the entire myocardial network. This is why the cardiac muscle is described as a syncytium (Guyton, 1986).

Automatic cells

Automaticity describes the ability of specialised cardiac tissue to initiate electrical impulses. The cells responsible are known as *pacemaker* or *automatic* cells. In the sino-atrial node, these will discharge spontaneously about 80 times per minute, although automatic cells elsewhere will have a slower discharge rate. In the atrioventricular node for example this may be 60 times per minute, and in the ventricles, 40 times per minute. This system of 'escape rhythms' exists to prevent rhythm failure should the SA node fail to discharge. Sometimes the rate of discharge will increase in places other than the SA node, and these then take over the pacemaker function of the heart. This is often seen following acute myocardial infarction (e.g. accelerated idionodal or idioventricular rhythms).

Both myocardial cells and automatic cells can transmit impulses, but the specialised conducting tissues are used preferentially since they allow a more rapid and ordered carriage of impulses through the heart.

Cardiac electrophysiology

The electrolyte concentrations within cardiac cells and in the extracellular fluid are of major importance for electrical stimulation of the heart. The ions primarily involved in the generation of a cardiac action potential are sodium (Na^+), potassium (K^+) and calcium (Ca^{2+}). The predominant intracellular ion is potassium (K^+), and the predominant extracellular ions are sodium (Na^+) and calcium (Ca^{2+}). There are also negatively charged ions present; protein (Pr^-) within the cell and chloride (Cl^-) and bicarbonate (HCO_3^-) outside.

In the normal resting state, the potential across the myocardial cell membrane is about -90 mV. The relative concentration of Na^+ and K^+ and thus the electrical difference across the cell membrane is maintained by an active, energy-consuming, 'sodium pump'. The pump transfers K^+ ions into the cell up to five times more rapidly than it extrudes Na^+ ions. Within the cell, the concentrations of potassium and sodium are 140 and 10 mmol/l respectively, whereas outside the concentrations are 4 and 140 mmol/l. This ionic imbalance helps maintain the resting membrane potential at -90 mV, and the cells are then said to be 'polarised'. Should an electrical stimulus reach the cell membrane, permeability is altered allowing a change in ionic concentrations and depolarisation of the cell.

There are distinct phases of electrical activity in myocardial cells during the generation of an action potential (figure 2.7).

1. *Polarisation (phase 4):* In the resting (inactive) state, where the cell has a membrane potential of -90 mV, the cell is said to be polarised. The cell interior is negatively charged with respect to the exterior.

2. *Depolarisation (phase 0):* When electrical activation of the cell occurs, changes in the cell membrane permeability result in marked shifts in ionic concentrations. There is a rapid influx of positively charged Na^+ into the cell (the fast sodium current) until

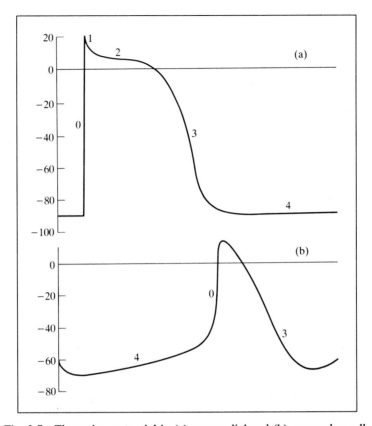

Fig. 2.7   The action potential in (a) myocardial and (b) pacemaker cells

a threshold potential of $-60\,\text{mV}$ is reached. At this critical potential, membrane permeability is further increased, with a secondary rapid intracellular passage of Na^+ ions, accompanied by a moderate but more sustained influx of Ca^{2+} ions. Depolarisation is represented by the upstroke or spike on the action potential curve.

It can be seen that, after excitation, the polarity of the membrane has been reversed, the membrane potential changing rapidly from $-90\,\text{mV}$ to a slightly positive value of $+20\,\text{mV}$. The cell now has a net positive intracellular charge and negative extracellular charge (figure 2.8). Since this is the reverse pattern to that of the surrounding cells a potential difference exists, and an electrical current will flow from one cell to the next, and so on.

3. *Repolarisation (phases 1–3)*: Repolarisation is the process whereby the cell is returned to its normal resting state. This has three phases, the first of which is the 'overshoot' when chloride ions re-enter the cell, and there is a slow fall in intracellular charge to $+10\,\text{mV}$ (phase 1 of the action potential). After the initial spike the membrane remains depolarised (for 0.15 second in atrial muscle; 0.3 second in ventricular muscle), exhibiting a plateau, followed by the abrupt descent which represents repolarisation. The plateau phase (phase 2) of the action potential reflects a moderate

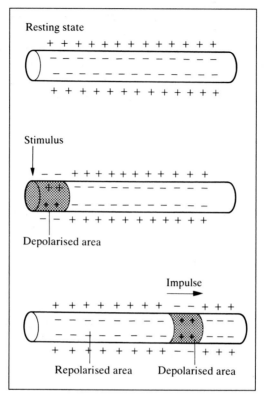

Fig. 2.8 Myocardial cell transmembrane potential (a) at rest, (b) during depolarisation and (c) during repolarisation

and sustained slow influx of Ca^{2+} which accompanies the more marked but less sustained influx of Na^+. The calcium entry into the cell is essential for excitation–contraction coupling (see below). The calcium and sodium influx is balanced by an efflux of K^+. Thus, the net effect is a relative balance of positive charges which gives rise to the plateau.

The downstroke of phase 3 represents the rapid efflux of K^+ from the cell, when membrane permeability to K^+ increases markedly.

Following repolarisation, phase 4 recovery ensues whereby sodium is actively pumped out again and potassium inwards so that the cell becomes repolarised. The transmembrane potential returns to its resting level of $-90\,mV$ and the action potential ends.

Once depolarisation has started, it is inevitably transmitted along the length of the cell to the adjacent cells. In this manner a single electrical stimulus can depolarise the whole heart.

The action potential in automatic cells

The action potential in automatic cells differs from that in myocardial cells. The specialised fibres of the conduction system have the inherent ability to initiate an electrical impulse spontaneously without external influence. Because these cells are responsible for initiating the electrical impulse, phase 4 of the action potential does not properly exist, and the cells have an unstable resting phase with slow spontaneous phase 4 (diastolic) depolarisation (figure 2.7). This slow depolarisation is produced by a slow continuous movement of sodium ions into the cells during diastole, which reduces the intracellular negative charge until a threshold potential is reached, and full depolarisation takes place.

The refractory period

The myocardium is normally refractory to restimulation during the initial phase of systole. The normal *effective refractory period* of the ventricle is 0.25 to 0.3 second, and occurs when the potential lies at about $-55\,mV$. Stimulation, no matter how strong, does not produce an action potential. Certain antidysrhythmic agents act by lengthening or shortening this refractory period.

Following the effective refractory period there is a *relative refractory period* of about 0.05 second during which the muscle can be stimulated, but with difficulty. Just after this is a vulnerable period when even a very weak stimulus can evoke a potential.

The normal refractory period of the atrium is about half that of the ventricles, and the relative refractory period is an additional 0.03 second. As a result, the atria can beat much faster than the ventricles.

Myocardial contraction

The mechanism by which the action potential causes the myofibrils to contract is known as *excitation–contraction coupling*. Electrical excitation produces mechanical activation, leading to myocardial contraction.

Electrical excitation

The function of the automatic cells is to regulate the contraction of the myocardial cells by providing the initial electrical stimulation. Their contractile elements are sparse and do not contribute significantly to the cardiac contraction.

Normally the activating impulse spreads from the sinus node in all directions. It travels at a rate of about 1 m/s, thus reaching the most distant parts of the atrium in only 0.08 second. A delay of approximately 0.04 second in AV transmission occurs during passage through the node, which allows atrial systole to be completed. From the atria, the wave of electrical excitement passes rapidly along the specialised muscle fibres of the AV bundle, bundle branches and peripheral ramifications of these branches. The spread of excitation causes contraction of the ventricular musculature.

Mechanical activation and myocardial contraction

The unit of contraction is the sarcomere, which contains the two contractile proteins, actin and myosin (see above). The contractile process is initiated when the nerve impulse reaches the cardiac cell and travels along the sarcolemma. A series of fine branching T-tubules (the *sarcoplasmic reticulum*) run from the sarcolemma to the inner contractile elements. These allow any electrical changes occurring at the cell membrane to be rapidly transmitted to the myofibrils, and provide the link between the electrical and mechanical activities of the heart.

When an action potential reaches the cardiac muscle membrane, it spreads to the interior of the cell via the sarcoplasmic reticulum. This releases calcium ions from pouches (*cisternae*) in the T-tubules. These diffuse into the myofibrils to catalyse a chemical reaction which activates the sliding of the actin and myosin filaments along each other to effect contraction. The strength of myocardial contraction is dependent upon the concentration of Ca^{2+} ions, as well as the rate of ATP production. At the end of contraction, the calcium ions in the sarcoplasm are rapidly pumped back into the cisternae.

The cardiac cycle

The function of the heart is to maintain a constant circulation of blood through the body. It acts as a pump whose cyclical contraction (*systole*) and relaxation (*diastole*) is known as the *cardiac cycle*. This cyclical activity is normally initiated by spontaneous generation of an action potential at the SA node. The impulse travels at about 1 m/s through the atrial muscle to produce atrial systole. Tissues at the atrioventricular groove prevent transmission from atrial to ventricular muscle, and conduction can take place only through specialised tissues in the AV junction. The duration of the cardiac cycle is about 0.8 second, producing an average heart rate of 75 beats per minute. Provided the heart receives excitation along the normal pathways, the heart rate remains constant; each successive cardiac cycle follows the same pattern of systole and diastole.

The duration of atrial systole is about 0.1 second and that of ventricular systole 0.3 second. Thus, the combined duration of atrial and ventricular systole is approximately 0.4 second. The timing remains fairly constant at fast heart rates, so that any increase in heart rate decreases diastolic timing. Complete cardiac diastole normally lasts 0.4 second, but as the pulse rate increases, the diastolic interval decreases. Since coronary perfusion takes place in diastole, fast heart rates may critically impair the myocardial blood supply.

Atrial function

Atrial diastole lasts for 0.3 second, during which venous blood drains into the atrium which act as a reservoir, storing the blood. The AV ring moves upwards at the end of ventricular systole, causing a rise in atrial pressure (the '*v*' *wave*). The AV valves then open and the ventricles rapidly begin to fill, allowing the valve cusps to float upwards into opposition. The atria then contract (the right usually very slightly before the left), a process taking 0.1 second. Blood is forced through the AV valves into the

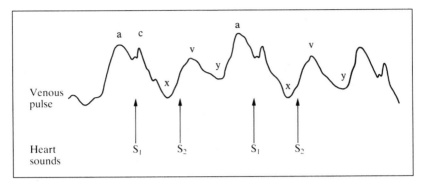

Fig. 2.9 The venous pulse waveform

ventricles, increasing ventricular filling by about 10 to 20 per cent, and priming the ventricles for contraction.

Since there are no valves between the right atrium and the venae cavae, some blood is also expelled backwards during atrial contraction, causing a transient rise in the central venous pressure: the *'a' wave* (figure 2.9). The delay of electrical transmission at the AV node allows the atria to empty completely before ventricular contraction starts.

Ventricular function

The pressure of blood in the ventricles begins to rise while that in the relaxing atria is falling. The cusps of the AV valves snap shut (causing the first heart sound, *S1*), and are held in opposition by the pull of the papillary muscles on the chordae tendineae. After closure of the AV valves the blood pressure rises because of isometric contraction of the ventricular muscle. During this phase, the ventricles alter their shape (becoming shorter and fatter), though not their volume (this is called isovolumetric contraction). This momentarily causes a backward bulging of the AV valve cusps into the atria and produces a transient increase in atrial pressure (the *'c' wave*).

When the rising ventricular pressure exceeds the pressure in the aorta and pulmonary artery, the semilunar aortic and pulmonary valves open. The isotonic phase of contraction then begins, and the ventricular contents are ejected. Descent of the AV ring during ventricular systole causes a fall in right atrial pressure (the *'x' descent*).

As the ventricular muscle relaxes and the pressure falls below that in the aorta and pulmonary artery the semilunar valves close (the second heart sound, *S2*), producing the dicrotic notch on arterial pressure traces. The aortic valve closes slightly before the pulmonary valve. Simultaneously, blood enters the atria, and the intra-atrial pressure gradually rises, so that when the AV valves open, blood flows rapidly from the atria to the ventricles, producing the third heart sound (*S3*) heard in some children and young adults.

Haemodynamics

The circulation is a continuous circuit, although it is often conveniently subdivided into the systemic and pulmonary circuits.

The pulmonary circulation

The pulmonary circuit is a low-pressure system with short, wide, thin-walled vessels and a small capacity (500 to 900 ml). The mean pressure in the circuit in the adult is approximately 15 mmHg – less than one-sixth of that in the systemic circulation. It circulates all the blood from the right ventricle to the left atrium. As blood is carried through the pulmonary vascular bed, carbon dioxide diffuses outwards into the lungs, and oxygen is absorbed.

The pulmonary trunk carrying deoxygenated blood passes upwards from the right ventricle and divides into two main *pulmonary arteries,* one passing to each lung. Within the lungs, the arteries divide and subdivide to form the pulmonary capillary bed where gaseous exchange takes place. Eventually these capillaries join up to form two main *pulmonary veins* carrying oxygenated blood to the left atrium.

The systemic circulation

The systemic circuit is a high-pressure system which supplies all the tissues of the body (except the lungs) with blood. The aorta is elastic in nature which helps it function both as a reservoir for blood during the rapid ejection phase from the left ventricle, and as a compression chamber to help propel the blood forward. As the branches arising from the aorta divide, the total cross-sectional area of the arteries, arterioles and capillaries increases, and the average velocity of blood flow decreases. The arterioles offer the largest resistance to flow. In the capillary bed there is often stasis of flow in some capillaries and an active flow in others. The normal systemic capillary pressure is about 24 to 25 mmHg, and the normal systemic capillary blood volume at rest is about 5 per cent of the total volume (250 ml).

Coronary blood flow

The primary function of the coronary circulation is to provide an adequate supply of oxygen to support the metabolic demands of the heart. The rate of oxygen consumption is the major factor that determines coronary blood flow. Myocardial oxygen consumption (MVO_2) is related to myocardial work in response to exercise or other stimuli, including drugs such as adrenaline, noradrenaline, calcium, thyroxine and digitalis.

About 4 per cent of cardiac output passes into the coronary vessels (about 225 ml/min) which fill in diastole. During systole, the coronary vessels are compressed so that the resistance to flow at that time is sharply increased. Coronary blood flow is largely determined by the calibre of the coronary arteries themselves, and is regulated almost entirely by the local metabolic needs of the working cardiac muscle.

Regulation of myocardial function

The normal adult blood volume is about 5 litres; about 3.5 litres are in the systemic (predominantly venous) circulation. The volume in the heart is about 0.6 litre, bringing the total central circulation in the heart and lungs to about 1.5 litres. Not all blood is expelled from the left ventricle at the end of systole. The residual volume, the *left ventricular end diastolic volume* (LVEDV), is about 140 ml. The quantity of blood ejected during ventricular systole (the *stroke volume*) is only about 80 ml, and hence the *ejection fraction* (EF) is approximately 80/140 = 60 per cent. If the heart rate is 70 beats per minute, then:

$$\text{Cardiac output} = \text{Heart rate} \times \text{Stroke volume}$$
$$\text{(beats/min)} \quad \text{(ml/beat)}$$
$$= \text{about 5.6 litres}$$

The cardiac output may increase up to 20 litres during heavy exertion. To alter cardiac output to meet changing bodily demands for tissue perfusion the heart rate or stroke volume (or both) must be altered. These mechanisms normally operate together to increase the cardiac output as required.

The main determinants of cardiac output are stroke volume and heart rate. If the stroke volume is constant, cardiac output will linearly follow heart rate. However, stroke volume varies constantly, and thus the heart rate must alter to maintain the cardiac output.

Stroke volume is determined by:

● Preload (filling of the heart during diastole)
● Afterload (resistance against which the heart must pump)
● Contractility of the heart muscle.

Preload

Preload is the tension exerted on cardiac muscle at the end of diastole, usually expressed as the *left ventricular end diastolic pressure* (LVEDP). This is determined by the volume of blood in the left ventricle at the end of diastole (LVEDV). The Frank–Starling law of 1918 states that, within physiological limits, increases in LVEDV are accompanied by an increase in stroke work. Hence, although the volume of blood passing through the heart may vary considerably, cardiac muscle fibres can contract more forcefully to cope with increased loads. This intrinsic ability of the heart to adapt to changing loads of inflowing blood may be shown graphically (see figure 2.6), and is approximately linear. Unfortunately, once the load increases beyond physiological limits, the heart begins to fail. Preload can be estimated by measurement of left and right atrial pressures. Clinically, this is done either by a central venous pressure (CVP) line in the right atrium, or by a Swan–Ganz catheter measuring the pulmonary capillary wedge pressure to approximate the pressure in the left atrium.

Afterload

Afterload is the force opposing ventricular ejection and is a function of both arterial pressure and left ventricular size. Two major determinants of left ventricular afterload are the resistance of the aortic valve and systemic vascular resistance. Conditions that increase afterload include those causing obstruction to ventricular outflow (e.g. aortic stenosis) and those causing high systemic vascular resistance (e.g. hypertension).

Contractility

Contractility is an intrinsic property of the heart, and exists independently of loading. The speed and force of contraction can be increased by sympathetic nervous stimulation or drugs such as adrenaline, noradrenaline or dopamine. These improve the speed and strength of contraction (i.e. they have positive inotropic and chronotropic effects) by increasing ATP production and calcium (Ca^{2+}) fluxes. Myocardial hypoxia, ischaemia or beta-blocking agents have the reverse effect, and decrease cardiac contractility (negative inotropic and chronotropic effects). The contractile state can be gauged by the size of the *ejection fraction* (EF). The normal EF is 0.60 to 0.75, i.e. the left ventricle ejects about 60 to 75 per cent of its contents during systole. This may be estimated by echocardiography, nuclear scanning or at cardiac catheterisation. Using the Frank–Starling graphs, contractility can be represented by different curves; higher degrees of contractility displace the curve upwards and to the left (figure 2.10).

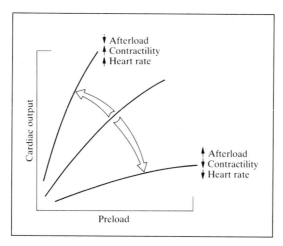

Fig. 2.10   Ventricular function (Starling's) curves showing the effects of preload, afterload, contractility and heart rate

Blood pressure

Blood pressure may be defined as the force or pressure that the blood exerts upon the vessel walls. When the ventricle contracts blood is forced into an already full aorta, and the pressure wave produces a systolic blood pressure of about 120 mmHg (16 kilopascals [kPa]). During complete cardiac diastole, the arterial pressure falls to about 80 mmHg (11 kPa).

Blood pressure is maintained through many variables, including:

- Cardiac output
- Blood volume
- Peripheral resistance
- Elasticity of the vessel walls
- Venous return

Cardiac output is controlled by pulse rate and stroke volume. An increase in cardiac output raises both systolic and diastolic blood pressure, but an increase in stroke volume increases the systolic pressure to a greater degree. Blood volume is obviously important as can be seen by the fact that blood pressure falls in shock. This may be due to an absolute loss of blood volume (e.g. haemorrhage) or a relative loss of circulating volume when there is widespread vasodilatation (e.g. septicaemic shock).

Peripheral resistance is controlled via sympathetic vasoconstrictor nerves originating in the vasomotor centre of the medulla oblongata. Normally, the artery walls are in a state of mild constriction, giving rise to 'resting tone'. Selective vasoconstriction and vasodilatation can take place around the body to ensure a constant blood supply to the vital organs, especially the heart and brain.

The elasticity of the arterial walls is important to propel the blood forwards. Distension and recoil occur throughout the arterial system. During diastole, arterial recoil maintains the diastolic blood pressure. As the arterial tree ages, atheromatous deposits cause 'hardening of the arteries'. Elasticity is lost and the systolic blood pressure rises, since the arterial walls are unable to buffer the effect of the ventricular systolic shock wave.

Venous return via the superior and inferior venae cavae also plays an important role in maintenance of the blood pressure. The force of the left ventricle is not sufficient on its own to force blood round the body. It is therefore assisted by muscular contraction and respiration. Contraction of skeletal muscle puts pressure on the veins and squeezes blood forwards. Backward flow is prevented by valves. The negative intrathoracic pressure caused by inspiration also helps by sucking blood into the heart. In addition, diaphragmatic movement raises the intra-abdominal pressure, squeezing blood out of the abdominal vessels.

References

Guyton A C (1986) *Textbook of Medical Physiology*. Philadelphia: W B Saunders.
Starling E H (1918) *The Linacre Lecture on the Law of the Heart*. London: Longmans Green.
Thompson D R (1983) Specialised internodal pathways. *International Journal of Cardiology*, **4**: 393–396.

3

The Pathology and Epidemiology of Ischaemic Heart Disease

Ischaemic heart disease (IHD) is the single major cause of death in the Western world, and accounts for over 163 000 deaths in England and Wales each year (figure 3.1). Thirty per cent of all male deaths and 22 per cent of female deaths are attributable to IHD, and well over a third of these occur in people aged less than 70 years. In addition, there are about 115 000 patients discharged from hospitals in England and Wales every year who have been diagnosed as suffering from ischaemic heart disease (Mann and Marmot, 1987).

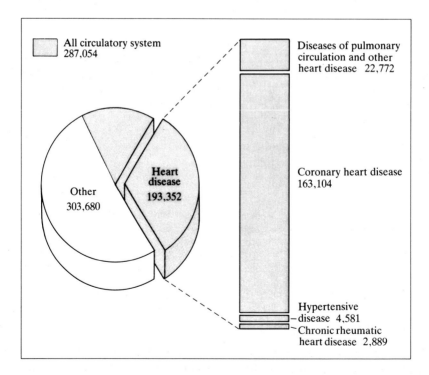

Fig. 3.1 Mortality in England and Wales in 1985 (From Wells, 1987. Reproduced by kind permission of the Office of Health Economics)

The term ischaemic heart disease is used to describe the effects of impaired or absent blood supply on the myocardium. In the majority of cases this is caused by atheromatous obstruction of the coronary arteries (Davies, 1987). Epidemiological and clinical studies have consistently linked the presence of atherosclerosis in patients with IHD (Alpert and Braunwald, 1980; Bulkley, 1986; Factor and Kirk, 1986), and coronary angiography reveals atherosclerotic changes present in over 97 per cent of patients with acute myocardial infarction (Pichard et al, 1983).

Although coronary atheroma is responsible for virtually all cases of IHD, many more people have coronary atheroma than have clinical evidence of myocardial ischaemia, which suggests that the association between coronary atherosclerosis and the clinical manifestations of IHD is not direct. In addition, the severity of symptoms has a poor correlation with the severity of coronary atherosclerosis. About 10 per cent of patients with angina pectoris or myocardial infarction have either normal coronary arteries or exhibit no critical stenoses in their coronary arteries. This is often the case in young patients (Betriu et al, 1981).

It therefore appears that the clinical manifestations of IHD are precipitated by additional, transient factors which interfere with coronary blood supply, occurring against a background of varying degrees of coronary atherosclerosis (Maseri, 1982).

THE PATHOGENESIS OF ISCHAEMIC HEART DISEASE

Essentially, myocardial ischaemia results from an imbalance between myocardial oxygen demand and supply. Critical restriction to ordinary flow occurs when the diameter of the lumen is reduced by more than 50 per cent (equivalent to a 75 per cent stenosis if the vessel is circular), usually resulting in angina pectoris. If sudden occlusion causes an abrupt diminution or even total loss of coronary blood supply acute myocardial infarction results.

Oxygen demand depends mainly upon heart rate, the strength of myocardial contraction and left ventricular wall tension.

1. *Heart rate:* When the heart rate increases, systolic timing does not alter by very much, and the increased heart rate shortens diastole. As a result, there is a reduction in coronary perfusion time (which takes place in diastole) despite the higher demands placed upon it by the increased heart rate.

2. *Force of myocardial contractility:* Sympathetic stimulation leads to an increase in heart rate and force of contraction, both of which increase myocardial work.

3. *Myocardial wall tension:* Wall tension is determined by intracardiac pressures and volumes. These are usually determined by preload and afterload. Increased wall tension increases myocardial work.

In general, the delivery of oxygen to the myocardium varies with coronary blood flow, which is in turn determined by perfusion pressure. Perfusion pressure may be compromised by abnormalities of the vessel wall, abnormalities in blood flow or abnormalities in the blood itself.

1. *Abnormalities of the coronary vessel wall:* Coronary blood supply may be impaired by fixed or reversible lesions. Atheroma is the commonest cause of coronary stenosis, although congenital lesions such as coronary ectasia may be responsible. In most cases of stable angina, there is 50 per cent stenosis in one or more of the coronary arteries, and in between one-half and two-thirds of cases the original lumen is replaced by several smaller channels where recannalisation has occurred in a previous thrombosis. Coronary artery spasm gives rise to intermittent, reversible stenoses, and is the underlying abnormality in 'variant angina', described by Prinzmetal et al (1959).

Both spasm and atheroma are usually always present in patients with symptomatic IHD, although their precise contribution in impairing myocardial perfusion at any given time will differ (Maseri, 1982). For example, many patients with variant angina show little or no atheroma on angiography. It is now accepted that temporary occlusion of coronary flow by spasm, even in the absence of atheroma, can lead to angina or even myocardial infarction. However, the usual situation is for spasm and fixed stenosis to act in combination, that is, vascular contraction takes place around a fixed obstruction causing a critical reduction in flow which leads to regional ischaemia (figure 3.2). The coronary vessel wall may rarely be involved by inflammatory diseases such as systemic lupus erythematosus (SLE) and polyarteritis nodosa (PAN), which cause narrowing of the blood vessels.

2. *Abnormalities in blood flow:* Aortic valve disease, especially aortic stenosis, will obstruct blood flow from the left ventricle and reduce perfusion of the coronary arteries. Mitral stenosis can also do the same.

3. *Abnormalities in the blood:* Anaemia will prevent adequate oxygen carriage and may provoke angina. Hyperviscosity syndromes such as polycythaemia and myeloma may result in myocardial ischaemia by slowing blood flow.

Myocardial infarction and unstable angina often occur at times when there is little or no demand placed upon the heart (at rest or during minimal exertion). The precipitating cause would therefore seem to be decreased oxygen supply to the heart,

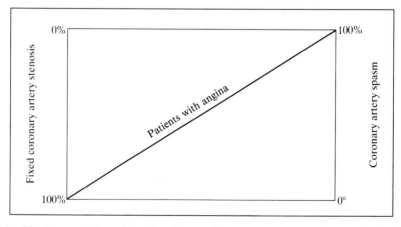

Fig. 3.2 The inter-relation of fixed and reversible coronary artery obstruction in chronic stable angina. The graph shows that different combinations of atheroma and coronary arterial spasm can produce angina

rather than increased oxygen demand. High-grade stenoses of the coronary arteries are associated with a higher risk of acute myocardial infarction than are low-grade stenoses (Haft and Bachik, 1984), but the rapid onset of symptoms suggests that there is a precipitating event occurring in the presence of advanced coronary atherosclerosis. It is now known that several mechanisms – atherosclerosis, platelet adhesion, coronary thrombosis and coronary artery spasm – interact in the pathogenesis of ischaemic heart disease and its clinical manifestations (angina pectoris, acute myocardial infarction and sudden death).

ATHEROSCLEROSIS

Atherosclerosis is a complex disease characterised by focal proliferation of smooth muscle cells and accumulation of lipid within the intima of large and medium arteries. An important feature is the focal distribution of the lesion as plaques. There is a predilection for these plaques to occur around branching vessels or areas of arterial curvature, suggesting that haemodynamic stresses may play an important initiating role (Ross, 1986).

Atherosclerotic plaques are generally classified into three types.

1. *Fatty streaks:* The process of atherosclerosis begins in childhood with the development of flat, lipid-rich lesions termed *fatty streaks.* These consist of lipid-laden macrophages and smooth-muscle cells within the intima. The lesions are yellowish in appearance, and cause little or no obstruction of the affected artery. They are thought to be benign in themselves, but may be precursors of advanced atheromatous lesions.

2. *Fibrous plaques:* These are white lesions which become elevated so that they protrude into the lumen of the artery. They are uncommon in the first 20 or 30 years of life. During the development of the plaque there is a proliferation of smooth-muscle cells to form a *fibrous cap.* The deposition of a new connective tissue matrix and the accumulation of lipids lead to layers of varying amounts of extracellular lipid and cell debris. The fibrous plaque often progresses with potential for luminal narrowing, or it may degenerate.

3. *Advanced (complicated) lesions:* These are degenerative lesions composed of fibrous tissue, fibrin, intracellular and extracellular lipid and often extravasated blood. The necrotic lipid-rich core increases in size and often becomes calcified. The atheromatous plaques cause narrowing of the lumen, and may become fissured. The cause of plaque fissuring is unknown, but could be arterial spasm. Fissures in the fibrous cap allow blood to dissect inwards forming a platelet-rich thrombus within the intima. If the fissure heals, a large plaque-containing thrombus remains which partially or completely occludes the coronary lumen. Alternatively, fresh thrombus may extend into the lumen and may cause complete obstruction. This dynamic process occurs over a period of hours to days preceding an acute coronary event. Alternatively, spontaneous resolution may take place due to thrombolysis. Up to 60 per cent of patients with stable angina, and 85 per cent of those with previous myocardial infarction and angina, have segments of artery in which the original channel is replaced by several small channels, suggesting recannalisation through a previous occlusive thrombus.

Although several theories have been postulated to explain the pathogenesis of atheroma, the aetiology remains unclear. The role of repeated endothelial injury is generally assumed to be central in the initiation and progression of atherosclerotic plaques. Causes of endothelial injury include raised low-density lipoprotein (LDL-cholesterol) levels, toxins (e.g. from smoking), vasospasm and other haemodynamic stresses. Endothelial injury exposes subendothelial collagen, and causes adenosine triphosphate (ATP) and adenosine diphosphate (ADP) to be released from damaged cells. This activates platelets, causing them to adhere to the vessel wall. In turn, these platelets release thromboxane A2 and ADP which cause a secondary aggregation of platelets and contraction of vascular smooth muscle. Platelet-derived growth factor (PDGF) is also released which stimulates smooth-muscle cells to migrate from the arterial media into the intima, and then proliferate. If the injury is minor and brief, the endothelium will heal and regress leaving an irregular and slightly thickened intima. Repeated injury, however, may lead to lipid accumulation and further pro-liferation of smooth muscle cells.

Plaque rupture with thrombosis seems to be a common pathogenic mechanism in many acute coronary events including sudden death, unstable angina, non-transmural and transmural myocardial infarction (Davies and Thomas, 1985). Plaque fissuring is a random and unpredictable event, occurring in response to mechanical stresses, coronary artery spasm or other factors acting on the coronary vasculature. Plaque rupture exposes collagen which triggers platelet activity and initiates thrombosis.

NON-ATHEROSCLEROTIC CAUSES OF ISCHAEMIC HEART DISEASE

The heart can be rendered ischaemic by mechanisms other than fixed atherosclerotic lesions in the coronary arteries. In about 10 per cent of patients with acute myocardial infarction, transient coronary artery spasm may serve to adversely alter the balance between myocardial supply and demand. Acute infarction may occur in patients with Prinzmetal (variant) angina, where coronary artery spasm is the underlying abnor-mality. Coronary artery spasm occurs in about one-third of patients with unstable angina. It may also complicate Raynaud's disease or follow the withdrawal of nitrate therapy.

Inflammation of the coronary vessels can occur in the collagen diseases (e.g. polyarteritis or rheumatoid arthritis), leading to coronary insufficiency, and there is usually evidence of arteritis in other parts of the body. Coronary artery emboli may arise from the left atrium or ventricle (e.g. from atrial myxomas, bacterial endocar-ditis or mitral valve disease), and coronary obstruction may complicate aortic or coronary dissection, especially following cardiac catheterisation. Mechanical obstruction of blood flow to the coronary arteries may also be a feature of aortic stenosis and hypertrophic obstructive cardiomyopathy (HOCM).

CORONARY HEART DISEASE AND RISK FACTORS

There are many regional and national differences in the incidence and mortality from coronary heart disease (Keys, 1980). Epidemiological studies have sought associations between the occurrence of coronary heart disease and physical, biochemical and environmental characteristics of populations and individuals. As a result, predictive variables or 'risk factors' have been defined which have been shown to associate with the development of coronary heart disease; for example, male gender, increasing age and a positive family history of coronary heart disease (Shaper et al, 1985). These of course are unavoidable. However, many other treatable risk factors have been described, the most important of which are hyperlipidaemia, cigarette smoking and hypertension. In addition, diabetes mellitus is an important risk factor for both small and large vessel disease. An important feature of the different risk factors is that, where they occur together, the cumulative risk is not just additive, but synergistic (Criqui, 1986), with one factor multiplying the risk of another (figure 3.3)

Although by definition each risk factor associates positively with the risk of ischaemic heart disease, it by no means follows that risk factors are causal in producing disease (Burch, 1980). Indeed, it is important to remember that a significant number, perhaps the majority, of patients presenting with ischaemic heart disease do not have identifiable risk factors. In addition, there is no relationship between particular risk factors and the severity or extent of atheroma.

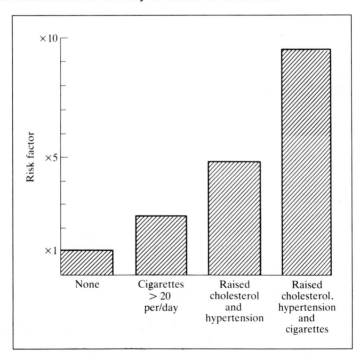

Fig. 3.3   The synergistic effect of risk factors on the chances of a first major coronary episode, where blood cholesterol level is greater than 6.5 mmol/l and blood pressure is greater than 160/95 mmHg

Oliver (1987) points out that the risk factors are weak predictors of coronary heart disease for individuals, and there are probably many other mechanisms which can precipitate the clinical syndromes of ischaemic heart disease.

Genetic predisposition

There have been marked changes in the morbidity and mortality from coronary heart disease over the last few decades. During the ten year period from 1968 to 1977, the age-adjusted cardiovascular death rate in the USA fell by 24 per cent, and it still continues to fall. This decline in cardiovascular deaths can only be explained by changes in environmental or nutritional factors. Alterations in the genetic structure of such populations cannot have taken place sufficiently fast to account for such dramatic changes. Nevertheless, extensive work has shown that genetic influence is of importance in the aetiology of coronary heart disease. It is not uncommon to find that coronary heart disease aggregates in families, especially in those with maternal histories of illness (Rissanen and Nikkila, 1979). The presence of coronary heart disease in a first-degree relative with onset before the age of 55 years is a very strong risk factor. Studies of identical and non-identical twins (De Faire, 1974; Berg, 1983) indicate that coronary heart disease is more often found in both identical twins than in both non-identical twins, which supports the evidence for the genetic influence. Genetic factors affecting this susceptibility to coronary heart disease may operate through known risk factors which run in families, such as hyperlipidaemia, diabetes and hypertension, or through as yet undefined genetic mechanisms.

Smoking

Smoking is the only risk factor that is almost certainly causally related to coronary heart disease (Dawber, 1980). It is probably the most important risk factor for both first and subsequent heart attacks. Each year about 10 000 men and women under the age of 65 die from coronary heart disease attributable to smoking. It is directly implicated in 25 per cent of coronary deaths in patients under the age of 65 years, and 80 per cent of men under the age of 45 years. Those with additional risk factors, such as hypertension and diabetes, are especially at risk. Myocardial infarction and sudden death occur two to four times more frequently in smokers than in non-smokers (Friedman et al, 1979) and, overall, the risk of death from coronary heart disease is twice that of non-smokers. Those who start smoking before the age of 20 years and those smoking more than 20 cigarettes per day increase their risk by three to five times (Ball and Turner, 1974).

Smoking additionally contributes to the 24 000 deaths due to bronchitis and to the 38 000 lung cancers occurring annually in the UK.

Tobacco smoke is a complex aerosol containing (in addition to tar) the two implicated cardiovascular toxins, nicotine and carbon monoxide. Nicotine absorption varies from about 5 to 100 per cent, depending upon smoking patterns. A heavy smoker may absorb about 100 mg of nicotine per day. Its pharmacological action is to stimulate catecholamine release which raises the heart rate, blood pressure and force of myocardial contraction, leading to increased myocardial work. There is additionally a thrombogenic action caused by inhibition of fibrinolysis, release of free fatty acids and an increase in platelet aggregation and stickiness.

Carbon monoxide is a cellular poison and makes up about 3 to 6 per cent of inhaled cigarette smoke, which is eight times the maximum air pollution allowed in industry. Carbon monoxide binds 200 times more readily to haemoglobin than does oxygen (which it displaces), thus forming carboxyhaemoglobin. Typically, a heavy smoker will have 20 per cent of his haemoglobin carboxylated, which shifts the oxygen dissociation curve to the left, thereby impairing oxygen release in tissues. Oxygenation is therefore reduced despite increased myocardial requirements due to nicotinic stimulation. Carbon monoxide may additionally increase endothelial permeability.

Pipe and cigar smoke have identical effects if inhaled, but smoking patterns in this group of patients usually differ, with a reduced intake of smoke into the lungs. However, this does not mean that the medical profession should sanction it. Former cigarette smokers who switch to these forms of smoking maintain an increased risk of cardiovascular events; this probably relates to the smoking pattern with the tendency to inhale. It is worth noting that self-reports on the depth of inhalation are extremely inaccurate.

Hyperlipidaemia

The major lipids are triglycerides and cholesterol. The former are found predominantly in adipose tissue as stored energy reserves, and cholesterol is a cell membrane component. They are insoluble in water and in order for them to be transported in blood are converted to water-soluble complexes called *lipoproteins*. The main lipoproteins are chylomicrons, low-density lipoprotein (LDL), very low-density lipoprotein (VLDL) and high-density lipoprotein (HDL).

Chylomicrons are the largest lipoproteins and consist mainly of exogenous (dietary) triglyceride which has been absorbed from the small intestine. *VLDL* is a small triglyceride-rich (50 per cent) lipoprotein bearing lipids synthesised mainly in the liver. *LDL* is the main transport vehicle for cholesterol, and high levels of LDL-cholesterol (and hence total cholesterol) form an independent risk factor for coronary heart disease. *HDL* is the smallest lipoprotein, comprising two subfractions: HDL2 and HDL3. These contain cholesterol which is transported away from cells to the liver. High levels of HDL, particularly HDL2, are negatively correlated with atheromatous disease. Raised levels are often found in premenopausal women, joggers and moderate, regular drinkers of alcohol.

The hyperlipidaemias are a common group of metabolic disorders which affect more than 10 per cent of the population of Western industrialised countries. They may be subdivided into either primary (idiopathic) or the more common secondary forms. The former are often familial and should only be diagnosed by exclusion of known underlying causes, the commonest of which are diabetes, thyroid disease, renal disease, cholestasis, alcohol and other drugs. Patients may have either raised cholesterol levels, raised triglyceride levels, or both. Typical 'normal' lipid levels for the UK are shown in table 3.1.

The hyperlipidaemias have been classified into six types by the World Health Organisation (Beaumont et al, 1970). This classification is shown in table 3.2.

Table 3.1. 'Normal' plasma lipid concentrations.

	Normal range (mmol/l)
Cholesterol	4.0–6.5
Triglycerides	0.5–1.8
HDL-cholesterol: men	1.0–1.5
women	1.2–1.8

LDL-cholesterol can be estimated by:

$$\text{Total cholesterol} - \left(HDL + \frac{\text{Triglyceride}}{2.2} \right)$$

There is a clear correlation between raised serum cholesterol levels and the risk of coronary heart disease (Rose and Shipley, 1980), and the relationship is virtually linear (figure 3.4). Although 'normal' ranges for cholesterol are usually quoted as up to 6.7 mmol/l, the optimum serum cholesterol level is 4–4.5 mmol/l. Above this level there is a direct proportional rise in atherosclerotic cardiovascular events, notably coronary heart disease. Atheromatous plaques progress more quickly in the presence

Table 3.2. Classification of the hyperlipidaemias.

Type	Other names	Incidence in UK (%)	Lipoprotein increased	Plasma cholesterol	Plasma triglycerides	Plasma appearance (4 °C/12 h)
I	Exogenous hypertrigly-ceridaemia	0.1	Chylomicrons	+	+ + +	Milky with clear infranatant
IIa	Monogenic and polygenic hypercholes-terolaemia	20–25	LDL	+ + +	N	Clear
IIb	Familial combined hyperlipidaemia	20–25	LDL VLDL	+ +	+	Turbid
III	Floating or broad beta disease	2–5	Abnormal LDL	+ +	. + +	Turbid
IV	Essential or carbohydrate-induced hypertrigly-ceridaemia	35–50	VLDL	N/+	+ +/+ + +	Turbid
V	Exogenous and endogenous hyperlipidaemia	2–3	VLDL Chylomicrons	N/+	+ +/+ + +	Milky with turbid infranatant

N	= normal levels	+ + +	= elevated
+	= slight elevation	+ + +	= marked elevation

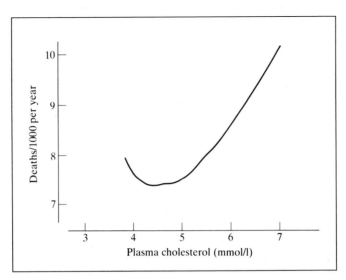

Fig. 3.4 Relationship of plasma cholesterol concentrations to mortality, based on a $7\frac{1}{2}$ year follow-up of 17 718 men in the Whitehall study (data from Rose and Shipley, 1980)

of a high serum cholesterol, and recent evidence has shown that successful lowering of the cholesterol level leads to regression of atheroma (Glueck, 1986). Reducing very high cholesterol levels may additionally reduce the incidence of coronary heart disease, coronary death, myocardial infarction, angina and the need for coronary artery bypass surgery (Oliver, 1984). The role of hypertriglyceridaemia in the aetiology of coronary heart disease is a little harder to interpret (Riemersma, 1984), but hypertriglyceridaemia can cause acute pancreatitis or may draw attention to other cardiovascular risk factors such as diabetes.

The main influence upon plasma cholesterol levels is diet. The elevating effect comes mostly from the ingestion of saturated fats. Eating cholesterol is generally less influential, but there appears to be individual sensitivity. Between 1963 and 1977, the American nation reduced its consumption of dairy produce and other saturated fats by 47 per cent, with a concomitant increased intake of vegetable fats and oils of 58 per cent. It is likely that this (along with changes in smoking habits and better treatment of hypertension) has contributed to the falling incidence of coronary heart disease.

Hypertension

Our attitude to hypertension has changed dramatically over the last 30 years, and is reflected in terms of awareness, screening, investigation and management. The justification for regarding hypertension as a disease requiring therapy is that (as for hyperlipidaemia) the upper limits of the population distribution of blood pressure are associated with increased morbidity and mortality.

The distribution of blood pressure values in the population is a continuum, and the cut-off point above which patients are considered hypertensive is arbitrary. Blood pressure rises with age, and usually accelerates after the age of 45 years. Guidelines from the World Health Organisation (WHO/International Society of Hypertension, 1983) state that a single (seated) blood pressure greater than 160/95 is abnormal, values below 140/90 are normal and readings between are borderline. Of course this definition does not allow for the population being screened, the age of the patient or gender. Generally, Western populations have higher blood pressures than populations in underdeveloped countries, and estimated incidences of about 35 per cent have been quoted for the Western industrialised populations. About half of these will have diastolic blood pressures between 90 and 99 mmHg; 28 to 42 per cent will lie between 100 and 129 mmHg and about 2 per cent will be above 130 mmHg (Bannan et al, 1980). Unfortunately, not all people know that they are hypertensive; hypertension is usually asymptomatic.

Life insurance tables show that the higher the blood pressure, the higher the risk of dying. The Framingham study provided evidence of higher risks of stroke (seven-fold), heart failure (four-fold) and coronary heart disease (three-fold) with increases in blood pressure. The risk is not uniform, but higher in those with other risk factors such as smoking and hypercholesterolaemia. The systolic blood pressure seems to be equally as important as the diastolic but is not emphasised so much (Kannel et al, 1971).

Diabetes

There is a linear trend between carbohydrate intolerance and subsequent development of ischaemic heart disease. Whilst part of this risk is mediated by the association of diabetes with hypertension and hyperlipidaemia, it is clear that diabetes itself increases the cardiovascular risk independently. The incidence of coronary heart disease in diabetics is approximately twice that of the age-matched population, and it is even higher in diabetic women, who seem to lose the protection that their gender normally affords. Even those patients with impaired glucose tolerance (IGT) run twice the risk of developing large vessel atheroma when compared to those with normal glucose tolerance (figure 3.5). (See also WHO Expert Committee on Diabetes Mellitus, 1980.)

Physical activity

It is perhaps inevitable that the availability of modern technology has been implicated in the rise in coronary deaths. Whereas the manual worker in the past was protected from the effects of a sedentary occupation, the advent of mechanical aids including the car, conveyor belts, lifts and other labour-saving devices has minimised the amount of exercise taken at work.

It is hard to demonstrate the benefits of exercise, since observations may simply reflect a generally healthier life-style in those who take regular exercise. However, those who engage in vigorous sports and keep-fit exercises have half the incidence of fatal and non-fatal coronary events, compared with those who do not (Morris et al, 1980). This remains the case, regardless of age or the presence of other risk factors.

Exercise favourably influences lipid levels (raising HDL values) and fibrinolytic activity, and helps combat obesity. Physical fitness is also psychologically beneficial.

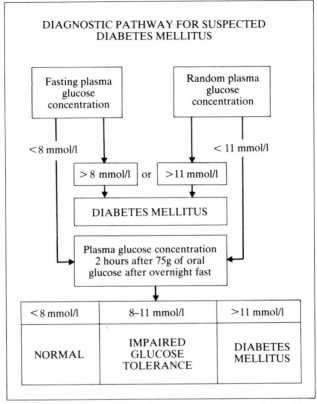

Fig. 3.5 Diagnostic pathways for suspected diabetes mellitus (Reproduced by kind permission of Current Medical Literature Ltd.)

Unfortunately, it probably does not influence prognosis following acute myocardial infarction. There is no evidence that it prevents progression of the disease, promotes coronary collateral circulation or reduces the risk of further heart attacks.

Obesity

The association between coronary heart disease and obesity is complex. Hypertension and hypercholesterolaemia vary with obesity in a continuous manner, and both of course are major coronary risk factors. The effect of obesity in general is to increase blood pressure, blood volume, resting cardiac output, left ventricular filling pressure and vascular resistance. All these factors will lead to an increased cardiac workload. Other risks of obesity are diabetes (135 per cent increase), cerebrovascular disease (53 per cent), coronary heart disease (35 per cent), accidents (18 per cent) and cancer (16 per cent). Other coexisting problems that frequently occur are hypertension, respiratory disease, arthritis, varicose veins, hernias and gall-stones.

Obesity may be assessed by the *body mass index* (BMI) given by:

$$BMI = \frac{Weight\ (kg)}{[Height\ (m)^2]}$$

BMI values for non-obese individuals lie between 20 and 25. Obesity is viewed as starting at a value of 30, and gross obesity at 40. About 6 per cent of men and 8 per cent of women are obese (i.e. BMI greater than 30), which is equivalent to nearly 3 million people in the UK.

Abdominal fat seems to relate more strongly to coronary heart disease than does fat on the limbs or hips. The waist–hip ratio may be a better predictor of cardiovascular mortality than the body mass index (Jarrett, 1986).

Stress

Although stress probably plays a major role in the genesis of coronary heart disease, it is very difficult to quantify. Certainly acute mental stress, anger or excitement can precipitate angina or dysrhythmias, which could lead to myocardial infarction, heart failure or sudden death. Stressful life-events often precede admission to coronary care (Solomon et al, 1969).

The influence of personality factors on coronary heart disease has become a subject of increasing interest. Among the personality traits related to ischaemic heart disease are aggression, hostility, ambition and anxiety (Rissanen and Nikkila, 1979). Research in this area has focused mainly on the 'Type A' behaviour pattern originally described by Friedman and Rosenman (1959). This behaviour is characterised by intense striving for achievement, competitiveness, time urgency, being easily provoked, impatience, hostility, abruptness of gesture and speech, tenseness of facial muscles, overcommitment to vocation or profession and excessive drive. 'Type B' behaviour, in contrast, is characterised by a relaxed, unhurried, satisfied life-style. Neither are fixed personality traits.

The Type A behaviour pattern may constitute an independent risk factor for coronary heart disease although there is no relation between Type A behaviour and the course of ischaemic heart disease following acute myocardial infarction (Case et al, 1985). In addition, Type A behaviour has not been found to relate to new cardiac events in British men, although it is more common in those with ECG or questionnaire evidence of coronary heart disease (Johnston et al, 1987). It may be that Type A behaviour confers a risk only in collaboration with other behavioural or psychological factors that result in increased sympathetic (catecholamine) activity.

Socioeconomic and geographical factors

There are marked international differences in the occurrence of ischaemic heart disease, even allowing for the differences made in disease classification by different countries. In the 'seven countries' study (Keys, 1980), the incidence of coronary heart disease varied between 0.15 per cent in Japan and 1.98 per cent in Finland, and mortality rates were similar. Migrants who move from low-risk to high-risk areas increase their rates of ischaemic heart disease to those of the host country.

Ischaemic heart disease is more common is wealthy as opposed to poor countries, although within these communities there is an inverse relationship between ischaemic heart disease and the social class; coronary heart disease is more common in social classes IV and V (Rose and Marmot, 1981). Smoking and dietary habits differ in these lower socioeconomic groups, and there is a tendency to higher blood pressure, obesity and heavier smoking habits. However, this probably does not account for all the observed increased risk.

Other factors

A high blood uric acid level (with or without gout) is possibly an independent risk factor. However, those prone to this are usually overweight, with hyperlipidaemia and glucose intolerance. Alcoholics and heavy drinkers have an increased cardiac mortality, although moderate drinkers (particularly of wine) appear to be less prone than even those who do not drink. This may be because alcohol ingestion raises HDL levels, and can ameliorate stress.

Data on the relationship between oral contraceptives and cardiovascular disease continues to accumulate. The study from the Royal College of General Practitioners (1974) found that the incidence of myocardial infarction was three times higher in women taking the oral contraceptive pill, the problem being greater in those with other risk factors, particularly smoking. This may in part be due to alteration of plasma lipid concentrations or perhaps changes in blood clotting factors; raised levels of factors VII and VIII and fibrinogen have been found to be predictors of ischaemic heart disease mortality.

THE MANIFESTATIONS OF ISCHAEMIC HEART DISEASE

The main clinical manifestations of ischaemic heart disease are:

● Angina (stable or unstable)
● Myocardial infarction (non-transmural and transmural)
● Sudden death

Cardiac failure and acute dysrhythmias are also usually attributable to myocardial ischaemia.

Angina

Angina is a symptom and not a disease. It may be broadly defined as:

● A discomfort located in the chest or adjacent areas which is
● Caused by myocardial hypoxia secondary to inadequate coronary blood flow and is
● Not associated with myocardial necrosis

Post-mortem studies on patients with stable angina usually reveal more than 75 per cent stenosis (cross-sectional) of two or more coronary vessels. In life, however, patients with angina show much less evidence of atheroma, and the myocardium is usually, remarkably, spared.

In patients with unstable angina the vessels show plaques undergoing fissuring with thrombus, and those with previous histories of angina at rest are most likely to have arterial spasm in association with the areas of atheromatous stenosis.

Myocardial infarction

Myocardial infarction refers to necrosis of myocardial cells caused by cessation or reduction in their blood supply. It is usually associated with an occlusive thrombus in one or more of the coronary arteries superimposed on a discrete and fissured atherosclerotic plaque (*Lancet*, 1985).

Coronary occlusion quickly leads to transmural myocardial ischaemia. After 20 minutes, necrosis begins and progresses in a wavefront from endocardium to epicardium. The infarcted area is at first red because of 'stuffing in' of the red cells (*infarct* = 'stuffed in'). The area later becomes pale as the necrotic muscle swells and squeezes out the extravasated blood. Finally, the infarcted area is gradually replaced by fibrous scar tissue over the course of one week to three months.

Although occlusive thrombi are found in up to 90 per cent of cases of patients immediately following myocardial infarction, this figure may fall in the later hours because of spontaneous thrombolysis (Rentrop, 1985; Mandelkorn et al, 1983). The speed with which some arteries reopen suggests that spasm may play an important role. About 1 per cent of patients with acute myocardial infarction have normal coronary arteriograms, and the cause of the infarction remains speculative (Arnett and Roberts, 1976).

Sudden death

A sudden death is one occurring from natural causes, where the patient dies within six hours of developing symptoms (and often immediately). Ischaemic heart disease is responsible for about 70 per cent of sudden deaths, but about half will have had no previously recognised heart disease. If a coronary artery is ligated experimentally, histological changes do not occur for four to six hours, so that patients who die suddenly often do not have firm morphological, enzyme or electrocardiographic evidence of myocardial infarction.

Sudden death has two major underlying causes: vascular (haemorrhagic or thromboembolic) and dysrhythmic. These may occur alone or, more commonly, together. Ambulatory electrocardiography in patients dying suddenly suggests that an acute ventricular dysrhythmia is the most common cause of death (Milner et al, 1985). Most cases are presumed to be initiated by an acute event such as coronary artery spasm, acute plaque fissuring or perhaps coronary emboli arising from ulcerated plaques, producing distal 'microinfarcts'. Post-mortem evidence usually shows plaque fissuring, often in association with fresh coronary thrombus. In 40 per cent of cases, this would have led to myocardial infarction if the victim had lived longer. About a third of cases have smaller intraluminal thrombosis, which seems to embolise distally, creating microinfarcts, rather like transient cerebral ischaemic attacks (Stehbens, 1985). In 20 per cent of cases, there is a fissure associated with intra-intimal thrombus, which may be responsible for initiating spasm, or intraluminal coronary thrombosis. In those with no evidence of fissures or acute coronary artery thrombosis, the cause of the dysrhythmias is probably left ventricular dysfunction secondary to myocardial ischaemia (Glover and Littler 1987).

References

Alpert J S and Braunwald E (1980) Pathological and clinical manifestations of acute myocardial infarction. In: *Heart Disease: A Textbook of Cardiovascular Medicine,* ed. Braunwald E, p. 1309. Philadelphia: W B Saunders.

Arnett E N and Roberts W C (1976) Acute myocardial infarction and angiographically normal coronary arteries: an unproven combination. *Circulation,* 53: 395–400.

Ball K and Turner R (1974) Smoking and the heart. The basis for action. *Lancet,* ii: 822–826.

Bannan L T, Beevers D G and Wright N (1980) Hypertension: the size of the problem. *British Medical Journal,* 281: 921–923.

Beaumont J, Carlson L A, Cooper G, Fejfar Z, Fredrickson D S and Strasser T (1970) Classification of the hyperlipidaemias and the hyperlipoproteinaemias. *Bulletin of the World Health Organisation,* 43: 891–915.

Berg K (1983) The genetics of coronary heart disease. In: *Progress in Medical Genetics,* Vol. V, eds. Steinberg A G, Bearner A G, Motulsky A G and Childs B. Philadelphia: W B Saunders.

Betriu A, Pare J C, Sanz G A, Casals F, Magrina J, Castaner A and Navarro-Lopes F (1981) Myocardial infarction with normal coronary arteries: a clinical-angiographic study. *American Journal of Cardiology,* 48: 28–32.

Bulkley B H (1986) Pathology of coronary atherosclerotic heart disease. In: *The Heart,* ed. Hurst J W, 6th edn., pp. 839–856. New York: McGraw-Hill.

Burch P R J (1980) Ischaemic heart disease; epidemiology, risk factors and cause. *Cardiovascular Research,* 14: 307–338.

Case R B, Heller S S and Case N B (1985) Type A behaviour and survival after acute myocardial infarction. *New England Journal of Medicine,* 312: 737–741.

Criqui M H (1986) Epidemiology of atherosclerosis: an updated overview. *American Journal of Cardiology,* 57: 18C–23C.

Davies M J (1987) Pathology of ischaemic heart disease. In: *Ischaemic Heart Disease,* ed. Fox K M, pp. 33–68. Lancaster: MTP Press.

Davies M J and Thomas A C (1985) The cause of acute myocardial infarction, sudden ischaemic death and crescendo angina. *British Heart Journal,* 53: 363–373.

Dawber T R (1980) *The Framingham Study. The Epidemiology of Atherosclerotic Disease.* Cambridge, Massachusetts: Harvard International Press.

De Faire U (1974) Ischaemic heart disease in death discordant twins. *Acta Medica Scandanavica* (Suppl.) 568: 1–109.

Doll R and Peto R (1976) Mortality in relation to smoking. *British Medical Journal,* 2: 1525–1536.

Factor S M and Kirk E S (1986) Pathophysiology of myocardial ischaemia. In: *The Heart,* ed. Hurst J W, 6th edn., p. 856. New York: McGraw-Hill.

Friedman M and Rosenman R H (1959) Association of specific overt behaviour pattern with blood and cardiovascular findings. *Journal of the American Medical Association,* 169: 1286–1296.

Friedman D G, Dales L G and Ury H K (1979) Mortality in middle aged smokers and non-smokers. *New England Journal of Medicine,* 300: 213–217.

Glover D R and Littler W A (1987) Factors influencing the survival and mode of death in severe ischaemic heart disease. *British Heart Journal,* 57: 125–132.

Glueck C J (1986) Role of risk factor management in progression and regression of coronary and femoral atherosclerosis. *American Journal of Cardiology,* 57: 35G–41G.

Haft J I and Bachik M (1984) Progression of coronary artery disease in patients with chest pain and normal or intraluminal disease on arteriography. *American Heart Journal,* 107: 35–39.

Jarrett R J (1986) Is there an ideal body weight? *British Medical Journal,* 293: 493–495.

Johnston D W, Cook D G and Shaper A G (1987) Type A behaviour and ischaemic heart disease in middle aged British men. *British Medical Journal,* 295: 86–89.

Kannel W B, Gordon T and Schwartz M G (1971) Systolic versus diastolic blood pressure and risk of coronary heart disease. The Framingham Study. *American Journal of Cardiology,* **27:** 335–346.

Keys A (1980) *Seven Countries.* London: Harvard University Press.

Lancet (1985) Treatment of coronary thrombosis. *Lancet,* **i:** 375–376.

Mandelkorn J B, Wolf N M, Singh S, Shechter J A, Kersh R I, Rodgers D M, Workman M B, Bentivoglio L G, LaPorte S M and Meister S G (1983) Intra-coronary thrombus in non-transmural myocardial infarction and in unstable angina pectoris. *American Journal of Cardiology,* **52:** 1–6.

Mann J I and Marmot M G (1987) Epidemiology of ischaemic heart disease. In: *Oxford Textbook of Medicine,* eds. Weatherall D J, Ledingham J G G and Warrell D A, 2nd edn., p.13.143. Oxford: Oxford Medical Publications.

Maseri A (1982) Expanding views on ischaemic heart disease: a perspective for the 1980s. *Clinical Science,* **62:** 119–123.

Milner P G, Platia E V, Reid P R and Griffith L P C (1985) Ambulatory electrocardiographic recordings at the time of fatal cardiac arrest. *American Journal of Cardiology,* **56:** 588–592.

Morris J N, Everitt M G, Pollard R, Chave S P W and Semmence A M (1980) Vigorous exercise in leisure time: protection against coronary heart disease. *Lancet,* **ii:** 1207–1210.

Oliver M F (1984) Hypercholesterolaemia and coronary heart disease: an answer. *British Medical Journal,* **288:** 423–424.

Oliver M F (1987) Problems and limitations. In: *Screening for Risk of Coronary Heart Disease,* eds. Oliver M F, Ashley-Miller M and Wood D, pp. 3–9. Chichester: John Wiley & Sons.

Pichard A D, Ziff C, Rentrop P, Holt J, Blanke H and Smith H (1983) Angiographic study of the infarct-related coronary artery in the chronic stage of acute myocardial infarction. *American Heart Journal,* **106:** 687–692.

Prinzmetal M, Kennamer R, Merliss R, Wada T and Bor N (1959) Angina pectoris. I. A variant form of angina pectoris: preliminary report. *American Journal of Medicine,* **27:** 375–388.

Rentrop K P (1985) Thrombolytic therapy in patients with acute myocardial infarction. *Circulation,* **71:** 627–631.

Riemersma R A (1984) Coronary heart disease: raised cholesterol or triglycerides? *International Journal of Cardiology,* **5:** 193–194.

Rissanen A M and Nikkila E A (1979) Aggregation of coronary risk factors in families of young men with fatal and non-fatal coronary heart disease. *British Heart Journal,* **42:** 373–380.

Rose G and Marmot M G (1981) Social class and coronary heart disease. *British Heart Journal,* **45:** 13–19.

Rose G and Shipley M J (1980) Plasma lipids and mortality: a source of error. *Lancet,* **i:** 523–526.

Ross R (1986) The pathogenesis of atherosclerosis – an update. *New England Journal of Medicine,* **314:** 488–500.

Royal College of General Practitioners (1974) *Oral Contraceptives and Health.* London: Pitman.

Shaper A G, Pocock S J, Walker M, Phillips A N, Whitehead T P and Macfarlane P W (1985) Risk factors for ischaemic heart disease: the prospective phase of the British Regional Heart Study. *Journal of Epidemiology and Community Health,* **39:** 197–209.

Solomon H A, Edwards A L and Killip T (1969) Prodromata in acute myocardial infarction. *Circulation,* **40:** 463–471.

Stehbens W E (1985) Relationship of coronary artery thrombosis to myocardial infarction. *Lancet,* **ii:** 639–642.

Wells N (1987) *Coronary Heart Disease: The Need for Action.* London: Office of Health Economics.

WHO/International Society of Hypertension (1983) Memorandum: Guidelines for the treatment of mild hypertension. *WHO Bulletin,* **61:** 53–56.

WHO Expert Committee on Diabetes Mellitus (1980) *Second Report.* WHO Technical Report Series No. 646. Geneva: WHO.

Patient Assessment

The initial contact with a patient suspected of having coronary artery disease may be either in an outpatient department or following an acute admission to hospital. Clinical appraisal will include taking a history, making an examination and carrying out special investigations.

These initial steps frequently take place on the coronary care unit and may necessarily have to be brief. The immediate decisions to be made are: does he have a cardiovascular illness, and if so what needs to be done (either therapeutically or diagnostically)? As many as two-thirds of patients admitted to coronary care may be later shown not to have suffered a myocardial infarction, so that the coronary care unit has a diagnostic as well as a therapeutic role.

In the medical clinic, patients may present with many symptoms other than chest pain. Equally, not all patients presenting with chest pain will be found to have coronary heart disease. Although the diagnosis of myocardial ischaemia may be easy, this is frequently not the case. The physician must be aware of clinical methods available for confirming or refuting the diagnosis. If coronary artery disease is suspected, full assessment is required to plan therapy and predict prognosis.

Assessment may be divided into:

- Defining symptoms
- Demonstration of clinical signs
- Organising appropriate investigations

SYMPTOMS OF HEART DISEASE

Chest pain and breathlessness are two of the commonest complaints that lead to a patient seeking medical advice. Causes of chest pain are many and diverse (table 4.1). Patients suspected of having acute myocardial infarction are admitted to coronary care in the belief that the short-term prognosis may be improved by early intensive care, with particular reference to control of fatal dysrhythmias (Adgey et al, 1971). Nevertheless, the coronary care unit can be a dangerous place for patients who have non-cardiac chest pain, and all medical staff should consider differential or concomitant diagnoses. All too often it is assumed that ill patients attached to cardiac monitors have had a heart attack. The frequency with which non-cardiac pain appears on coronary care demonstrates how difficult it is to determine the origin of chest pain (table 4.2).

Chest pain can originate from most tissues in the chest, including the heart and pericardium, the lungs and pleura, the oesophagus, the vertebrae and ribs, and the

Table 4.1 Some causes of chest pain.

Cardiovascular causes	Non-cardiac causes
Myocardial ischaemia	Herpes zoster
Coronary artery spasm	Oesophageal reflux
Myocardial infarction	Oesophageal spasm
Pericarditis	Hiatus hernia
Dissecting aortic aneurysm	Pneumonia
Pulmonary embolism	Pneumothorax
Mitral valve prolapse	Pleurisy
	Peptic ulceration
	Gall-bladder disease
	Musculoskeletal pain
	Da Costa's syndrome (cardioneurosis)

skin. Diagnosis is often difficult, because the pain can originate from more than one of these tissues. For example, many patients presenting with angina often have concurrent oesophageal reflux.

Chest pain is often described in atypical ways, and normal findings on physical examination do not exclude a diagnosis. When signs are elicited, they are often those caused by the pain (hypotension, sweating) and not by the underlying disease.

Table 4.2 Primary discharge diagnosis in patients admitted to coronary care (Leicester General Hospital, 1985).

	Percentage
Cardiovascular (78.9%)	
Myocardial infarction	37.3
Angina	18.4
Dysrhythmias	12.8
Left ventricular failure	5.7
Pericarditis	2.4
Post cardiac arrest	2.3
Non-cardiac (21.1%)	
Chest pain of uncertain origin	6.7
Gastrointestinal causes	2.1
Respiratory tract infection	2.0
Musculoskeletal	2.0
Viral infection	1.7
Pulmonary embolus	1.3
Anxiety/hyperventilation	0.9
Cerebrovascular accident	0.7
Aortic dissection	0.4
Asthma	0.3
Others – pancreatitis, pneumothorax, carcinoma of lung, anaemia, gastrointestinal haemorrhage, constipation, cervical spondylitis, Munchausen's syndrome, etc.	< 0.5

Sudden onset of severe chest pain should be managed as myocardial infarction until proved otherwise. Fifty per cent of deaths from heart attacks occur in the first two hours: 25 per cent immediately or within 15 minutes, 15 per cent in the next 45 minutes, and 10 per cent in the second hour. Rapid admission to hospital is usually indicated, and most coronary care units offer an open policy whilst accepting that many admissions may be inappropriate. Unfortunately, this can lead to abuse of the service, which is unavoidable if lives are going to be saved.

Chest pain

The most important diagnosis not to be missed is coronary artery disease, but the differential diagnosis of chest pain must always be considered.

Myocardial ischaemia

About half the patients presenting with myocardial infarction suffer from angina or will have had a previous heart attack. This is useful diagnostically, since the patient is often able to identify the cause of his pain correctly. The differentiation of angina from myocardial infarction is often difficult unless the pain is particularly severe or accompanied by sweating, faintness and vomiting. It is therefore wise to assume that myocardial infarction has occurred if the pain lasts longer than half an hour, or does not respond to two active glyceryl trinitrate (GTN) tablets. The action of GTN takes only a few seconds or at most two to three minutes. The tablets have a limited active life, and any carried in pockets for years will not relieve any sort of pain.

Anginal pain is usually described as a constricting ache in the chest frequently radiating to the jaw, the neck, the back and one or both arms. It is precipitated by exercise (including sexual intercourse), particularly in the cold. It is relieved quickly by the rest and GTN. Nocturnal angina (angina decubitus) is often relieved by sitting up. Angina is often atypical and 10 per cent of patients do not have central chest pain as a leading symptom. The origin of anginal pain is probably the myocardium itself, with a phenomenon analogous to cramp taking place. The impulses travel from the myocardium via sympathetic fibres to the thoracic sympathetic ganglia to nerve roots T1–5. These spinal nerves supply the anterior chest wall and the inner aspect of the arm and hand. For that reason the pain is felt in the region bounded by these thoracic nerves. Even in its atypical presentation, ischaemic pain rarely extends beyond the region between the lower jaw and the epigastrium (roots C3–T6). The location is never so sharply localised that it may be identified with a pointing finger.

Pericardial pain

Pain is the usual presenting feature of pericarditis and arises from the parietal pericardium (the visceral pericardium being insensitive). Pericardial pain is sharp, aching and usually made worse by lying back or swallowing. The diagnosis is confirmed by the presence of a pericardial friction rub. The commonest underlying cause is acute myocardial infarction. The next most frequent cause is a viral infection, especially in the young patient who has often had a recent flu-like illness. Other causes include connective tissues disorders (e.g. systemic lupus erythematosus or sarcoidosis), tuberculosis and renal failure. The ECG classically (but not always) shows widespread concave ST segment elevation.

Aortic dissection

The chest pain of aortic dissection classically radiates through to the back, and presents with shock and loss of peripheral pulses. Myocardial infarction may result if blood tracks round to occlude the coronary arteries, and pericarditis as well if blood leaks through to the pericardium. The mixture of pains coming from these different tissues can make diagnosis difficult.

Chest pain from the lungs

Pleural pain is localised and associated with respiration (especially deep inspiration), and usually complicates pneumonia or viral chest infections.

Pulmonary emboli cause dyspnoea, pleuritic pain and haemoptysis, but large emboli may mimic myocardial infarction, presenting with shock and central chest pain. It is worth remembering that patients with pulmonary emboli may also have critical myocardial ischaemia. The embolus may cause so much additional strain upon the heart that angina may be the presenting complaint.

A left-sided pneumothorax can be confused with myocardial pain, particularly in tension pneumothorax when shock is present.

Oesophageal pain

Oesophageal pain ('indigestion and heartburn') is the commonest mistaken origin of myocardial pain, and is the commonest cause of chest discomfort in the general population. Post-mortem examination of patients dying from acute myocardial infarction usually reveals one or two antacid tablets in the stomach, taken shortly before death by a mistaken patient. The main problem is that about one-third of the population has a degree of oesophageal reflux, and symptoms are bound to coexist with other causes of chest pain.

Mucosal (Mallory–Weiss) tears may occur after bouts of vomiting, as may oesophageal rupture. Both present with chest pain, and the latter with shock. Other gastrointestinal disorders such as peptic ulceration and gall-bladder disease often cause difficulty with differential diagnosis. An upper gastrointestinal bleed may present with lower chest pain and shock.

Musculoskeletal pain

Fractures of the ribs, vertebral collapse and other muscular strains can cause chest pain. Bornholm's disease (intercostal myalgia) and Tietze's syndrome (sternal costochondritis) may be severe and are usually associated with a flu-like illness in the younger patient.

Skin

Herpes zoster often presents with pain a day or two before the rash appears. If this affects a thoracic nerve root, chest pain which is often indistinguishable from the pain of myocardial infarction may be the leading symptom.

Chest pain of unknown origin

This is a proper diagnosis which may be applied to a patient presenting with chest pain in whom myocardial ischaemia seems unlikely and no other cause can be found. The typical patient is a middle-aged male presenting with chronic, intermittent stabbing pain in the left breast lasting for a few seconds, often radiating down the left arm. GTN has usually been tried and, although claimed to be useful, only works after 30 minutes. The problem is how far to investigate these patients, and many end up having coronary angiography.

Dyspnoea

Dyspnoea means difficulty with breathing and is entirely subjective. Many patients who are obviously short of breath at rest will not complain of respiratory difficulties, yet others claim to be short of breath on exertion, but are able to complete exercise stress tests with apparent ease. Breathlessness is usually due to a cardiorespiratory disorder, obesity or anaemia. Dyspnoea caused by cardiac disease is probably due to a combination of factors.

Left ventricular failure is the classical cardiac cause of acute breathlessness, with pulmonary oedema causing increased lung rigidity and decreased oxygen transfer. Respiration will therefore require greater effort, which is not helped by oedematous narrowing of the larger airways. Dyspnoea may also be caused by a raised left atrial pressure alone, which causes pulmonary venous congestion with few physical signs. The venous congestion reduces vital capacity and stimulates pulmonary stretch receptors which cause the shortness of breath.

Orthopnoea is difficulty with breathing when lying flat. It is often an early symptom of left ventricular failure, but may not be volunteered by the patient who learns to sleep propped up with three or four pillows. The increase in venous return in the recumbent patient reduces vital capacity and lung compliance. Patients with chronic obstructive airways disease often complain of waking with dyspnoea and wheezing. Orthopnoea in this instance is actually due to the loss of the diaphragmatic component of their respiratory pattern, corrected by sitting up. Hence it can be seen that orthopnoea does not automatically indicate heart failure.

Paroxysmal nocturnal dyspnoea (PND) may be viewed as a delayed form of orthopnoea. Dyspnoea is probably precipitated by the patient sliding down the bed into a horizontal position. The increase in pulmonary congestion leads to dyspnoea, which is reversed by the patient sitting up or standing. Typically the patient jumps out of bed to an open window, gasping for breath.

In patients with right ventricular failure, an enlarged liver and ascites may contribute to orthopnoea by diaphragmatic splinting.

Cheyne–Stokes Breathing

John Cheyne (1818) and William Stokes (1846) described this well-known abnormality of respiration independently. It consists of a respiratory cycle beginning with hardly perceptible respiratory efforts gradually increasing in depth (rather like the sound of a wood-saw) until very much exaggerated. The effort then dies away until breathing ceases for a period of about 20 to 30 seconds. The whole cycle is then repeated, lasting for between one and three minutes. The mechanism is quite complex, but essentially the pauses in respiration allow the levels of arterial carbon dioxide to rise, which stimulates the respiratory centre to set off a fresh cycle of breathing. Cheyne–Stokes breathing is common in the elderly, especially during sleep. However, it is also found in those with chronic chest disease or following a stroke. In cardiac patients it is common in heart failure or may be associated with heart rhythm disturbances, such as junctional rhythms and heart block.

Syncope

Syncope is a transient loss of consciousness resulting from inadequate cerebral blood flow, leading to cerebral ischaemia. There are many causes of syncope, and only a few are due to cardiac causes. Cerebral blood flow is kept remarkably constant and is not influenced by autonomic control. Vasovagal attacks are the most common cause of syncope, and occur following prolonged standing or in response to emotion or pain. The face is pale, the pupils dilated and the pulse and respiration are slow. Peripheral pulses are often impalpable, leading to the frequent diagnosis of cardiac arrest.

Carotid sinus syncope may result from stimulation of the carotid sinus, either during carotid massage, or if the patient's neck-wear is too tight.

Micturition syncope occurs in old men with nocturia who lose consciousness whilst voiding. This is either because straining reduces venous return and subsequently cardiac output (Valsalva manoeuvre), or because sudden decompression of an over-dilated bladder causes reflex vasodilatation.

Exertion syncope is a characteristic feature of aortic stenosis, when the cardiac output through the narrow valve cannot meet the demands of increased activity.

Dysrhythmia-induced syncope may result from heart rates which are too slow or too fast to maintain cerebral blood flow. Stokes–Adams attacks may be missed if the ECG is normal between attacks. The attack may terminate in a convulsion leading to an erroneous diagnosis of epilepsy. However, there is no aura and recovery is prompt and accompanied by flushing as the blood flows again through vessels dilated by hypoxia. The desire to sleep does not occur and headache is not so common.

Paroxysmal tachycardias (supraventricular or ventricular) often lead to a marked fall in cardiac output with resulting syncope.

Oedema

Oedema is an abnormal accumulation of fluid in the interstitial tissues, and is usually preceded by weight gain from 3 to 5 kg of extracellular fluid. It is a relatively late manifestation of heart failure. Oedema will collect preferentially in loose tissues, and the distribution of fluid is determined by both gravity and the degree of ambulation. In most patients the legs and feet are affected, but in those who are confined to bed the fluid accumulates over the sacrum. Greater degrees of oedema will gradually affect the whole of the lower extremities, extending to the torso and eventually the face (*anasarca*). The oedema characteristically pits when pressure is applied (*pitting oedema*).

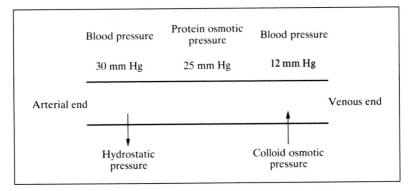

Fig. 4.1 Changing pressures within a capillary

Normally, fluid is exuded into the tissues because arterial capillary pressure (30 mmHg) exceeds plasma oncotic pressure (25 mmHg). However, the fluid is forced back into circulation at the venous end of the capillaries because pressure here (12 mmHg) is exceeded by the oncotic pressure (25 mmHg). If the venous pressure rises (as in heart failure), the resorption of fluid is impaired and oedema results (figure 4.1). Effusions into the chest and abdomen (ascites) occur later in the course of heart failure for the same reasons.

Haemoptysis

Coughing up blood is not an uncommon symptom in cardiac disease. When related to circulatory pathology, it is small in amount and the sputum is usually only streaked. When haemoptysis is related to exercise or is heavy, it usually indicates mitral stenosis with pulmonary veins rupturing under high pressure. However, frank haemoptysis usually indicates pulmonary disease (such as bronchial carcinoma or tuberculosis) or pulmonary infarction.

Palpitations

Palpitation is an awareness of the heart beat, familiar to those awaiting examinations! Most normal people are aware of their heart beat at some time, especially at night when lying on the left side. As such, palpitation is a common symptom regardless of any underlying heart disease. It may be felt and described in many different ways. Some complain of a racing heart, whilst others of thumping or feeling a missed beat. In a hyperdynamic circulation (in pregnancy or thyrotoxicosis, for example) the symptoms are more prominent.

Palpitation is an important complaint in those with cardiac rhythm disturbances, but the description frequently does not help with diagnosis.

A thumping or pounding heart is the commonest complaint and is usually the awareness of normal beats, sometimes exaggerated in strength and speed by sympathetic overactivity (e.g. stress and anxiety). They frequently occur for prolonged periods, and on a daily basis.

Dropped beats are probably the next commonest complaint, and these are more frequent if basic sinus rhythm is slow. Ectopic activity and sinus thumping is more frequent during hyperdynamic circulatory states (pregnancy, fevers or thyrotoxicosis), and when the heart is overstimulated by drugs (for example tobacco, caffeine, alcohol, bronchodilators and nasal decongestant sprays).

Racing of the heart is usually abnormal if the pulse rate exceeds 120 beats per minute and may be due to supraventricular, junctional or even ventricular tachycardia. The history may go back for many years, although attacks are usually infrequent.

If the heart is giving irregular flutters, it is usually due to paroxysmal atrial fibrillation. Frequent ectopic beats may produce the same feeling, and both are common in the elderly.

SIGNS OF HEART DISEASE

Cyanosis

Cyanosis describes the blue (cyan) discoloration imparted to the skin and mucous membranes due to low oxygen content of the blood. It seems to become visible only when there is greater than 5 per cent of reduced (i.e. oxygen-depleted) haemoglobin in the blood of the vessels being considered. Cyanosis is either peripheral or central.

Peripheral cyanosis

Peripheral cyanosis is observed in the peripheries, the fingers and toes, and is caused by a higher degree of oxygen extraction at these sites. For example, most people are aware that their fingers go blue in the winter. When the weather is cold peripheral circulation shows down, allowing the blood to spend longer in the fingers and toes, with a resulting greater degree of deoxygenation. The same applies to patients with low cardiac output (e.g. mitral stenosis or shock).

Central cyanosis

Central cyanosis is due either to inadequate oxygenation of the blood as it passes through the lungs (as in pulmonary disease) or to more than 30 per cent of left ventricular output by-passing the lungs altogether. If, for instance, there is a congenital heart lesion such as a patent ductus arteriosus, most of the blood will pass from the pulmonary to the systemic circulation before it reaches the lungs (so-called right-to-left shunting), producing central cyanosis. The patients' fingernails are frequently clubbed, and warm mucous membranes (e.g. mouth and lips) as well as the peripheries are blue.

Rarely, central cyanosis can be produced by certain drugs leading to the formation of methaemoglobin and sulphaemoglobin which do not carry so much oxygen.

Arterial pulses

Arterial pulses should be examined for rate, rhythm, volume and the character of the waveform. Although the rate and rhythm are usually assessed by palpating the right radial artery, an artery closer to the heart (e.g. the carotid) is usually better for appreciating pulse width and waveform. In clinical practice, all features can most easily be felt in the right brachial artery. All other peripheral pulses should of course be sought at some time during physical examination to determine presence and strength. This is especially important soon after admission to the coronary care unit, so that a missing pulse is not later explained by a peripheral embolus arising as a complication of myocardial infarction. The cardiac output at the time of examination must be borne in mind. An absent pulse may be due to low cardiac output in the acute stage of myocardial infarction which will later reappear as perfusion improves. Arterial bruits should also be listened for.

The characteristics of the arterial pulse are as follows.

Rate

The pulse should be counted over 30 or 60 seconds. This will enable irregular pulses to be counted more accurately, and pauses and ectopics to be appreciated. The normal adult pulse rate varies between 60 and 100 beats per minute. Sinus bradycardias (less than 60 beats per minute) are frequent following inferior myocardial infarction or in those taking beta-adrenergic blocking agents. Slow pulse rates may also be due to junctional rhythm or heart block. Rates in excess of 100 beats per minute are often due to anxiety or pain. Heart rates of over 120 beats per minute usually indicate an abnormal tachydysrhythmia.

Rhythm

The normal pulse is regular, or may exhibit the gentle slowing and quickening of a sinus arrhythmia. This can often best be appreciated by studying the RR intervals in ECG rhythm strips during respiration. The heart will quicken on inspiration and slow on expiration. On inspiration, venous return to the heart increases because of the negative intrathoracic pressure. The heart rate therefore increases to cope with the increased load. During expiration, venous return falls and the heart slows again. An occasional irregularity in an otherwise regular pulse suggests ectopic beats, which may arise from either the atria or the ventricles. An 'irregularly irregular' pulse is found in atrial fibrillation or with multiple ectopic beats. The two may be differentiated by an ECG strip or clinically by exercising the patient. As the heart rate increases, ectopic beats will be abolished, resulting in a regular pulse. There is no change in the pulse if the rhythm is atrial fibrillation.

Pulse volume

Pulse volume (width or amplitude) is an appreciation of the difference between systolic and diastolic blood pressures (*the pulse pressure*), and should be described as normal, small volume or large volume. It is not difficult to appreciate if

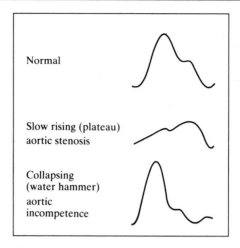

Fig 4.2   Sample arterial pulse waveforms

comparison is made with the pulse in a patient who is shocked and in another who is pregnant. The former will have a low-volume pulse and the latter will have a high-volume pulse. Low-volume pulses are often found following myocardial infarction, in mitral stenosis and in constrictive pericarditis. Large-volume pulses are found in anaemia, aortic incompetence and thyrotoxicosis.

Character of the pulse wave

This is not easy to appreciate, but may aid diagnosis (figure 4.2). The terms widely used and heard on the coronary care unit are:

1. *The plateau pulse*   Low volume, slow rise and slow fall (e.g. aortic stenosis).

2. *The collapsing pulse*   Large volume, rapid rise and rapid fall (e.g. aortic incompetence, thyrotoxicosis and heart block).

3. *Pulsus paradoxus*   Pulse volume decreases with inspiration (e.g. chronic obstructive airways disease, asthma and cardiac tamponade).

4. *Pulsus alternans*   Alternate high-volume and low-volume beats (e.g. left ventricular failure).

5. *Absent pulse*   Missing pulses are usually due to atherosclerosis. However, in coronary care it is important to exclude peripheral embolisation and aortic dissection.

Blood pressure

The blood pressure is an accurate predictor of morbidity and mortality, and is therefore one of the most important clinical observations. However, there is still considerable confusion over the correct way to measure it. Blood pressure is usually measured with an aneroid or mercury sphygmomanometer, although precise measurement of arterial blood pressure requires invasive monitoring. Mercury sphygmomanometers are widely available in hospital practice and are more useful than the aneroid type which need frequent recalibration.

The correct selection and application of the pressure cuff is important, especially in obese patients (Geddes and Whistler, 1978). The width of the cuff should be 40 per cent of the arm's circumference, and the inflatable bag should cover more than two-thirds of the circumference of the arm. Hence a typical 'normal' cuff should measure 13 × 35 cm. The cuff should be applied firmly 2 cm above the antecubital fossa, and must not be twisted or in contact with the patient's clothing (Swales, 1979). The patient should be comfortable, and the forearm supported, slightly extended and externally rotated.

The cuff should be inflated whilst the brachial pulse is first palpated to determine the systolic pressure. The cuff should then be fully deflated and reinflated to 30 to 40 mmHg above the systolic pressure. The mercury column should be observed at eye level, and allowed to fall until a faint tapping sound is heard with the stethoscope placed firmly over the brachial artery. This is phase 1 of the Korotkoff sounds (Nicolai Korotkoff, 1905) and is equivalent to the systolic blood pressure. It should be measured to the nearest 2 mmHg.

There is then often a silent gap (phase 2) until sounds are heard again (phase 3). The sounds then become faint (phase 4) until they completely disappear (phase 5). Phase 4 and phase 5 have been used to indicate diastolic blood pressure in the past. These days, phase 5 should be universally used unless sounds are heard down to zero. In this instance, both phase 4 and phase 5 pressures should be recorded.

Normally, diastolic pressure rises a little on standing, and the systolic blood pressure falls slightly. In patients with autonomic failure or shock, there may be a very large fall (*postural hypotension*). There is little difference between sitting and lying blood pressures. It is normal to measure the blood pressure twice, recording the second reading. The arm used for measurement should be recorded, and blood pressure should always initially be taken in both arms so that subclavian stenosis is not missed.

There are certain occasions on which blood pressure estimation is difficult (table 4.3). This is particularly so in severe hypotension, when indirect readings with a sphygmomanometer are inaccurate, and invasive monitoring is then preferable. In atrial fibrillation, the blood pressure may vary from beat to beat, and an average of several estimations may then be required.

Jugular venous pressure (JVP)

The pulsation and level of the internal jugular vein is used to assess the central venous pressure (CVP), and may be seen in front of the sternomastoid muscle. With a normal CVP, pulsation of the internal jugular vein is usually visible only when the patient lies flat. When observing for CVP elevation, the height above the sternal angle should be measured with the patient lying at 45°. Confirmation of the level may be made by pressing on the abdomen which increases the CVP transiently (by increasing venous return to the heart). Much has been written about pulsation in the jugular vein, but clinically it is difficult to appreciate. Sometimes 'a' and 'v' waves may be seen which correspond to atrial and ventricular contraction. The most important abnormalities of the JVP are:

Table 4.3. Problems in measuring blood pressure.

Problem	Cause	Reasons
False high reading	Cuff too small	Small cuff does not adequately disperse the pressure over the arterial surface
	Bladder not centred over the brachial artery	More external pressure is needed to compress the artery
	Cuff not applied snugly	Uneven and slow inflation results in varying tissue compression
	Arm positioned below heart level	Hydrostatic pressure imposed by weight of blood column above site of auscultation additive to arterial pressure: reposition arm to appropriate level
	Very obese arm	Cuff too small for large arm will cause too little compression of the artery at the suitable pressure level: apply a large thigh cuff to the upper arm if necessary
False low reading	Cuff too large	Pressure is spread over too large an area and produces a damping effect on the Korotkoff sounds
	Arm positioned above heart level	Hydrostatic pressure in the elevated arm causes resistance to pressure generated by the heart

1. *Elevation,* due to a high right-sided heart pressure (e.g. heart failure, cor pulmonale).

2. *Large 'a' waves* associated with tricuspid stenosis, pulmonary stenosis and complete heart block. In the last condition, the atrial contractions are not synchronised with ventricular contractions. Every so often the atria contract against a closed tricuspid valve, and the force of contraction produces a huge *cannon wave*. There will be no 'a' wave in atrial fibrillation, since the atria do not contract.

3. *Large 'v' waves* occur in tricuspid regurgitation, usually secondary to heart failure when the distended right ventricle makes the tricuspid valve leak.

Examination of the JVP should always be followed by examination of the liver.

Palpation of the liver can be used to transiently elevate the JVP (*hepatojugular reflux*). Liver enlargement (as in heart failure) and pulsation (as in tricuspid incompetence) can also be appreciated.

The apex beat and cardiac impulse

The *apex beat* (the maximal thrust of the left ventricle) is normally seen and felt just inside the midclavicular line in the 5th left intercostal space. It may be displaced by abnormalities of the heart, lungs or rib cage. Collapse of the right lung, for example, will move the mediastinum (and heart) to the right, and a thoracic scoliosis may move the mediastinum either way. Seeing or even feeling the apex beat is often difficult in the obese or in those with hyperinflated chests (e.g. in chronic obstructive airways disease and emphysema). Turning the patient to the left or leaning him forward may then help.

Forceful left and right ventricular contraction or *thrills* (palpable murmurs) may also be felt.

The left ventricle produces a sustained heaving or thrusting apex beat if hypertrophied, but when enlargement is due to dilatation it is weak and diffuse. It has a 'tapping' quality in mitral stenosis. If there is a left ventricular aneurysm, there may be a double apical beat (*rocking* or *dyskinetic impulse*). The right ventricular impulse is usually not palpable in health. When enlarged (owing to pulmonary hypertension or right-sided valve disease) the ventricle gives rise to a parasternal heave. More usually this is due to mitral incompetence.

Thrills

Thrills are palpable murmurs. The commonest are:

● *Apical systolic thrills* in mitral regurgitation and with ventricular septal defects (VSD)
● *A basal systolic thrill* in aortic stenosis
● *A systolic thrill* over the lower sternum in pulmonary stenosis
● *An apical diastolic thrill* in mitral stenosis

The heart sounds

The first sound

The first sound (S1) is related to closure of the mitral and tricuspid valves. The mitral component is louder (so it is best heard at the apex) and closes fractionally before the tricuspid valve. At the onset of ventricular systole, the valve cusps have been forced downwards into the ventricle by atrial contraction, and the sound seems to be related to it snapping back up again, the movement being checked by the chordae tendineae.

Loud first heart sounds will occur if the left atrial pressure is abnormally high (mitral stenosis), during fast heart rates, or if the atrium contracts very close to ventricular systole (i.e. with a short PR interval). A soft first heart sound occurs if the mitral valve is rigid (e.g. calcified) and does not move well, or if left ventricular contraction is poor.

When there is dissociated contraction of the atria and ventricles (as in complete heart block), the first sound varies in intensity depending on the position of the valve at the onset of ventricular systole.

The second sound

The second sound (S2) is related to closure of the pulmonary and aortic valves and is best heard in the second left intercostal space. It is louder in pulmonary or systemic hypertension. The sound is normally split because the aortic valve closes before the pulmonary valve on inspiration (the right ventricle takes longer to expel the increased venous return). The types of splitting are as follows.

1. *Wide splitting* is caused when the right ventricle is overloaded and the valve is unable to close quickly (pulmonary stenosis, cor pulmonale) or in right bundle branch block when there is delayed left ventricular depolarisation.

2. *Reversed splitting* (where the splitting is best heard on expiration) occurs if the ventricle is overloaded (aortic stenosis, left ventricular failure or systemic hypertension). It may also occur in left bundle branch block, because the right ventricle is prematurely activated.

3. *Fixed splitting* (which does not vary with respiration) occurs when increased venous return affects both ventricles (e.g. atrioseptal defect).

The third sound

The third sound (S3) is associated with the ventricles tensing during rapid filling, and implies heart failure or a widely open mitral valve. (It cannot therefore occur in severe mitral stenosis.) It is low pitched and best heard at the apex. It may occur normally in the young and in pregnancy, but is usually abnormal in patients over the age of 40 years.

The fourth sound

The fourth sound (S4) is heard late in the cardiac cycle (just before the first sound) and is probably produced by rapid atrial emptying into a non-distending ventricle, as may be caused by hypertrophy or myopathy. It is never heard in health, and is usually found in left ventricular hypertrophy or cardiomyopathy (HOCM).

Gallop rhythm

This is often heard in heart failure. The addition of a third heart sound with a tachycardia makes the sounds resemble a galloping horse. If both third and fourth heart sounds are present, it is called a *summation gallop*.

Other heart sounds

Ejection clicks occur immediately after the first heart sound at the time of aortic and pulmonary valve opening and are usually associated with stenosis of the valves.

The opening snap of the mitral valve occurs at the time of mitral opening, and cannot be heard if the valve is heavily calcified. It may be confused with a third heart sound, but is much more widely conducted.

Heart murmurs

Murmurs are sounds caused by turbulent blood flow. This may be either because the blood flow is more rapid or because it is passing through an obstructed pathway. The significance of any such murmur may be:

- *Innocent:* minor turbulance unassociated with disease or structural abnormality
- *Physiological:* as in pregnancy, thyrotoxicosis, fever or anaemia (hyperdynamic flow)
- *Pathological:* indicative of a structural or functional cardiac abnormality

Innocent and physiological murmurs are sometimes referred to as *functional murmurs,* and are benign.

Murmurs are either systolic or diastolic, and their intensity is classed as grades 1 to 6 for systolic murmurs and 1 to 4 for diastolic murmurs. The higher the number, the louder the murmur. Clues to the origin of the murmur may be found by determining when the murmur occurs in the cardiac cycle, where and how it is best heard, how loud it is and, finally, where it radiates to.

1. *Systolic murmurs*   These are either pan-systolic (i.e. heard throughout systole) or mid-systolic (loudest in mid-systole). The latter are sometimes called *ejection systolic murmurs,* as they are usually associated with outflow through a stenosed pulmonary or aortic valve.

Innocent and physiological murmurs are virtually always systolic.

2. *Diastolic murmurs*   These are either early diastolic, mid-diastolic or late diastolic (pre-systolic). They are always low pitched.

3. *Continuous murmurs*   These start in systole and continue into diastole, but not necessarily throughout the whole cardiac cycle.

Features of the different murmurs are shown in figure 4.3.

Functional murmurs

Functional murmurs are very common in children and most disappear at or about puberty. Others that are most frequent are:

1. *Pulmonary systolic murmur*   This short 'blowing' murmur is often found in young adults. It may be heard down the left sternal edge and apex. A number of patients will be noted to have a sternal depression or an abnormally straight back ('straight back syndrome'). The mediastinum presumably squashes the heart from front to back, altering blood flow patterns. Although previously considered to be a form of pseudo-heart disease, it may be a familial condition and associated with mitral valve prolapse (Davies et al, 1980).

2. *Aortic ejection murmur*   In the middle-aged and elderly patient, aortic sclerosis and dilatation of the ascending aorta (especially in hypertension) are frequent. The murmur is usually easy to differentiate from aortic stenosis, since the pulse character is normal, and there is no evidence of left ventricular hypertrophy unless the patient has hypertension.

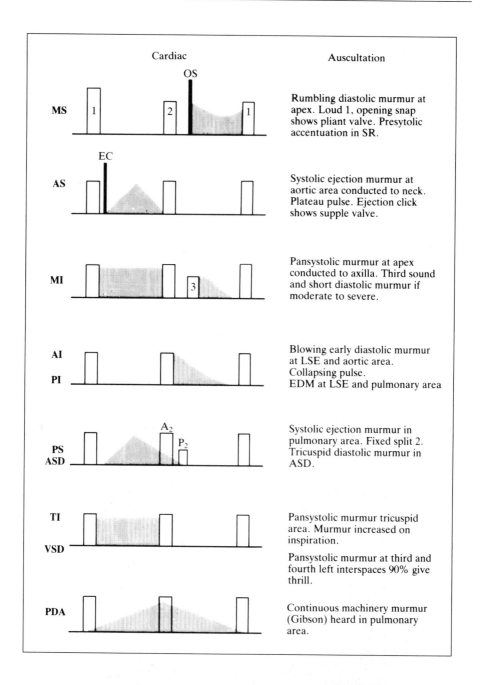

Fig. 4.3 Representation of cardiac murmurs heard on auscultation
MS = mitral stenosis; AS = aortic stenosis; MI = mitral incompetence; AI = aortic incompetence; PI = pulmonary incompetence; PS = pulmonary stenosis; ASD = atrial septal defect; TI = tricuspid incompetence; VSD = ventricular septal defect; PDA = patent ductus arteriosus; 1, 2 = first and second heart sounds

3. *Mitral systolic murmur* Fibrosis and calcification of the mitral ring is common in the elderly, and produces a murmur identical to mitral incompetence. In young women, a short late systolic murmur is fairly common, and may be due to prolapse of a mitral cusp into the left atrium at the end of ventricular systole. The prognostic significance of this is debatable (Oakley, 1984).

Pericardial friction rub

This is a scratchy sound (rather like sandpaper) produced by the inflamed visceral and parietal pericardia rubbing against each other. It may be localised, generalised, long lasting or transient. It is best heard with the patient sitting forward.

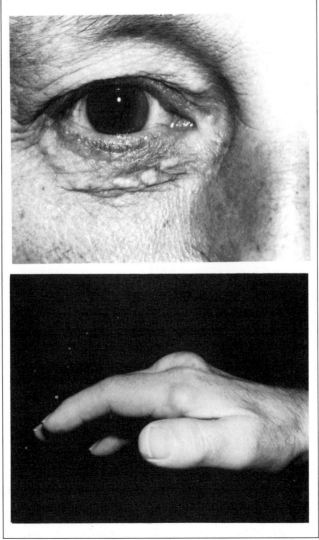

Fig. 4.4 Cutaneous signs of high blood lipids: (a) xanthelasma (b) tendon xanthoma

Signs of hyperlipidaemia

There are three common cutaneous signs of high blood fats.

1. *Arcus lipidis (senilis)*   A white ring surrounding the cornea is very common in the elderly due to degenerative changes. However, in patients under the age of 45 years it is frequently associated with high blood cholesterol levels.

2. *Xanthelasma*   These are small raised yellow plaques on the eyelids which contain cholesterol (figure 4.4).

3. *Tendon xanthomata*   Tendon xanthomata are hard nodules found over the knuckles (figure 4.4), the patella and in the Achilles tendon. They are an important sign of familial hypercholesterolaemia (FH), a condition associated with a very high incidence of early and severe coronary heart disease.

References

Adgey A A J, Allen J D, Geddes J S, James R G G, Webb S W, Zaidi S A and Pantridge J F (1971) Acute phase of myocardial infarction. *Lancet,* **ii:** 501-504.
Davies M K, Mackintosh P, Clayton R M, Page A J F, Shiu M F and Littler W A (1980) The straight back syndrome. *Quarterly Journal of Medicine,* **49:** 443-460.
Geddes L A and Whistler S J (1978) The error in indirect blood pressure measurement with the incorrect size of cuff. *American Heart Journal,* **96:** 4-8.
Oakley C M (1984) Mitral valve prolapse: harbinger of death or variant of normal. *British Medical Journal,* **288:** 1853-1854.
Swales J D (1979) The assessment of the hypertensive patient. In: *Clinical Hypertension,* pp. 138-141. London: Chapman and Hall.

5

The Investigation of
Coronary Artery Disease

Investigation of patients with coronary heart disease may be required for diagnostic, therapeutic and prognostic reasons. The screening of asymptomatic patients is usually unrewarding, and attention is therefore directed at those with cardiac symptoms, predominantly chest pain and dyspnoea (Petch, 1986). The sequence of investigation may be:

1. *Preliminary (General Practice)* Blood tests should be carried out to exclude anaemia and to measure blood sugar, lipids and urate. A chest radiograph and resting electrocardiogram should also be performed.

2. *Intermediate (District General Hospital)* This includes exercise electrocardiography, echocardiography and nuclear scanning.

3. *Specialist (Regional Cardiac Centre)* Specialist investigation usually involves left heart catheterisation, left ventricular angiography and coronary angiography.

THE ELECTROCARDIOGRAM

The normal electrical impulse originates in the sino-atrial (SA) node and is conducted as a wave over the atrium. This wave activates the atrioventricular (AV) node and is then transmitted to the ventricles by the bundles of His. The left bundle perforates the intraventricular septum, and both bundles carry the impulse onwards, the septum being activated from left to right. The impulse then spreads over the endocardial surface of the ventricles via the Purkinje fibres and spreads through the ventricular myocardium from endocardium to epicardium.

The electrical forces generated by the heart travel in multiple directions simultaneously. The electrocardiogram (ECG) is designed to record these electrical impulses, and the generated waveform has been labelled as P, Q, R, S, T and U waves. The *P wave* represents atrial activation, and the *QRS complex* ventricular activation. The *T wave* represents ventricular repolarisation but the atrial repolarisation wave (T_a) is usually not seen, being buried in the QRS complex.

The signals are amplified and (by convention) the display is arranged so that impulses moving towards a surface electrode give rise to an upward (positive) deflection, whilst impulses moving away from the electrode a downward (negative) one. To help interpret the electrical movement patterns, electrocardiography is carried out in

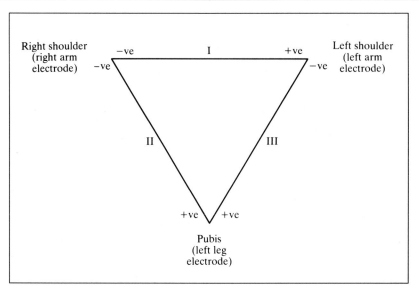

Fig. 5.1   The Einthoven triangle (named after Willem Einthoven, 1860–1927, Professor of Physiology, University of Leiden)

different planes. The three major planes are recorded via electrodes on the right arm (RA), left arm (LA) and left leg (LL). A fourth electrode is traditionally placed on the right leg, but this is not used for recording and serves as a ground (earth) electrode. An electrical triangle is formed by the three planes, with the heart in the centre (figure 5.1). These three different views of the heart are designated standard leads I, II and III.

The normal electrocardiogram (ECG) consists of recordings from 12 leads. In addition to the three main standard limb leads there are three 'augmented' bipolar leads (aVR, aVL and aVF). Six unipolar chest (V) leads complete the standard 12-lead ECG, and view the heart electrically from the front as shown in figure 5.2.

Positioning of the leads

The standard (limb) leads are not often confused as they are usually clearly marked on the electrodes. However, positioning of the chest leads can easily vary between serial recordings, and it is important that the correct surface marking is used to prevent artefactual ECG changes between recordings.

- V1: Fourth intercostal space immediately to the right of the sternum
- V2: Fourth intercostal space immediately to the left of the sternum
- V3: Mid-way between V2 and V4
- V4: Fifth intercostal space, midclavicular line
- V5: Anterior axillary line, on the same horizontal line as V4
- V6: Midaxillary line, also horizontal with V4

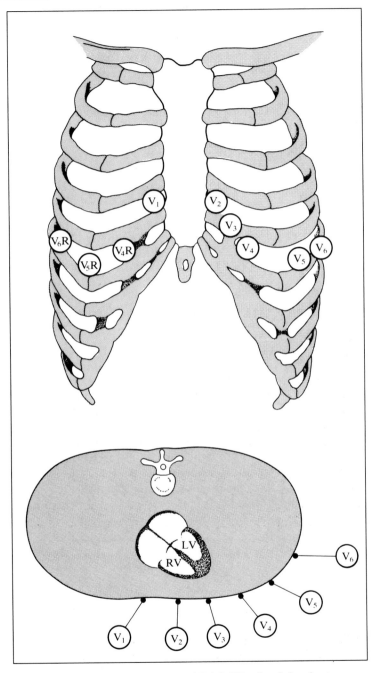

Fig. 5.2 The positioning of ECG V leads of the chest

Many other additional placements can be used to demonstrate particular aspects of the heart (Marriott, 1983) such as V7 and V8 (further laterally), or V3R and V4R (V3 and V4 positions on the right side of the chest).

Assessing the quality of the recording

Before analysing an electrocardiogram, it is essential to ensure that the recording was obtained correctly. Errors in lead placement or connection, paper speed selection, standardisation and incorrect lead labelling are very common. Hence, the technical quality of the recording should first be assessed.

1. *Standardisation*   A potential of 1 mV should be represented by a 10 mm vertical deflection. A standard deflection should be recorded at the start and finish of a 12-lead recording.

2. *Speed*   Recordings are usually made at 25 mm/s. Ensure that the machine has not been running at 50 mm/s.

3. *Correct lead placement and labelling*   The net electrical movement in the heart is from lead aVR towards lead II. Hence, in the normal ECG, the complex should be totally positive in lead II (upright P, QRS and T waves), and totally negative in aVR.

4. *Clear tracings*   Too little or too much stylus heat will produce too faint or too thick a tracing. Mains interference may produce a fuzzy trace, as may patient movement caused by cold, shock or fear.

Analysing the ECG

If a standard approach is made towards an ECG (Schamroth, 1977), important changes will not be missed. The sequence should be: rate, rhythm, axis, waveform.

Rate

The ECG is recorded at 25 mm/s on standard ECG paper which has fine lines at 1 mm intervals, and heavier divisions at 5 mm. Each millimetre therefore represents 0.04 second and each large division is 0.2 second.

To calculate the rate, the number of large squares between two successive complexes should be measured, and divided into 300. If the heart rhythm is irregular, a greater number of complexes should be assessed. Special rulers (often provided by manufacturers of cardiac drugs) can simplify the calculation of rate, and also give anticipated values for the QT interval.

Rhythm

Normal sinus rhythm should show a normal P wave preceding each QRS complex, with a constant PR interval. If this is not the case, a dysrhythmia is present (dysrhythmias will be discussed later).

Axis

The cardiac axis represents the net electrical direction the impulse takes as it spreads through the myocardium. It does not represent the anatomical position of the heart; right-axis deviation does not mean that the heart has swivelled around such that is pointing over the right shoulder!

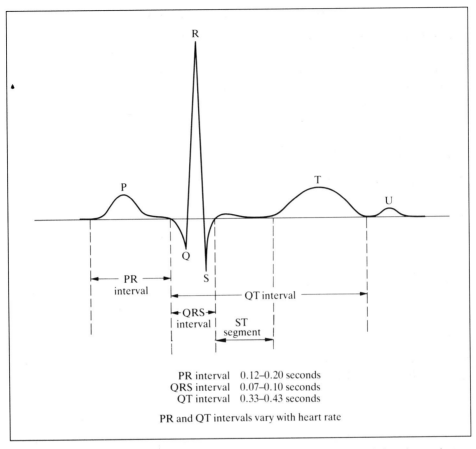

PR interval   0.12–0.20 seconds
QRS interval   0.07–0.10 seconds
QT interval   0.33–0.43 seconds

PR and QT intervals vary with heart rate

Fig. 5.3   The electrocardiographic cycle showing nomenclature and time intervals

Axis is usually assessed in the frontal plane with lead I designated 0°, and the 360° circle surrounding the heart divided into +180° (clockwise) and −180° (anti-clockwise). Normally the cardiac axis lies between −30° and +110°, and can be quickly determined in the following manner:

1. Which lead has an equally positive and negative QRS component? This will be at right angles (90°) to the cardiac axis. However, the impulse could be in either direction, which leads to a further question.

2. Which lead has the predominant QRS vector? The net electrical movement must be in this direction as movement towards a surface electrode gives a positive deflection.

Waveform

The size of the different waves and the intervals between them are all precisely defined, and are subject to biological variability such as heart rate, age and sex. Values are shown in figure 5.3.

P wave

The normal P wave results from the spread of activity from the sinus node across the atria. This electrical movement is from right to left so that the P wave will be upright in leads I, II and aVF, and inverted in aVR. It should not be greater than 0.1 second in duration and should not be taller than 3 mm in the standard leads, or 2.5 mm in the V leads.

Abnormalities may be:

1. *Inversion*   This means the atria are being depolarised from an unusual site, and not the sino-atrial node (unless there is dextrocardia). The origin may be elsewhere in the atrium, in the AV node or even below this.

2. *Excessive height*   A tall peaked P wave results from right atrial enlargement. Because this is often secondary to pulmonary hypertension the wave is sometimes referred to as *P pulmonale*.

3. *Excessive width*   With left atrial enlargement, the P wave becomes broad and notched like the letter M. Because this often results from mitral valve disease, the wave is known as *P mitrale*. Often the P wave is biphasic in lead V1.

4. *Absent*   The P wave is missing during AV nodal rhythm, or may be replaced by flutter or fibrillation waves.

PR interval

This represents the time taken for atrial activation and AV nodal delay, and increases with age. It is measured from the start of the P wave to the beginning of the QRS complex and is normally 0.12 to 0.20 second long (three to five little ECG strip squares). A shortened PR interval is seen when the impulse originates in junctional tissue or when there are accessory conduction pathways (e.g. Wolff-Parkinson–White syndrome). The PR interval lengthens if there is atrioventricular block.

QRS interval

This represents ventricular activation and is measured from the onset of the Q to the end of the S wave. A value greater than 0.12 second (three little squares) is abnormal and usually indicates an intraventricular conduction disorder.

QT interval

This represents the complete electrical activity time of ventricular stimulation and recovery (depolarisation and repolarisation). This is measured from the beginning of the QRS complex to the end of the T wave and varies with heart rate (the QT interval shortens as the heart rate increases). The corrected QT interval (QT_c) may be calculated by the formula:

$$QT_c = \frac{QT}{\sqrt{RR}}$$

where QT is the QT interval and RR is the RR interval. Practically, the QT interval should be less than 50 per cent of the preceding cycle length and seldom exceeds 0.44 second.

The QT interval lengthens in heart failure, following myocardial infarction and with hypocalcaemia. It is shortened in hypercalcaemia and hyperkalaemia.

T wave

The *T wave* results from repolarisation of the ventricles, and might therefore be assumed to produce a negative deflection. However, because repolarisation takes place in the opposite direction to depolarisation, i.e. from epicardium to endocardium, the T wave is usually positive, and has the same axis as the QRS complex. The T wave may be inverted in leads V1 and V2 in healthy individuals, and in V3 in negroes.

T waves are normally no greater than 5 mm tall in the standard leads (10 mm in the V leads), but may be taller in hyperkalaemia, myocardial infarction or ischaemia. Flattening or slight inversion is a non-specific abnormality, but may reflect hypothyroidism or a low serum potassium. T wave inversion may be found in myocardial infarction, ventricular hypertrophy or bundle branch block.

ST interval

The ST segment is measured from the *J point* (at the junction of the S wave and the ST segment) to the start of the T wave. It is very slightly curved upwards, but isoelectric. ST displacement or changes in shape are of major importance in electrocardiographic interpretation. Horizontal displacement beyond 1 to 2 mm upwards or 0.5 mm downwards is abnormal. ST elevation typically occurs in myocardial infarction (when the segment is convex upwards) and pericarditis (when the segment is concave upwards). ST depression is found in myocardial ischaemia and with digoxin therapy.

Frequent mistakes in interpretation of ST morphology are:

1. *High ST take-off* This frequently occurs in young patients, particularly negroes, and can be up to 2 mm in leads V1 and V2. It is often accompanied by a slight notch on the downstroke of the preceding R wave.

2. *ST depression*
    a. ST sag during digoxin therapy.
    b. Downward sloping from the J point during sinus tachycardia. Erroneous diagnoses of myocardial ischaemia may be made during exercise stress tests if the ST shift is not measured 40 ms from the J point.
    c. Ventricular hypertrophy leads to ST depression over the relevant ventricle.

U wave

These are low-voltage, broad waves following the T wave. Their origin is not known, but they are especially prominent in hypokalaemia and during digoxin therapy.

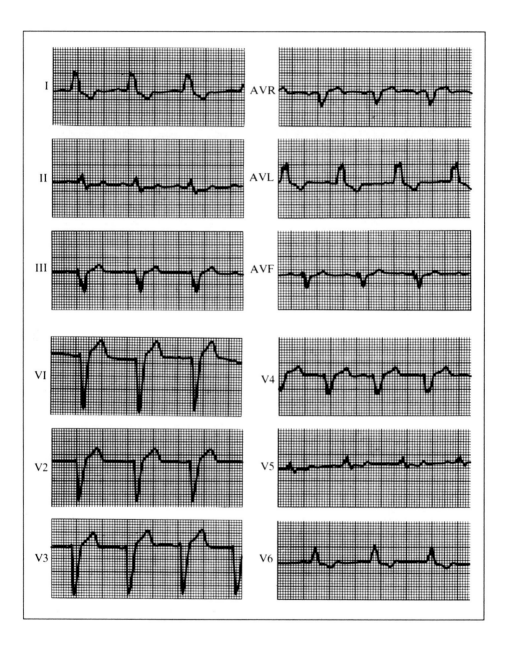

Fig. 5.4 ECG: left bundle branch block (see page 80)

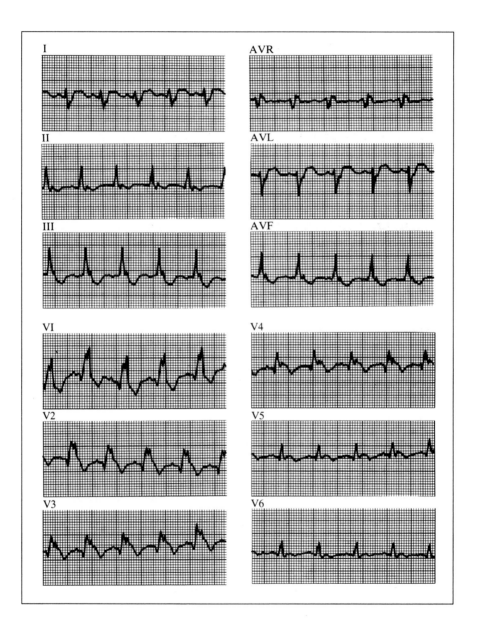

Fig. 5.5 ECG: right bundle branch block (see page 80)

Intraventricular conduction blocks

Intraventricular conduction blocks (IVCBs) are frequently found in patients with cardiac disease. The term IVCB refers to an impairment or block of conduction in one or more of the fascicles of the conducting tissue distal to the bundle of His.

Bundle branch block

Left bundle branch block

When the left bundle is blocked, septal depolarisation is activated from right to left instead of the normal left to right. Hence, the initial q wave in the left ventricular leads is lost, and is replaced by a small upward r wave. The right ventricle is depolarised before the left, producing an R wave in V1 and an S wave in V6. The left ventricle then depolarises, producing an S wave in V1 and a second R wave (R') in V6. The depolarisation time is therefore prolonged and the QRS duration is greater than 0.12 second.

Characteristically, the morphology of the QRS produces a W-shaped complex in lead V1 and an M in V6 (see figure 5.4 above).

Right bundle branch block

Although depolarisation takes place in the normal direction across the septum, depolarisation of the right ventricle is delayed, producing a late R' wave in right chest leads and a deep S wave in left chest leads. The genesis of the widened QRS is the reverse of left bundle branch block, and an M is produced in lead V1, and a W in V6 (figure 5.5 above).

Hemiblocks

The left bundle divides into two hemifascicles, an anterior one running superolaterally, and a posterior fascicle running inferomedially. Each of these may be blocked individually or in addition to the main left or right bundle.

Electrocardiographically the QRS duration is very slightly increased (0.02 second), although it will still be in the normal range. The commoner left anterior hemiblock is manifest as left-axis deviation ($< -30°$), and should be suspected when unexplained left-axis deviation is found. Left posterior hemiblock is much less common, and manifests as right-axis deviation ($> +110°$). An rS pattern may be seen in lead I and a qR in III (the reverse being seen in left anterior hemiblock).

Incomplete bundle branch block

This term is commonly used when the morphology of the QRS complex is similar to that observed in established bundle branch block, but the QRS duration is within normal limits (i.e. less than 0.12 second). These changes probably do not indicate actual block, but are due to ventricular enlargement (Goldman and Mervin, 1979).

Ventricular hypertrophy

Ventricular hypertrophy increases the amplitude of the QRS complex. Hypertrophy of the left ventricle increases the height of the R waves in the left chest leads, while that of the right ventricle increases the height of the R waves in the right ventricular leads. Septal hypertrophy produces a large, narrow Q wave in the left chest leads.

Unfortunately, many factors can influence the magnitude of the QRS complex, including age, thickness of the chest wall, expanded chests (in chronic obstructive airways disease), hypothyroidism and pericardial effusions. However, the following measurements are useful for the diagnosis of ventricular hypertrophy on voltage criteria:

1. *Left ventricular hypertrophy*
   a. The R wave in V5 or V6 is greater than 25 mm.
   b. The R wave in V5 or V6 plus the S wave in V1 is greater than 35 mm (40 mm in the young).
   c. The R wave in aVF is greater than 20 mm.
Confirmatory evidence is provided by left-axis deviation ($< 0°$), ST depression and T wave inversion in V4–V6 and possible P mitrale.

2. *Right ventricular hypertrophy*
   a. An R > S wave in V1, and measures more than 5 mm.
   b. The R wave in V1 plus the S wave in V5 or V6 is greater than 10 mm.
Confirmatory evidence is right-axis deviation ($> +110°$), ST depression and T wave inversion in V1–V3, and possible P pulmonale.

THE CHEST RADIOGRAPH

The plain chest radiograph or X-ray (Jefferson and Rees, 1980) is one of the most important aids to the diagnosis of cardiovascular disease. The alveolar air provides an excellent radiographic contrast medium upon which to outline the heart, the great vessels and the pulmonary vasculature. The standard postero-anterior (PA) chest radiograph is taken at full inspiration, with the patient standing facing the film which is 1.5 m from the X-ray tube focus. High-kilovoltage exposures (120 to 150 kV) are often preferable for visualising the mediastinum and lung vasculature, although conventional kilovoltage (70 to 80 kV) allows the bony skeleton and calcified lesions to be seen. In the standard PA view, the right border of the heart consists (from top to bottom) of superior vena cava, the ascending aorta and the right atrium. The left border is formed by the aortic arch, the descending aorta, the pulmonary artery and its left main branch, and the left ventricle (figure 5.6). Standard PA chest films are desirable whenever possible because:

● The diaphragm is flattened, and allows the bases of the lungs to be seen
● The erect position lowers hydrostatic pressure in the low-pressure pulmonary vascular tree
● The scapulae are slid away from the lung fields
● The PA projection reduces magnification of the heart shadow

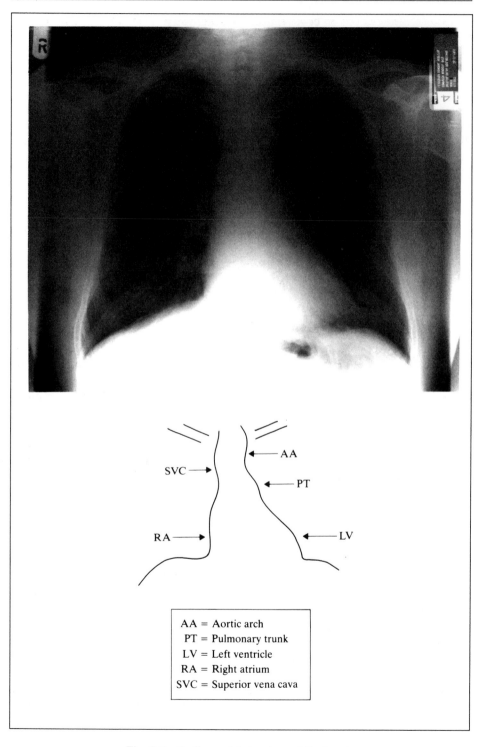

Fig. 5.6   Radiographic borders of the heart

However, the patient on coronary care is often too ill to stand, and a recumbent portable AP film is usually taken with consequent interpretation problems, as might be anticipated from the preceding remarks.

Interpretation

The film should first be correctly identified and orientated. The radiograph should then be assessed in a routine method so that nothing is missed. The order is not important, but one suggested sequence is:

- Technical quality
- Cardiac shadow
- Lung fields
- Diaphragm
- Mediastinum
- Bones
- Upper abdomen

Technical quality

All films should be correctly identified and dated. Right and left markers will avoid a missed diagnosis of dextrocardia. If the film is taken straight, the medial ends of the clavicles should be equidistant from the midline (marked by the spinous processes of the vertebrae). Too low a kilovoltage will underpenetrate the film and enhance lung markings. This is particularly common in the obese patient, often leading to an erroneous diagnosis of pulmonary congestion. It is important to note what kilovoltage has been employed, particularly in coronary care where interpretation of pulmonary congestion is important. A change to a higher kilovoltage on a subsequent chest film will show the apparent clearing of pulmonary oedema.

The heart

The cardiac size is assessed by determining the cardiothoracic ratio (CTR). This is given by the ratio of the widest part of the heart shadow to the widest transverse thoracic diameter (measured from the inner surface of the ribs). The CTR should be less than 0.5 in adults. This method of assessing cardiac size is not infallible, however. For example, in aortic valve disease, left ventricular enlargement is towards the diaphragm, and the cardiac diameter is not affected.

Enlargement of the cardiac shadow may be due to pericardial effusion, cardiac dilatation or hypertrophy. Cardiomegaly is common in athletes and does not necessarily indicate dilatation or hypertrophy.

The diagnosis of pericardial effusion is not always easy on the standard chest film because it cannot readily be distinguished from other causes of cardiac enlargement. If it has formed rapidly, cardiac dilatation may be seen on consecutive films. Large effusions make the heart outline globular; small effusions are hard to detect radiologically and are best detected by echocardiography.

The most frequent cause of cardiac enlargement is dilatation due to volume overload. Hypertrophy normally leads to a volume reduction within the heart chambers, so that the overall cardiac diameters are only very slightly increased. Dilatation and hypertrophy frequently coexist, and are probably best differentiated by echocardiography.

Although a good knowledge of radiographic anatomy is useful to distinguish which part of the heart is responsible for the cardiac enlargement, the same final picture can be produced by different underlying processes. Enlargement of the left atrium is the most easy to recognise, gives a projection of 2 cm below the left pulmonary artery shadow, and causes a convex bulge immediately below the left main bronchus. In extreme enlargement, the left atrium will protrude above the right atrium causing a double density at the right border of the heart. Right atrial enlargement simply makes the right border look more prominent, and it produces a long continuous convexity of the right heart border.

Enlargement of the ventricles may be difficult to distinguish on the conventional chest radiograph. Left ventricular enlargement pushes the cardiac shadow downwards and outwards below the cupola of the left diaphragm, and is found in association with hypertension, aortic valve disease and mitral incompetence. The right ventricle enlarges forwards, reducing the retrosternal air space. A normal left ventricle is sometimes pushed posteriorly by right ventricular enlargement (due to pulmonary hypertension or pulmonary stenosis), and the cardiac apex is rounded and lifted up, above the left diaphragm.

The lung fields

The normal pulmonary artery divisions can be traced to within about a centimetre of the lung edge. The pulmonary veins are large and horizontal in the lower lung fields, but are seen as smaller linear opacities draining towards the left atrium in the upper lung fields.

Increased pulmonary capillary pressures and diminished cardiac output are the final common pathways for the production of pulmonary oedema. As pressure in the pulmonary veins rises, radiological manifestations follow a specific pattern until a critical pressure of about 30 mmHg is reached:

- 18–20 mmHg: onset of pulmonary congestion
- 20–30 mmHg: increasing congestion
- >30 mmHg: onset of pulmonary oedema

Radiological evidence of pulmonary oedema occurs first in the lower pulmonary veins where perivascular interstitial oedema develops. This results in local hypoxia and reflex vasoconstriction in the affected vessels. The blood is then diverted to the upper lung vessels (upper lobe diversion) producing the characteristic radiological picture (figure 5.7). The interstitial oedema collects around hilar vessels to produce the 'bat wing' sign, and collection in and around the pulmonary lymphatics gives rise to thin linear opacities called Kerley lines. The *Kerley A lines* (engorged intralobular lymphatics) run from the periphery to the hilum, and the commoner *Kerley B lines* of interstitial oedema are short parallel lines which run horizontally at the lung peripheries, particularly in the costophrenic angles. As the pulmonary oedema worsens, fluid collects in the alveoli of the lower zones producing opacities, and later outside the lung to produce pleural effusions.

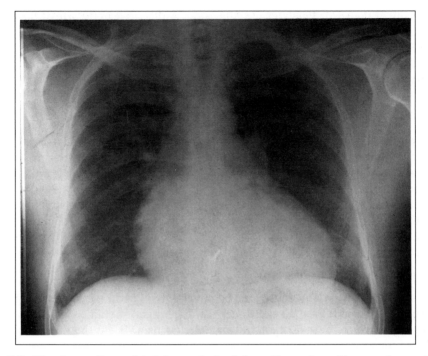

Fig. 5.7 The chest radiograph in left ventricular failure. Note enlarged heart and upper lobe diversion of blood

Rapid response to therapy in patients with early pulmonary congestion may produce a difference in clinical and radiological interpretation of the current haemodynamic position. Features are labile and may clear within a few hours of therapy. However, there may sometimes be a lag of up to 48 hours between haemodynamic stabilisation and resolution of radiological signs. In patients with long-standing pulmonary hypertension and heart failure, there may be thickening of the pulmonary vessel walls allowing substantial elevation of pulmonary capillary pressures without clinical congestion. Pulmonary oligaemia may be seen with large pulmonary emboli and emphysema.

The diaphragm

The diaphragm should expand to the level of the fifth rib anteriorly on full inspiration. Old chest disease may cause adherence of the diaphragm to the chest wall which may be falsely interpreted as a pleural effusion. A fat pad is sometimes seen adjacent to the cardiac border in the obese, and a slight hump of the right diaphragm is frequent in the elderly.

The mediastinum

The position and size of the aorta should be noted. Unfolding is common in the elderly and in the hypertensive patient. Other radiological abnormalities of the aorta commonly found in the elderly are due to degenerative changes and include calcification (especially of the aortic knuckle) and dilatation. An increase in the size of the aortic outline (particularly on serial films) may indicate aortic dissection, particularly in the presence of a small left pleural effusion. The shadow is often calcified.

The commonest causes of mediastinal masses are unfolding of the aorta, aortic aneurysm, hiatus hernia and enlarged lymph nodes.

Bones

The heart will be displaced if there is a thoracic scoliosis. Large aortic aneurysms may erode the anterior surface of adjacent vertebrae. Rib lesions (fractures or metastases) may be a cause of chest pain and should be looked for. Rib notching is a finding in coarctation of the aorta.

Sternal depression may displace the heart, and is the cause of a systolic murmur with apparent cardiac enlargement (the straight back syndrome). This may only be visible with a lateral chest film.

The neck and upper abdomen

Retrosternal extension of a goitre may be misdiagnosed as an aortic aneurysm. The presence of intraperitoneal air (air under the diaphragm) should be excluded, since peritonitis may present with chest and shoulder tip pain. Hiatus hernia or shadows of other congenital herniae may be seen in the mediastinum.

ECHOCARDIOGRAPHY

Ultrasound imaging (*echocardiography*) allows the heart to be studied non-invasively, and is a powerful tool for assessing cardiac anatomy, pathology and function. The echocardiogram uses a transducer which generates high-frequency pulses of short duration which travel through the body at different velocities (depending upon the tissues encountered) and are echoed back to be recorded by the same transducer. The two main techniques used are M-mode and two-dimensional (cross-sectional or real-time) echocardiography. The Doppler shift effect during ultrasound can be combined with these to provide information on the velocity and direction of blood flow. Contrast echocardiography (by injection of microbubbles) is also increasingly being used to define congenital abnormalities.

M-mode echocardiography

M-mode echocardiography is essentially a graph of depth of tissues against time. A single beam of ultrasound is directed towards the heart, usually from the fourth left intercostal space. By rotating the transducer, a sweeping view of many of the intracardiac structures may be obtained (figure 5.8). A suprasternal or xiphisternal position is occasionally used to promote views. The picture is recorded on rapidly moving paper, allowing measurement of intracardiac structures and timing of events. The sonic beam is only 1 to 2 cm wide, so that only small parts of the heart may be viewed at one time and structural/functional interrelationships cannot always be judged

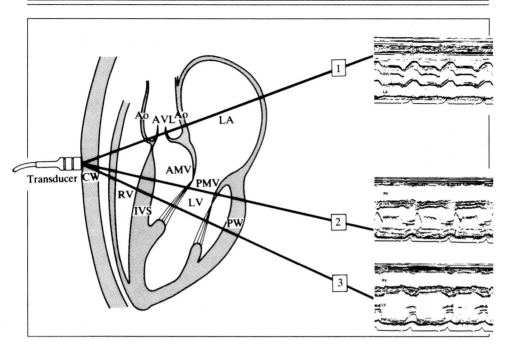

Fig. 5.8 Cardiac examination by M-mode echocardiography. (Reproduced by kind permission of the Department of Medical Illustration, Leicester Royal Infirmary)
CW = chest wall; RV = right ventricle; IVS = interventricular septum; LV = left ventricle; LA = left atrium; AMV = anterior leaflet of mitral valve; PMV = posterior leaflet of mitral valve; AVL = aortic valve leaflet; Ao = aorta; PW = posterior wall

Even with the best operators, technical difficulties may be encountered in up to 25 per cent of recordings.

The M-mode echo is useful for obtaining measurements of chamber size, wall thickness and assessing left ventricular function in patients who do not have areas of myocardial dysfunction. It may also be used to demonstrate mitral and aortic valve disease and pericardial effusions.

Two-dimensional echocardiography

These recorders generate multiple (30 to 40) echos, and scan the heart in sectors of up to 90°, usually from the apex and the parasternal regions. Up to 60 pictures are produced per minute to produce a moving real-time image which is anatomically recognisable. Multiple views from different sites are used to build up a complete picture of the heart. The images are stored on a computer floppy disk, and the computer can aid evaluation by accurately measuring ejection fractions and valve diameters.

Doppler echocardiography

These machines utilise the Doppler effect as applied to red cells. A continuous mode can resolve very high velocities through stenotic valves and a pulsed mode is used to measure flow at precise depths in conjunction with two-dimensional echocardiography. Doppler techniques have been enhanced by the use of colour digital flow analysis which allows real-time visualisation of cardiac blood flow superimposed upon a two-dimensional picture of the heart, for demonstrating valve lesions and congenital malformations.

Echocardiography in clinical practice

As a rule M-mode echocardiography can provide adequate diagnostic data for most routine indications, especially when enough clinical information has been submitted with the request for the investigation.

The aetiology of cardiomegaly

Clinical and radiological cardiomegaly may be due to ventricular dilatation and/or hypertrophy, a left ventricular aneurysm or pericardial effusion. Echocardiography is the best technique for identification of pericardial effusions and can also show thickening or calcification of the pericardium. M-mode echocardiography is superior to two-dimensional mode in determining myocardial hypertrophy because it allows precise ventricular measurements to be made. However, since two-dimensional echocardiography shows larger portions of the heart at one time, it can reveal paradoxical or patchy dyskinetic motion following myocardial infarction, or presence of a ventricular aneurysm.

Valvular disease

The echocardiogram is able to provide adequate diagnostic information about valvular disease in over two-thirds of patients without resort to cardiac catheterisation. Asymptomatic systolic murmurs are sometimes shown to have important underlying causes, such as atrioseptal defects, hypertropic cardiomyopathy or a bicuspid aortic valve. The haemodynamic severity of aortic stenosis cannot be accurately assessed with conventional echocardiography, but Doppler studies allow direct estimation of the transvalvular pressure gradient.

Other conditions

1. *Subacute bacterial endocarditis (SBE)*   Vegetations may be demonstrable in over half the patients with SBE. They are best shown on two-dimensional echocardiography, when they appear as rapidly oscillating masses attached to or replacing normal cardiac tissue.

2. *Cardiac source of arterial emboli*   If clinical examination is normal, the echocardiogram will only rarely show a source for arterial emboli. Occasionally, however, occult valvular disease, vegetations, ventricular aneurysms or an atrial myxoma will be found. Mitral valve prolapse is common (4 per cent of the population), and can be identified by echocardiography. It has recently attracted attention as a cause of asymptomatic systolic murmurs, paroxysmal dysrhythmias and as an important source of emboli in the younger adult (Oakley, 1984).

Table 5.1. Comparative values of M-mode and two-dimensional echocardiography.

M-mode echocardiography	Two-dimensional echocardiography
Advantages	
Cheap and more commonly available	Shows larger picture of heart
Easy measurement of wall thickness and chamber diameter	Reveals structure/function interrelationships
Event timing is easier	Visually easy to interpret
Useful in left-sided valvular disease	Allows direct measurement of mitral and aortic valves
	Can show: right-sided valvular disease
	lesions of the aortic root
	ventricular dyskinesis
Disadvantages	
Allows only small views to be seen at any one time	Expensive and not widely available
Often difficult to interpret	Not good for measurement of wall thickness and chamber size
Not very good at showing right-sided valvular disease	

3. *Congenital heart disease* Echocardiography can be used to precisely define cardiac anatomy in many types of congenital heart disease.

The comparative advantages of two-dimensional and M-mode echocardiography are considered in table 5.1.

EXERCISE STRESS TESTING

Many patients with cardiac disease have no signs, symptoms or abnormal investigations at rest, and exercise stress testing may reveal hitherto undocumented abnormalities. Demonstrating electrocardiographic changes on exertion is one of the most important and valuable non-invasive diagnostic investigations of patients with known or suspected cardiovascular disease. The procedure has a low complication rate although any investigation of patients with myocardial disease runs a risk of cardiac arrest or myocardial infarction. It is therefore usual for such tests to be carried out by trained staff, with a doctor in attendance and with resuscitation facilities immediately available. Sudden death may occur up to two hours after the test, although in a series of 20 000 tests in Seattle there were only six cases of ventricular fibrillation, all of which occurred in the first five minutes following cessation of the test (Irving et al, 1977). All had clinical myocardial disease, were hypotensive during exercise and were fortunately resuscitated. Close monitoring of patients with highly abnormal tests is therefore required, with overnight admission to hospital if necessary.

Despite a wealth of experience and a great deal of published work on the investigation, controversy still surrounds the interpretation of the test. For example, if ST depression of 1 mm is used to diagnose ischaemia, the false positive rate may be as high as 64 per cent (Epstein, 1978). It is more important perhaps to look at symptoms, pulse and blood pressure response and the recovery time following exercise.

In general, early onset of angina, marked and widespread ST depression, slow recovery and a poor blood pressure response are indicative of severe ischaemic heart disease.

Cardiac function during exercise

The cardiovascular system must be able to adapt to exercise in order to supply increased amounts of oxygen to working tissues. This is achieved by:

- Increased heart rate
- Increased stroke volume
- Changes in blood pressure and distribution
- Increased oxygen extraction from the blood in tissues

Heart rate

The heart quickens almost immediately with exercise because of increased sympathetic drive and reduced vagal tone. It rises with the level of exertion until a maximum rate is reached (approximately equal to 220 minus the patient's age). At this heart rate, the potential for further exercise is limited.

Stroke volume

The heart size decreases during exercise and there is a concomitant increase in ejection fraction and cardiac output. This is brought about by increased sympathetic stimulation which increases myocardial contractility and heart rate.

Changes in blood pressure and distribution

The systolic blood pressure rises with exercise, while the diastolic pressure falls slightly. Higher systolic blood pressures are found with increasing age. There is a reduction in systemic vascular resistance with generalised vasodilatation to supply working muscle. In contrast, splanchnic blood flow virtually ceases.

Oxygen extraction

The normal myocardium is very efficient at oxygen extraction both at rest and during exercise. Increased oxygen demand by the heart during exercise is therefore met by coronary vasodilatation. With increasing coronary atheromatous deposits, this mechanism is progressively inhibited.

Abnormal responses to exercise

Fatigue is a normal response to exercise, but this is often premature in patients with cardiac disease. Dyspnoea and chest pain are other common symptoms, and claudication is often a limiting factor in those with widespread arterial disease. The majority of cardiac patients are able to maintain an adequate cardiac output at rest, but the diseased myocardium does not respond normally to exercise. Although they are

Table 5.2. Contraindications for ECG stress testing.

Cardiac
Unstable angina
Severe hypertension
Myocarditis or pericarditis
Aortic stenosis
Serious dysrhythmias

Non-cardiac
Anaemia
Elderly or infirm patient
Gross obesity
Severe respiratory disease

Drugs/electrolytes
Digoxin toxicity
Electrolyte imbalance
Unstable antidysrhythmic therapy

usually able to produce a tachycardia to increase cardiac output, the left ventricle dilates instead of shrinking. This not only worsens regional ischaemia, but left ventricular function is impaired such that there may be only a small rise, or even a fall in blood pressure. Failure to attain a systolic blood pressure of more than 130 mmHg during exercise, or a fall of more than 10 mmHg, are poor prognostic signs.

Stress testing

The original step tests have now been replaced by treadmill and bicycle tests, the choice largely being determined by cost and available space. There are several contraindications to stress testing, which are shown in table 5.2.

The different recommended lead systems for detecting regional myocardial ischaemia employ from two to 20 electrodes. The simplest and most useful lead for recording is MCL5 (positive lead in the V5 interspace and the negative on the manubrium), which will demonstrate up to 90 per cent of detectable abnormalities. However, the commonest lead system utilises the normal 12–lead recording positions. The torso rather than the limbs is used for the limb leads to prevent entanglement and to reduce movement artefact. Precordial mapping techniques employing greater than 12 leads are really only research tools. There are many different protocols designed for different circumstances and available equipment (Pollock et al, 1976). The ideal protocol should offer:

- An appropriate work load for the patient which will not cause excessive stress
- A gradually increasing work load with enough time at each level to attain steady state
- Continuous ECG, heart rate and blood pressure recording
- Medical supervision and resuscitation facilities

The commonest tests employ the Bruce protocol (Bruce et al, 1963; table 5.3) suitable for routine use, and the Naughton protocol (Naughton et al, 1964; table 5.4) suitable following myocardial infarction.

Table 5.3. Bruce protocol for exercise (treadmill) ECG test.

Stage	Speed (m.p.h.)	Grade (%)	Duration (min)	METs (units)	Total time elapsed (min)
1	1.7	10	3	4	3
2	2.5	12	3	6–7	6
3	3.4	14	3	8–9	9
4	4.2	16	3	15–16	12
5	5.0	18	3	21	15
6	5.5	20	3	—	18
7	6.0	22	3	—	21

There are various parameters that can be observed and assessed during an exercise test. These may be:

● *Symptomatic:* onset of symptoms and relationship to exercise
● *Haemodynamic:* changes in blood pressure and heart rate
● *Electrocardiographic:* changes in the ST segment and cardiac rhythm

Table 5.4. Naughton protocol for exercise (treadmill) ECG test.

Stage	2.0 m.p.h. Grade (%)	3.0 m.p.h. Grade (%)	3.4 m.p.h. Grade (%)	Duration (min)	METs (units)	Total time elapsed (min)
1	—	—	—	2	1.0	2
2	0.0	—	—	2	2.0	4
3	3.5	0.0	—	2	3.0	6
4	7.0	2.5	2.0	2	4.0	8
5	10.5	5.0	4.0	2	5.0	10
6	14.0	7.5	6.0	2	6.0	12
7	17.5	10.0	8.0	2	7.0	14
8	—	12.5	10.0	2	8.0	16
9	—	15.0	12.0	2	9.0	18
10	—	17.5	14.0	2	10.0	20
11	—	20.0	16.0	2	11.0	22
12	—	22.5	18.0	2	12.0	24
13	—	25.0	20.0	2	13.0	26
14	—	27.5	22.0	2	14.0	28
15	—	30.0	24.0	2	15.0	30
16	—	32.5	26.0	2	16.0	32

A standard resting ECG should be obtained before the test and current medication recorded. During the test, the patient should be encouraged to exercise for as long as possible, but signs of fatigue, pain and syncope should be noted, especially in the stoic patient. The systolic blood pressure should be recorded at the termination of each stage by palpation of the brachial artery. The diastolic blood pressure is difficult to measure and does not add to the value of the test.

Automatic ECG recorders will usually record a full 10 second ECG at predetermined time intervals (three leads recorded simultaneously for 2.5 seconds), and the test is continued until completion or another end-point has been reached (table 5.5).

Table 5.5.   End-points of the exercise stress test.

Absolute	Relative
Patient's request	Chest pain without ECG changes
Fall in blood pressure or heart rate	Less serious symptoms (anxiety, dizziness,
Sustained dysrhythmias	cramp)
Progressive angina	Attainment of predicted maximal heart rate
Severe dyspnoea, fatigue or faintness	Marked ST depression ($>$ 5 mm)
Equipment failure	Increasing ectopic activity or heart block
	Marked hypertension (SP $>$ 220 mmHg;
	DP $>$ 110 mmHg)

At the end of testing, the level of the test achieved (with timing) should be recorded with the reason for stopping. All symptoms and blood pressure readings should be recorded on the ECG.

Indications for stress testing

Chest pain

The main indications for exercise stress testing are in the diagnosis of chest pain and for indicating the extent of coronary artery disease in a patient with known myocardial ischaemia. Unfortunately, ST changes are not always present during exercise in patients with angiographically defined coronary artery disease, especially if lesions are limited to the circumflex and distal right coronary arteries. False negative tests may also be obtained if the patient is taking beta-blockers which limit cardiac work, or if exercise has been submaximal.

False-positive results may be obtained in up to 10 per cent of men and 25 per cent of women who have normal resting ECGs. There have been many explanations for these findings including ST changes due to hyperventilation or increased sympathetic tone. Such changes have been demonstrated during free-fall parachute jumps. *Vasoregulatory asthenia* is sometimes seen in young women with atypical chest pain. Multiple resting ST/T wave changes are found on the ECG which worsen (often dramatically) on exercise. Paradoxically, the changes are worse at the start of exercise, and improve as the test progresses.

Another peculiar syndrome describes angina in patients with angiographically normal coronary arteries (*Syndrome X*). Invasive studies often show abnormal myocardial contractility and the condition probably reflects an early form of cardiomyopathy.

Post-myocardial infarction

The prognosis of patients following acute myocardial infarction is affected not only by the site and size of the infarct, but also by circulation to the unaffected myocardium. Exercise testing has become routine in many hospitals to determine residual myocardial ischaemia for assessing prognosis. The correlation of ST changes with hypotension and chest pain are predictive of future cardiac events (Theroux et al, 1979; Akhras et al, 1982).

Other exercise-related symptoms

The aetiology of atypical anginal pain, dyspnoea, palpitations and dizziness may all be clarified by an exercise test. Occasionally, intermittent dysrhythmias may be recorded, and an exercise test should form part of the evaluation of patients with suspected cardiac rhythm abnormalities (Podrid and Graboys, 1984).

NUCLEAR SCANS AND NUCLEAR ANGIOGRAPHY

Radioisotope techniques for the assessment of myocardial disease and function have developed rapidly over the last 10 years. Nuclear scans can be used to define left ventricular size and wall motion, to measure cardiac output and to evaluate myocardial ischaemia. More recently, the importance of right ventricular dysfunction in low output states has been recognised, particularly following inferior and right ventricular infarction (Ferlinz, 1982). Nuclear scanning may be invaluable for examining these usually difficult areas of the heart. Ischaemic dysfunction which may only develop during exercise can also be easily visualised by nuclear angiography, usually seen as a fall in cardiac output with the development of regional contraction abnormalities (Dymond et al, 1984). A rarely needed use of scanning is in the diagnosis of myocardial infarction when conventional diagnostic methods are unhelpful.

The main nuclear scans performed in the investigation of cardiac disease (table 5.6) are:

- The thallium scan
- The pyrophosphate scan
- Nuclear ventriculography (first-pass and MUGA)

The thallium scan

Thallium-201 is a potassium analogue which concentrates in normal myocardial cells and can be used to demonstrate myocardial ischaemia and infarction. Abnormal tissue does not take up the tracer and therefore appears as a cold spot on the scan (*cold spot scanning*).

Thallium can also be injected during exercise to demonstrate myocardial perfusion abnormalities, and is especially useful in diagnostic problems of atypical chest pain where the ECG stress test is unhelpful. It is not widely used in the UK at present since the isotope is expensive and the information yielded is limited.

The pyrophosphate scan

In contrast to thallium scanning, *hot spot scanning* utilises technetium-labelled pyrophosphate which is taken up by damaged myocardial cells. This may be useful following recent myocardial infarction when traditional investigations (enzymes, ECG, etc.) are not helpful (see table 5.6).

Table 5.6. Uses of nuclear imaging.

MUGA scan
Diagnosis of ischaemic, infarcted or aneurysmal segments
Detection of right ventricular dysfunction
Evaluating wall dysfunction and cardiac output in response to exercise
Prognostic assessment following myocardial infarction

First pass
Demonstrating intracardiac shunts
Defining congenital defects
Evaluating left ventricular motion

Thallium scan
Evaluation of angina in the presence of
● bundle branch block
● equivocal ECG stress test
Evaluation of post-surgical infarcts

Pyrophosphate scan
Diagnosis of myocardial infarction
● when enzyme measurement is unhelpful
● when there is bundle branch block
● postoperatively
● when the infarct is posterior or affects the right ventricle

Radionuclide ventriculography

Radionuclide ventriculography is helpful in defining those patients with poor left ventricular function whose prognosis may be improved with surgery. There are two main techniques: *first-pass scanning* and *multigated acquisition (MUGA) scanning*.

First-pass scanning

A radiotracer (usually technetium-99m) is injected as a bolus into a peripheral vein and its radioactivity counted on its first passage through the heart. The chambers can be visually separated by its time of passage through the right and left heart, so that images of the right and left ventricles can be constructed. Wall motion of the anterolateral and inferior aspects of the left ventricle can also be demonstrated.

The MUGA scan

Technetium is used to label the patient's red cells, which are then re-injected. A period of equilibration is then allowed, and radioactivity is measured within the heart as it beats, and recorded frame by frame on a videotape activated by the ECG (one frame per cycle). This enables regional wall motion to be visualised (for defining dyskinetic segments and ventricular aneurysms) and can provide information on ventricular volumes, ejection fraction and cardiac output. In patients recovering from myocardial infarction, radionuclide ventriculography with technetium is an excellent way to identify poor left ventricular function, which is important prognostically (Kelly et al,

1985). Five-year mortality is 3 per cent in those with an ejection fraction greater than 40 per cent, but 33 per cent in those with an ejection fraction of less than 20 per cent (Fioretti et al, 1984).

CARDIAC CATHETERISATION AND ANGIOGRAPHY

Selective coronary angiography was introduced in 1959, and it is an invaluable specialist investigation for defining coronary circulation. Coronary obstruction is demonstrable in over 90 per cent of cases thought to have coronary heart disease. The extent and severity of the lesions with assessment of left ventricular function can be used to determine the patient's prognosis. However, the investigation is expensive and requires a minimum of five people (doctor, two nurses, radiographer and technician). The procedure takes about half an hour, and is performed under local anaesthesia. There is a small morbidity and mortality rate (due to myocardial infarction and dysrhythmias), but these days this is so low as to allow day-case investigation.

The investigation is carried out for four main reasons:

1. To record intracardiac pressures, and demonstrate pressure gradients

2. To measure cardiac output, and detect shunting (by measuring blood gases) at different levels

3. To identify anatomical and functional anomalies

4. To demonstrate pathology of the coronary arterial tree

The right heart is approached through a peripheral vein in the arm or leg, in the same way as for Swan–Ganz monitoring. The left heart is usually approached by the retrograde aortic method (via the femoral or brachial artery). Trans-septal perforation is an alternative approach to the left heart. A needle-bearing right heart catheter is positioned in the right atrium, perforates the atrial septum, and allows the catheter to be advanced into the left atrium.

Angiography is usually recommended:

1. For patients with stable angina whose symptoms are significantly affecting their life-style, to decide whether surgery is indicated

2. For patients with unstable angina following inpatient stabilisation

3. Following uncomplicated myocardial infarction. One per cent of patients are found to have left main stem stenosis, and 26 per cent have triple artery disease (Betriu et al, 1982). The remaining three-quarters do not have severe coronary artery disease, and do not need surgery to improve symptoms or prognosis. Those patients at risk may be defined by exercise stress testing and radionuclide angiography. Patients with poor exercise tests, post-infarction angina and large dyskinetic segments warrant angiography

HAEMODYNAMIC MONITORING

The ability to recognise and accurately assess serious circulatory changes in patients requiring intensive care or recovering from acute myocardial infarction is often of major importance, both diagnostically and for assessing therapy and prognosis (Swan, 1975). In recent years, many techniques have become available which permit easy bedside analysis of haemodynamic status and cardiac function (Daily and Schroeder, 1981). Cardiovascular haemodynamics may be correctly assessed clinically (e.g. using the Killip scale, table 5.7) in the majority of patients presenting with acute myocardial infarction (Killip and Kimball, 1967; George and Winter, 1985), and significant reductions in cardiac output are due to either left ventricular (pump) failure or hypovolaemia. However, in patients following myocardial infarction, these may coexist and distinction may be difficult (Shell et al, 1982). The presence of an elevated jugular venous pressure and peripheral oedema does not exclude hypovolaemia, and may be found in patients who additionally have chronic obstructive airways disease, pulmonary emboli, right ventricular myocardial infarction or acute respiratory failure.

Infarction of the right ventricle may complicate a third of inferior myocardial infarctions (Cintron et al, 1981), and may be associated with low left atrial pressures, despite elevation of the jugular venous pressure (Bradley, 1977). Indirect measurement of the left atrial pressure by determining the pulmonary artery wedge pressure (PAWP) allows the distinction between hypovolaemia failure (low PAWP) and left ventricular failure (high PAWP).

In patients with long-standing cardiac failure, the clinical signs may make interpretation of the cardiac status difficult. Selective peripheral vasoconstriction may mask a low cardiac output, and thickening of the pulmonary vessel walls allows a substantial rise in pulmonary capillary pressures without clinical signs of congestion. Hence, although a patient may be considered on clinical grounds to have only mild left ventricular failure, haemodynamically there might be a substantial reduction in the cardiac output with high pulmonary capillary pressures.

Haemodynamic monitoring on coronary care may include the measurement of the central venous pressure (CVP), pulmonary artery (PA) pressure, pulmonary artery wedge pressure (PAWP), systemic blood pressure and cardiac output. Typical indications for invasive monitoring are shown in table 5.8.

Table 5.7. The Killip scale.

Class	Description	Incidence (%)	Mortality (%)
I	No pulmonary crepitations or S_3	33	6
II	Bilateral basal crepitations which persist after cough, and/or an S_3	38	17
III	Crepitations over one half of the lung fields, with pulmonary oedema on chest radiography	10	38
IV	Pulmonary oedema with cardiogenic shock	19	81

Table 5.8.   Indications for invasive haemodynamic monitoring.

Cardiogenic shock
Moderate or severe heart failure
Unexplained hypotension
Suspicion or presence of:
* Pulmonary embolism
* Right ventricular infarction
* Severe hypertension
* Aortic dissection
* Mechanical heart defects (e.g. ruptured septum or mitral valve)

Central venous pressure monitoring

The central venous pressure (CVP) reflects right ventricular end-diastolic pressure (filling pressure or preload), and is usually measured in the right atrium or superior vena cava. The CVP is determined by blood volume, vascular tone and cardiac performance. Elevation of the CVP is common in acute myocardial infarction and reflects an elevated right ventricular pressure secondary to left ventricular failure. Other causes may be cardiac tamponade or tricuspid incompetence. Low CVP levels are usually due to hypovolaemia when infusion of fluids may lead to improved cardiac performance.

Measuring the central venous pressure

A CVP catheter is inserted percutaneously, usually into the subclavian vein, and advanced to lie in the superior vena cava or right atrium. The line is normally attached to a slow-running 5 per cent dextrose drip and a manometer (figure 5.9). The patient can be positioned at 45° or less during measurement of the CVP, but the zero point (normally the manubrium sterni) must remain constant. The manometer should be filled and then allowed to equilibrate through the CVP line. Normally the fluid falls freely, although it fluctuates with venous pulsation and respiration. The CVP should be measured at the end of expiration.

Intra-arterial pressure monitoring

In the clinically unstable patient, measurement of systemic blood pressure with a traditional cuff is often difficult, particularly if the patient is hypotensive. In shock, readings taken with the sphygmomanometer may differ from the actual arterial blood pressure by over 30 mmHg (Cohn, 1967). The insertion of an intra-arterial pressure line is useful for directly and continuously measuring systolic, diastolic and mean blood pressures. In addition, prolonged cannulation of an artery is less traumatic than multiple stabs when serial blood gas estimations are required.

Sites commonly utilised include the radial, brachial and dorsalis pedis arteries. Cannulation is performed percutaneously under local anaesthesia, using a 20-gauge Teflon catheter, which is attached to a T-connector and pressurised saline/heparin flushing system. This runs continuously at about 3–5 ml/h to minimise clotting,

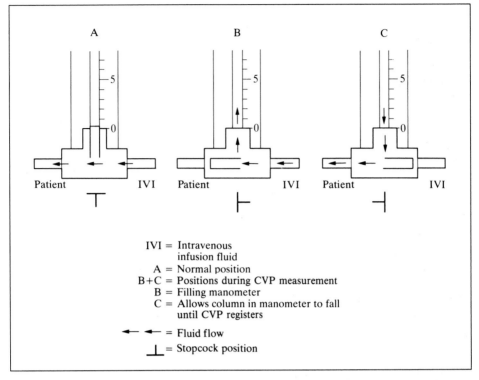

Fig. 5.9 Central venous pressure (CVP) monitoring, showing stopcock positioning

vasospasm and intimal damage. A transducer converts the pressures into a digital readout. Complications are not common but include:

- Obstruction (including spasm) leading to ischaemia
- Haemorrhage
- Air embolism
- Ecchymosis
- Sepsis

When the line is removed, pressure over the site should be maintained for at least 5 minutes, or longer if there are coagulation problems.

Pulmonary artery and pulmonary artery wedge pressures

The value of CVP measurement is limited because it basically reflects the functional state of the right ventricle, which does not always parallel that of the left ventricle. Information about left ventricular function is often essential for complete evaluation (Weisse et al, 1973).

Monitoring pulmonary artery and pulmonary artery wedge pressures may be useful following myocardial infarction, since it provides data to guide and evaluate therapy (Gold et al, 1971). One of the most important advances in haemodynamic monitoring has been the development of pulmonary artery flotation (Swan–Ganz) catheters

Table 5.9. Classification, therapy and mortality of patients following acute myocardial infarction.

Class	Cardiac Output	Index*	Wedge pressure (mmHg)	Therapy	Mortality (%)
No cardiac failure	Normal	>2.2	<18	Bed rest	3
Pulmonary congestion	Normal	>2.2	>18	Lower wedge pressure with: diuretics (blood pressure normal) vasodilators (blood pressure raised)	9
Peripheral hypoperfusion	Low	<2.2	<18	Plasma expanders	23
Pulmonary congestion and peripheral hypoperfusion	Low	<2.2	>18	Reduce wedge pressure with diuretics/ vasodilators If hypotensive, use inotropic agents	51

*Cardiac index (l/min/m^2) = cardiac output (litres) per minute per body surface area (metre^2) (From Forrester J S et al, 1976. Reproduced by kind permission of the *New England Journal of Medicine*)

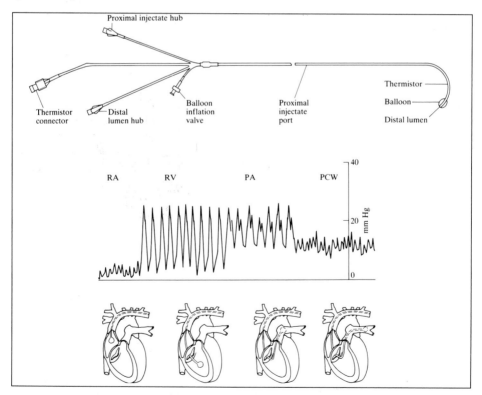

Fig. 5.10   The Swan–Ganz thermodilution catheter and typical pressures recorded during its passage through the heart (From Stokes and Jowett, 1985. Reproduced by kind permission of Churchill Livingstone)

(Swan et al, 1970). The Swan–Ganz catheter has been used to sub-classify patients following acute myocardial infarction by measurement of cardiac index and wedge pressures (Forrester et al, 1976). This enables prediction of short-term prognosis, and the selection of appropriate therapy (table 5.9).

The Swan–Ganz catheter (figure 5.10) is about 80 to 110 cm in length, marked at 10 cm intervals, and is available in three sizes: 5 FG (for children), 6 FG and 7 FG (for adults). The basic model has two lumina. The larger lumen terminates at the tip of the catheter and is used for recording intracardiac pressures, infusion of fluids and sampling of mixed venous blood. A smaller lumen serves to inflate the latex balloon which not only helps the catheter float through the right heart, but also allows repeated, reversible, pulmonary artery occlusion for recording wedge pressures. In the more complicated models, there is a third lumen terminating 30 cm proximal to the catheter tip, which enables simultaneous measurement of right atrial (RA) pressures, and a fourth channel which leads to a thermistor located close to the tip. These latter two channels are used together for calculation of right ventricular cardiac output by thermodilution (Forrester et al, 1972). Other types of catheter are available for pulmonary angiography and pacing, and all can be floated into the pulmonary artery by observing pressure tracings made during passage through the right heart, without requiring fluoroscopy. The catheter is normally inserted at the bedside under local anaesthesia via a peripheral vein (usually the subclavian or antecubital).

Uses of catheters

Measurement of PAW and PA pressures

PAWP is the pressure recorded when the Swan–Ganz catheter has been floated through the right heart and wedged into a peripheral pulmonary artery. The pulmonary arteries are end arteries and the pulmonary veins contain no valves. The catheter therefore registers the pressure transmitted retrogradely from the left atrium. The PAWP closely relates to the left atrial pressure (Connolly et al, 1954; Ibanez et al, 1984), and provides an indirect method of assessing left atrial pressure. Normal intracardiac pressures recorded by the Swan–Ganz catheter are shown in table 5.10.

Cardiac output

The measurement of cardiac output provides useful information about cardiac performance and response to therapy. Cardiac output may be measured at the bedside using the four-channel Swan–Ganz catheter by injecting 10 ml of 5 per cent dextrose

Table 5.10 Intracardiac pressures measured by the Swan–Ganz catheter

	Pressure (mmHg)
Right atrium	0–8
Pulmonary artery: systolic	15–30
diastolic	5–12
Pulmonary artery wedge pressure	5–12

at 4 °C or room temperature into the right atrium via the 30 cm port. A temperature drop of the blood is recorded by the thermistor at the tip of the catheter which lies in the pulmonary artery. From the recorded changes in temperature, a bedside computer can calculate the cardiac output (Swan, 1975). A mean of three serial readings is usually taken for the value of cardiac output.

Blood gas analysis

Blood gas analysis can be made on mixed venous blood, slowly aspirated via the tip port. Recently, another type of pulmonary artery flotation catheter became available (Opticath by Oximetrix of California) which has a separate channel containing two fibreoptic bundles for light transmission. By connecting these to an oximeter, continuous measurement of the Po_2 is possible.

Complications

Complications arising from the use of Swan–Ganz catheters are infrequent, but include the following:

1. *Dysrhythmias*   These include heart block and ventricular tachycardia (Sprung et al, 1981). They are caused by mechanical irritation of the endocardium or valves and are usually noted at the time of catheter insertion, manipulation or removal. Continuous ECG monitoring is therefore desirable, with special attention to the rhythm during catheter manipulation.

2. *Infection*   As with any centrally placed line, scrupulous asepsis is mandatory, not only during catheter insertion, but also when manipulating the catheter or during infusion of fluids. If the catheter is not secured to the skin, the non-sterile portion can migrate inwards and cause infection. A permanently indwelling introducer, with a flexible polythene sleeve, may be used to protect the proximal 30 cm of the catheter, and allow manipulation if the catheter needs repositioning.

3. *Pulmonary infarction*   This may be caused by frequent, prolonged or over-inflation of the balloon, or by thrombus formation around the catheter tip (Renke et al, 1975). With time, the catheter tends to migrate through the heart and to wedge spontaneously. If unnoticed, pulmonary infarction can result. Pressures should be displayed continuously on an oscilloscope, so that any pressure damping (indicating thrombus formation) or spontaneous wedging may be immediately recognised.

4. *Perforation of pulmonary artery*   Too rapid inflation of the balloon not only increases the risk of balloon rupture, but may also rupture the pulmonary capillary (Lemen et al, 1975). This is rare, but patients with pulmonary hypertension are at risk. Balloon inflation should therefore always be slow.

5. *Balloon rupture and air embolism*   Balloon rupture should be suspected when there is no resistance to attempted inflation and failure to wedge. It becomes more common the longer the catheter is left in place.

STATIC MONITORING

The continuous monitoring of cardiac rhythm is one of the most important aspects of cardiological investigation and forms a vital part of assessment of patients in coronary care and other high-dependency units. The major impact of the coronary care unit on the mortality from acute myocardial infarction has resulted from the detection and treatment of related dysrhythmias (Wagner, 1984; Brownlee, 1985). Static monitoring has provided the capability of anticipating the occurrence of potentially fatal dysrhythmias, with the opportunity for prompt treatment of other changes in rhythm likely to have adverse haemodynamic consequences.

These advances have become possible by the widespread availability of electronic oscilloscopes (monitors) which can continuously detect and display the electrical activity of the heart. As may be anticipated, the results of such monitoring vary according to whether all potentially serious dysrhythmias are recognised. Much 'manual' recording is limited by fatigue, boredom or distraction, but the recent introduction of computer-linked monitors can lead to detection of almost all serious dysrhythmias (Vetter and Julian, 1975).

Nurses from all wards and specialties are more frequently caring for patients attached to such monitors, and must therefore be familiar with electrode placement and monitor operation, as well as being able to recognise and distinguish normal and abnormal rhythms (Hubner, 1983).

Electrodes

Electrodes are small metal sensors which are fixed to the skin to allow cardiac electrical activity to be detected and conveyed to the monitor for visualisation. Great advances have been made in the design of these electrodes, and modern disposable, pre-gelled, self-adhesive electrodes usually obtain excellent skin contact with minimal or no skin preparation. Nevertheless, there are several steps which can be taken if the signal is poor.

1. Shaving of the skin will improve electrode contact, and earn the thanks of the patient when it is removed.

2. Wiping the skin with alcohol will remove excess body oil and sweat.

3. Rubbing the skin with dry gauze or a wooden spatula will remove loose, dry skin and aid contact.

The electrode site should be observed daily for allergic reactions, but otherwise there is no need to change the electrodes routinely. The monitor should be placed in good view, and not on a bedside table behind flowers and fruit. The monitor cable should be long and flexible enough to allow the patient to walk around the bed area and to use a commode. Time should be taken to inform the patient and relatives that, although the heart is being monitored, it does not necessarily mean that the patient is critically ill.

Monitoring

Standard electrocardiographic limb leads are recorded from the right arm, left arm and left leg to produce limb leads I, II and III (Schamroth, 1977). In order to help with patient mobility and reduce movement interference, monitoring on coronary care is usually via three chest electrodes. These are normally placed in the two infraclavicular spaces (right, negative; left, positive) and at the right sternal edge (earth), which are areas free from underlying muscular masses, thus minimising muscle potential artefact. In this configuration, a tracing similar to standard limb lead I is obtained. Additionally, a clear site is left for application of chest electrodes for full 12-lead ECG recording, defibrillation and external cardiac massage should they be required.

The ECG tracing should be observed for the following features:

● Rate
● Rhythm
● PR interval
● Ectopic beats

The exact configuration of the complexes is not important unless it is changing from beat to beat. It is the rhythm that is of importance.

Dysrhythmias may be recognised in any lead, but as a general rule monitoring the three lead equivalent of chest lead V1 is the best. This is because it clearly demonstrates the P wave, and usually allows clear differentiation between ventricular ectopic beats and those arising from the supraventricular region, but being conducted aberrantly. Aberration should be expected when the ectopic beat is preceded by a P wave different from that of a normal sinus beat, or is of a right bundle branch block pattern (RSR') in V1. This lead is also useful for diagnosing bundle branch block and for differentiating between left and right ventricular ectopic beats. In right bundle branch block, the left ventricle is depolarised before the right, and the net electrical movement is towards the V1 electrode, producing a predominant positive complex. This will also be seen in an ectopic beat arising in the left ventricle. In left bundle branch block and right ventricular ectopics the reverse is seen, with a predominantly negative V1 complex being recorded.

Although the V1 lead has all these undoubted advantages, it would seem to require fixation of four limb leads as well as a chest lead. Fortunately, a modified version of chest lead V1 has been described by Marriott (1983), designated MCL-1 (Modified Chest Lead 1), shown in figure 5.11. The positive (+) electrode is placed in the normal V1 intercostal space (fourth right), whilst the negative (−) and the earth (G) electrodes are located near the left shoulder and right shoulder respectively.

It must be noted that although routine monitoring by a familiar lead such as MCL-1 has obvious advantages, special leads are occasionally necessary to determine the origin of ectopic beats. A modified chest lead equivalent to V6 (MCL-6) is of particular value in differentiating between ventricular ectopy and aberration.

However, invasive techniques are sometimes necessary for precise assessment of a dysrhythmia. A lead passed into the oesophagus (in much the same way as for oesophageal pacing) is excellent for recording atrial activity, and the use of intracardiac catheter electrodes may help determine atrioventricular activation sequences.

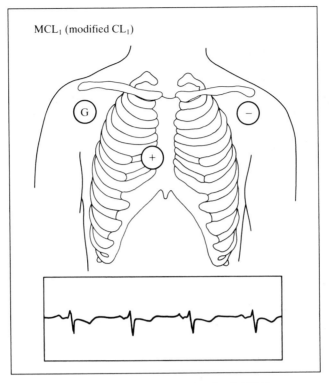

Fig. 5.11 Modified chest lead 1 (MCL1)
+ = positive electrode; − = negative electrode; G = ground electrode (From Jowett, Thompson and Bailey, 1985. Reproduced by kind permission of Churchill Livingstone)

Electrodes positioned in the region of the tricuspid value and right ventricle may then be used for recording electrical potentials in the bundle of His (Scherlag et al, 1969). These specialised techniques are of particular value in differentiating supraventricular from ventricular dysrhythmias, and in the identification of the site of block in atrioventricular conduction defects.

Computerised monitoring

Although visual observation of the oscilloscope by a trained observer is used on many units and on general medical wards, many dysrhythmias are missed. Over half of ventricular ectopic beats are not noticed, as well as between 5 and 10 per cent of multifocal ectopics (Romhilt et al, 1973). The use of computers for detection of dysrhythmias in acute care units and for review of rhythms over an extended period is therefore preferred (Knoebel and Lovelace, 1983). The simplest example of this is the rate detector alarm which will sound if preset heart rate limits are not met or are exceeded. Microchip technology has led to the development of an enormous number of computer-linked monitors which are able to recognise many dysrhythmias and sound alarms appropriately. Analysis can be performed at various levels of sophistication from simple dysrhythmia recognition to full reporting of standard

12-lead ECGs (MacFarlane, 1979). Using a storage mode, display of premature ventricular beat counts and trend analysis is possible for a 24-hour period. The complexity of the ECG signal and the frequent interference introduced by artefact have retarded the anticipated advances in this field. As a result, complex rhythm analysis is not usually feasible, and most systems are limited to determination of rate with recognition of pauses, premature ventricular complexes (PVCs) and tachycardias of both ventricular and supraventricular origin.

Problems with monitoring

The most frequent problem encountered with this form of monitoring is false alarm due to movement artefact, loose and disconnected electrodes, or too little electrode jelly. Very small or 'fuzzy' complexes, or even the appearance of asystole, may result on the screen (Conway, 1974). Electrical interference may also occur if there is insufficient grounding of the equipment, or from the use of other machinery (e.g. ventilators, electric razors or vaccuum cleaners) close by. Respiration or changing position in bed may affect the height of the complexes and may give rise to a wandering base line. It is important to ensure that T waves are not too large, as these may be counted and analysed by the machine as added beats.

Skin irritation sometimes occurs and signs of inflammation should be checked for periodically. Frequent electrode changes are required in patients who are perspiring profusely to ensure good electrical contact and to minimise skin irritation.

AMBULATORY MONITORING

Abnormalities of cardiac rhythm are common, and may affect patients with or without cardiac disease. Bradycardia is common in young people, and sinus pauses, nodal rhythm and first-degree block may also occur (Brodsky et al, 1977). Extrasystoles become commoner with increasing age, and ventricular ectopics affect 75 per cent of patients between the ages of 60 and 75 years (Bjerregaard, 1983). When the dysrhythmia is frequent, documentation is easily accomplished with brief periods of static monitoring. However, if the dysrhythmia is infrequent or transient, extended monitoring is required.

The standard 12-lead ECG provides little information about cardiac rhythm. The average ECG will record about 50 complexes, typically taken with the patient lying down and at rest. Static monitoring techniques (Jowett and Thompson, 1985; Jowett et al, 1985) clearly also have their limitations, and are unsuitable for detection of short rhythm disturbances, especially if induced by exertion or other factors in the daily life of the individual. Documentation of abnormal electrical activity therefore requires prolonged continuous recording during exercise (Antman et al, 1979).

Ambulatory ECG monitoring is designed to document transient rhythm and conduction disturbances, and aims to establish a relationship between symptoms and any accompanying disturbance in cardiac rhythm (Winkle, 1980). Most commonly this has been applied to the investigation of transient neurological symptoms which might be attributable to falls in cardiac output. For example, syncope and dizziness are often

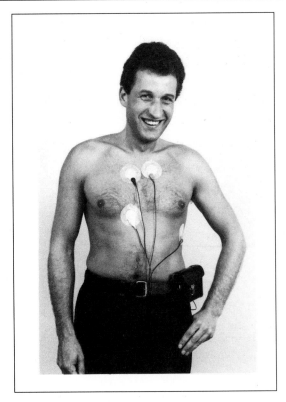

Fig. 5.12   The Holter monitor (Reproduced by kind permission of Reynolds Medical Limited)

found to be due to short-lived dysrhythmias. Other common referral symptoms are chest pain and palpitations.

Recorders are of two types:

● Continuous recorders
● Intermittent (sampling) recorders

The standard ambulatory monitor

Norman 'Jeff' Holter, an American, first put forward ideas for a portable ECG recorder in the late 1940s, and hence these recording machines are usually known as Holter monitors whatever their origin (Holter, 1961). From the initial bulky, short-duration machines, the monitors have been refined so that they are now small, light, strong and able to record the heart rhythm continuously for 24 to 48 hours.

The complete unit consists of a small tape recorder carried in a harness, which is worn by the patient as shown in figure 5.12. The recording electrodes are applied to the chest in the MCL-1 (V1) position which usually allows clear recording of the P waves and QRS complexes. A cassette tape is inserted into the machine, and the patient is told to carry out his normal day's activities. A detailed diary for the day should be kept by the patient to record activities (e.g. sleep, exertion or watching television) with clear descriptions of any symptoms, especially faintness, palpitations

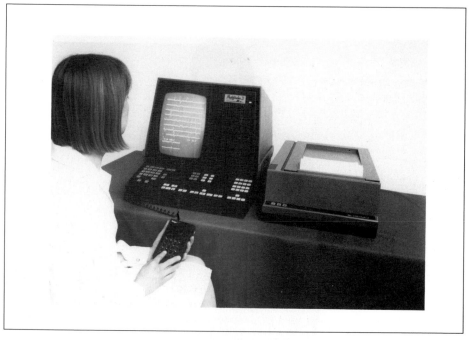

Fig. 5.13   High-speed electrocardioscanner (Reproduced by kind permission of Reynolds Medical Limited)

and dizziness. This diary, as well as the investigation referral note, is of major value during tape analysis and interpretation.

At the moment, ST segment analysis is not a routine use of ambulatory monitors, which are predominantly used for assessing cardiac rhythm. Faithful reproduction of ST segments and T waves usually requires specialised recorders and analysers for the diagnosis of myocardial ischaemia. Shift of the ST segment does not necessarily indicate ischaemia, and ST elevation may occur during nocturnal bradycardia in normal subjects (Deanfield et al, 1984). Intermittent ST depression, however, usually indicates impaired myocardial perfusion and is rare in normal individuals. Recently it has become apparent that there are many episodes of symptomless ischaemic episodes. The prognostic and therapeutic significance of this is unknown (Petch, 1985).

A typical 24-hour recording will provide about 100 000 complexes for analysis, but fortunately computerised scanning is available using high-speed electrocardioscanners, such as that shown in figure 5.13. The more advanced machines have automatic computer dysrhythmia recognition units, and are able to carry out ectopic counts or detailed rhythm analyses (Morris and Simpson, 1981). Most analysis systems require a skilled operator to oversee the equipment during replay of up to 120 times real speed. A 24-hour period may therefore be viewed in as little as 12 minutes, although selection of rhythm strips and paper printout make full processing a little longer. Presentation of the content of the complete recording is usually done in hourly blocks, with sample rhythms on standard ECG paper (figure 5.14). Other episodes of abnormal activity are also presented, with precise times enabling comparison with the patient's event diary of associated activities and symptoms.

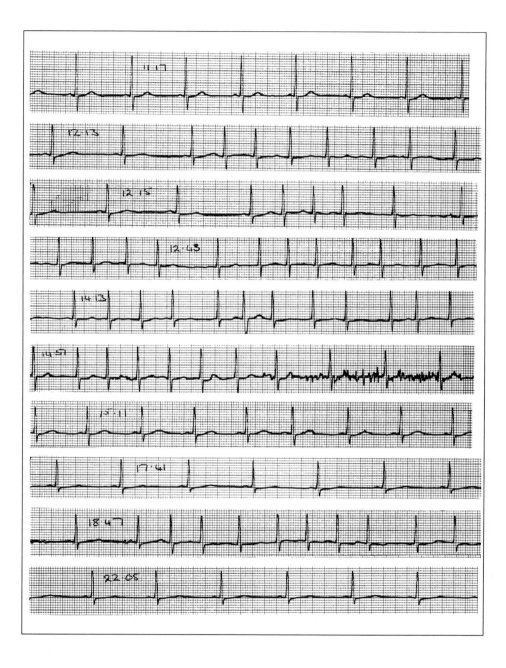

Fig. 5.14 Sample rhythms from a 24-hour Holter recording. The patient's diary is used to correlate symptoms and rhythm disturbances. The trace shows several short runs of paroxysmal atrial fibrillation

Other recording methods

Holter monitoring is limited by recording capacity and relies on events taking place during the period of study. Patients frequently complain that, 'It never happens when I'm attached to the monitor'. Fortunately, several modified recording systems have been developed which may aid the detection of dysrhythmias.

Event recorders

These are small recorders which are able to record for about 30 minutes duration. They can be manually activated by the symptomatic patient, or will activate automatically should any sudden change in rate or rhythm occur (according to preset criteria). Unfortunately, these will usually not show the onset of the dysrhythmia, which is often of importance in documenting the origin of the rhythm disturbance and for appropriate therapy.

Trans-telephonic recorders

These are small, hand-held recorders with chest electrodes fixed into the back. During an attack of palpitation, the patient presses the unit firmly over the heart and a short rhythm strip is automatically recorded. The signal may then be transmitted via the telephone to the coronary care unit. Here the signal is automatically decoded and printed out as a conventional ECG rhythm strip. The recorder can then be used again as many times as necessary, and is thus very useful for infrequent but recurrent symptoms.

Telemetric units

Telemetry is increasingly being used within hospitals for extended peri-infarction cardiac monitoring. The patient is fitted with standard chest electrodes, attached to a small transmitter carried in the pyjama pocket. The cardiac rhythm is transmitted continuously to a receiver (normally on the coronary care unit), where it is displayed, observed and analysed in the same way as the other patients on static monitors (Jowett and Thompson, 1985; Jowett et al, 1985). The advantage of this system is that patients can be mobilised in the early period following myocardial infarction, whilst still having the benefits of dysrhythmia monitoring.

The transmission range of these units is usually short, and thus relatively free from extrinsic radio interference. Longer-range transmission units have been developed for use by cardiac arrest teams. They may be of value both to junior staff in hospital (where advice on rhythm is immediately available from the more experienced staff on coronary care), and to ambulance crews and paramedics outside hospital, when administration of antidysrhythmic therapy can be recommended over the radio by the cardiac unit back at the hospital.

Recording artefacts

Whichever recording system is used, artefactual interference is often encountered and often makes interpretation difficult. Frequent causes are poor electrode contact, body movement and poor tape quality (due to tape stretch or inadequate erasure). Fortunately this is normally obvious during tape analysis, although many artefacts may closely resemble rhythm abnormalities. Hence, careful examination of related rhythm strips is often required to demonstrate that the recording is artefactual.

Men with nylon shirts or women with nylon underwear may also generate static electricity which can distort recordings, and should avoid wearing these articles of clothing during recording periods.

Using ambulatory monitoring

There are several major uses of ambulatory monitoring.

1. *Diagnosis of the aetiology of symptoms*   Confirmation of diagnosis requires the coincidence of symptoms and dysrhythmia. Asymptomatic recordings are usually of no help. Approximately 60 per cent of Holter recordings will show no abnormality, and a further 30 per cent will be normal despite symptoms being described during the recording (Zeldis et al, 1980). A positive diagnosis with concurrent dysrhythmia and symptoms will be made in only about 10 per cent of recordings (Clarke et al, 1980), whilst the remainder often show important asymptomatic dysrhythmias, such as ventricular tachycardia.

2. *Assessment of the incidence and frequency of previously identified rhythm disorders*   Rate-dependent conduction disturbances or dysrhythmias caused by metabolic changes are often detected this way.

3. *Immediate analysis of rhythm disturbance*   By the use of telemetric or transtelephonic recorders, immediate rhythm interpretation is available to the cardiac team. This facility is often used to assess pacemaker function and performance. Inpatient telemetry also allows extended ambulatory monitoring of the patient with recent myocardial infarction.

4. *Assessment of antidysrhythmic therapy*   The efficacy of a chosen antidysrhythmic drug cannot always be predicted. Electrophysiological testing (Weiner, 1982) may help appropriate selection of an agent, but as these techniques are not widely available, a therapeutic trial may have to be carried out. Comparison of tapes before and after drug therapy may indicate the value of a particular antidysrhythmic agent, or may give early warning of toxicity (e.g. bradycardia or heart block). Serial tapes have revealed the variability in the incidence of dysrhythmias on different days in the same patient. An important implication of this is that an antidysrhythmic drug may only be said to be effective if the number of extrasystoles is reduced by 80 per cent (Petch, 1985).

5. *Assessment of patients following cardiac arrest or cardiac surgery*   Continuous monitoring following a cardiac arrest may demonstrate frequent ventricular ectopic beats (PVCs), or short runs of ventricular tachycardia (Panidis and Morganroth, 1983). In some patients, these abnormalities may be a valuable guide for long-term therapy. Holter monitoring may also reveal advanced degrees of sino-atrial and atrioventricular block or the sick-sinus syndrome, which may have been the underlying cause of the cardiac arrest (Iseri et al, 1978). In evaluating possible dysrhythmia-related symptoms, the following sequence of investigation is useful:

a. Inpatient static or telemetric monitoring
b. Prolonged ambulatory Holter monitoring
c. Exercise stress (provocation) test (Podrid and Graboys, 1984)
d. Outpatient event recording
e. Electrophysiological studies

References

Akhras F, Upward J, Scott R and Jackson G (1982) Early exercise testing and coronary angiography after uncomplicated myocardial infarction. *British Medical Journal,* **284:** 1293–1294.
Antman E S, Graboys T B and Lown B (1979) Comparison of continuous to intermittent electrocardiographic monitoring during exercise testing for exposure of cardiac arrhythmias. *Journal of the American Medical Association,* **241:** 2802–2805.
Betriu A, Castaner A, Sanz G, Pare J C, Roig E, Coll S, Magrina J and Navarro-Lopez F (1982) Angiographic findings one month after myocardial infarction; a prospective study of 259 survivors. *Circulation,* **65:** 1099–1105.
Bjerregaard P (1983) Mean 24 hour heart rate, minimum heart rate and pauses in healthy subjects 40–79 years of age. *European Heart Journal,* **4:** 44–51.
Bradley R D (1977) *Studies in Acute Heart Failure.* London: Edward Arnold.
Brodsky M, Wu D, Denes P, Kanakis C and Rosen K M (1977) Arrhythmias documented by 24 hour continuous electrocardiographic monitoring in 50 male medical students without apparent heart disease. *American Journal of Cardiology,* **39:** 390–395.
Brownlee W T (1985) Acute arrhythmias. *British Journal of Hospital Medicine,* **33:** 138–145.
Bruce R A, Blackman J R, Jones J W and Strait G (1963) Exercise tests in adult normal subjects and cardiac patients. *Pediatrics,* **32:** 742–756.
Cintron G B, Hernandez E, Linares E and Aranda J M (1981) Bedside recognition, incidence and clinical course of right ventricular infarction. *American Journal of Cardiology,* **47:** 224–227.
Clarke P I, Glasser S P and Spoto E (1980) Arrhythmias detected by ambulatory monitoring: lack of correlation with symptoms of dizziness and syncope. *Chest,* **77:** 722–725.
Cohn J N (1967) Blood pressure measurement in shock. *Journal of the American Medical Association,* **199:** 972–976.
Connolly D C, Kirklin J W and Wood E H (1954) The relationship between pulmonary artery wedge pressure and left atrial pressure in man. *Circulation Research,* **2:** 434–440.
Conway N (1974) *A Pocket Atlas of Arrhythmias.* London: Wolfe Medical Books.
Daily E K and Schroeder J S (1981) *Techniques in Bedside Hemodynamic Monitoring,* 2nd edn. St. Louis: C V Mosby.
Deanfield J E, Ribiero P, Oakley K, Krikler S and Selwyn A P (1984) Analysis of ST-segment changes in normal subjects: implications for ambulatory monitoring in angina pectoris. *American Journal of Cardiology,* **54:** 1321–1325.
Dymond D S, Foster C, Grenier R P, Carpenter J and Schmidt D H (1984) Peak exercise and immediate post exercise imaging for the detection of left ventricular functional abnormalities in coronary artery disease. *American Journal of Cardiology,* **53:** 1532–1537.
Epstein S E (1978) Value and limitation of electrocardiographic response to exercise in the assessment of patients with coronary heart disease. *American Journal of Cardiology,* **42:** 667–674.
Ferlinz J (1982) Right ventricular function in adult cardiovascular disease. *Progress in Cardiovascular Diseases,* **25:** 225–267.

Fioretti P, Brower R W, Simoons M L, Das S K, Bos R J, Wijns W, Reiber J H, Lubsen J and Hugenholz P G (1984) Prediction of mortality in hospital survivors of myocardial infarction. Comparison of pre-discharge exercise testing and radionuclide ventriculography at rest. *British Heart Journal,* **52:** 292–298.

Forrester J S, Ganz W, Diamond G, McHugh T, Chonette D W and Swan H J (1972) Thermodilution cardiac output determination with a single balloon directed catheter. *American Heart Journal,* **83:** 306–311.

Forrester J S, Diamond G, Chatterjee K and Swan H J C (1976) Medical therapy of acute myocardial infarction by application of hemodynamic subsets. *New England Journal of Medicine,* **295:** 1356–1362.

George R J D and Winter R J D (1985) The clinical value of measuring cardiac output. *British Journal of Hospital Medicine,* **289:** 89–95.

Gold H K, Leinbach R C and Dunkman W B (1971) Wedge pressure monitoring in myocardial infarction. *New England Journal of Medicine,* **285:** 230–231.

Goldman L and Mervin (1979) *Principles of Clinical Electrocardiography.* California: Lange Medical Publications.

Holter N J (1961) New methods for heart studies. *Science,* **134:** 1214–1217.

Hubner P J B (1983) *Nurses Guide to Cardiac Monitoring.* London: Baillière Tindall.

Ibanez J, Raurich J M, Beltran X, Fiol M, Abizanda R, Marse P and Abadal J M (1984) Wedge pulmonary angiography to determine accuracy of pulmonary wedge pressure. *Critical Care Medicine,* **12:** 653–655.

Irving J B, Bruce R A and de Rouen T (1977) Variations in and significance of systolic pressure during maximal exercise (treadmill) testing. *American Journal of Cardiology,* **39:** 841–848.

Iseri L T, Humphrey S B and Siner E J (1978) Prehospital brady-asystolic cardiac arrest. *Annals of Internal Medicine* **58:** 741–745.

Jefferson K and Rees S (1980) *Clinical Cardiac Radiology.* London: Butterworths.

Jowett N I and Thompson D R (1985). Electrocardiographic monitoring. II: ambulatory monitoring. *Intensive Care Nursing,* **1:** 123–129.

Jowett N I, Thompson D R and Bailey S W (1985) Electrocardiographic monitoring. I: static monitoring. *Intensive Care Nursing,* **1:** 71–76.

Kelly M J, Thompson P L and Quinlan M F (1985) Prognostic significance of left ventricular ejection fraction after acute myocardial infarction: a bedside radionuclide study. *British Heart Journal,* **53:** 16–24.

Killip T and Kimball J (1967) Treatment of myocardial infarction in a coronary care unit. *American Journal of Cardiology,* **20:** 457–464.

Knoebel S B and Lovelace D E (1983) Symposium on arrhythmias. I – computers and clinical arrhythmias. *Cardiology Clinics,* **1:** 121–137.

Lemen R, Jones J G and Cowan G (1975) A mechanism of pulmonary artery perforation by Swan–Ganz catheters. *New England Journal of Medicine,* **242:** 211–212.

MacFarlane P W (1979) *Progress in Electrocardiography.* London: Pitman Medical.

Marriott H J L (1983) *Practical Electrocardiography.* Baltimore: Williams and Wilkins.

Morris J R W and Simpson A F (1981) ECG data analysis systems. In: *Clinical Ambulatory Monitoring,* ed. Littler W A. London: Chapman and Hall.

Naughton J, Balke B and Nagle F (1964) Refinements in methods of evaluation and physical conditioning before and after myocardial infarction. *American Journal of Cardiology,* **14:** 837–843.

Oakley C M (1984) Mitral value prolapse: harbinger of death or variant of normal. *British Medical Journal,* **288:** 1853–1854.

Panidis I and Morganroth J (1983) Sudden death in hospitalised patients: cardiac rhythm disturbances detected by ambulatory electrocardiographic monitoring. *Journal of the American College of Cardiology,* **2:** 798–805.

Petch M C (1985) Lessons from ambulatory electrocardiography. *British Medical Journal,* **291:** 617–618.

Petch M C (1986) Investigation of coronary artery disease. *Journal of the Royal College of Physicians,* **20:** 21–24.

Podrid P J and Graboys T B (1984) Exercise stress testing in the management of cardiac rhythm disorders. *Medical Clinics of North America*, **68**: 1139–1152.

Pollock M L, Bohannon R L, Cooper K H, Ayres J J, Ward A, White S R and Linnerud A C (1976) A comparative analysis of four protocols for maximal exercise testing. *American Heart Journal*, **92**: 39–46.

Renke R T, Higgins C B and Atkin J W (1975) Pulmonary infarction complicating the use of Swan–Ganz catheters. *British Journal of Radiology*, **48**: 885–888.

Romhilt D W, Bloomfield S S, Chou T C and Fowler N O (1973) Unreliability of conventional electrocardiographic monitoring for arrhythmia detection on coronary care units. *American Journal of Cardiology*, **31**: 457–461.

Schamroth L (1977) *An Introduction to Electrocardiography*. Oxford: Blackwell Scientific Publications.

Scherlag B J, Lau S H, Helfant R H, Berkowitz W D, Stein E and Damato A N (1969) Catheter techniques for recording His bundle activity in man. *Circulation,* **39**: 13–20.

Shell W E, Dewood M A, Peter T, Mickle D, Prause J A, Forrester J S and Swan H J C (1982) Comparison of clinical signs and hemodynamic state in the early hours of transmural infarction. *American Heart Journal,* **104**: 521–523.

Sprung C L, Jacobs L J, Caralis P V and Karpf M (1981). Ventricular arrhythmias during Swan–Ganz catheterisation of the critically ill patient. *Chest,* **79**: 413–415.

Swan H J C (1975) The role of hemodynamic monitoring in the management of the critically ill. *Critical Care Medicine,* **3**: 83–90.

Swan H J C, Ganz W, Forrester J S, Marcus H, Diamond G and Chonette D (1970). Catheterisation of the heart in man with the use of a flow-directed balloon catheter. *New England Journal of Medicine,* **283**: 447–451.

Theroux P, Waters D D, Haplon C, Debaisieux J C and Mizgala H F (1979) Prognostic value of exercise testing soon after myocardial infarction. *New England Journal of Medicine,* **301**: 341–345.

Vetter N J and Julian D G (1975) Comparison of arrhythmia computer and conventional monitoring in coronary care units. *Lancet,* **i**: 791–797.

Wagner C S (1984) Arrhythmias in acute myocardial infarction. *Medical Clinics of North America,* **68**: 1001–1008.

Weiner I (1982) Current applications of clinical electrophysiological study in the diagnosis and treatment of cardiac dysrhythmias. *American Journal of Cardiology,* **49**: 1287–1292.

Weisse A B, Narange R, Haider B and Regan T J (1973) Right and left heart pressures in acute myocardial infarction. *Cardiovascular Research,* **7**: 251–260.

Winkle R A (1980) Ambulatory electrocardiography and the diagnosis, evaluation and treatment of chronic ventricular arrhythmias. *Progress in Cardiovascular Diseases,* **23**: 99–128.

Zeldis S M, Levine B J, Michelson E L and Morganroth J (1980) Cardiovascular complaints: correlation with cardiac arrhythmias on 24-hour electrocardiographic monitoring. *Chest,* **78**: 456–462.

6

Nursing Assessment

Nursing consists essentially of helping people who are sick to perform activities which they would normally do for themselves (McFarlane, 1980). Unfortunately, on the coronary care unit, many nurses concentrate on understanding pathology, using technology and assisting with medical interventions, whilst placing relatively little emphasis on assessing and dealing with patient needs.

Nursing patients in coronary care is now increasingly complex because medical knowledge and technology have become more complex. There is less time for personal contact because the duration of the patient's stay in hospital is shorter, and because more disciplines are now involved in caring for the individual patient. It is therefore more difficult for the nurse to provide continuous and technically competent care which avoids depersonalisation of the patient and his family. An important aspect of nursing care is to enable the patient to regain his independence as quickly as possible, by the promotion of self-care (Henderson, 1960; Orem, 1980). Within coronary care, dependence on the nurse is usually of a temporary nature. Once recovered from the acute phase of myocardial infarction, patients usually regain their independence quite rapidly. What they do need, however, is advice on adjustments in their life-style, with health education and information on secondary prevention of coronary heart disease (see chapters 13 and 14). Education of the patient should be a fundamental and intrinsic function of nursing. Patients and their families need to understand about their illness and why certain treatments are necessary. This will aid maximum compliance in the future. To perform this role efficiently, the attending staff require the relevant knowledge, skills and experience. This requires constant updating of knowledge and the acquisition of new skills. These skills are not necessarily those relating to technical care, but perhaps psychological skills which may be utilised to speed recovery. Technical aspects of coronary care are important, but so are the emotional, social, spiritual and physical needs of the patient and his family.

PRIMARY NURSING

Primary nursing simply means that one nurse is responsible for one patient (Manthey, 1970, 1980). Admission, assessment, defining nursing problems, setting goals and planning appropriate care by an individual nurse on each shift is required to aid continuity of care. In the coronary care unit, as on the medical wards, it is important to appreciate that no two patients with the same illness react in the same way. It therefore seems only logical and sensible for nurses to provide individualised care.

The concept of primary nursing together with systematic problem solving establishes a form of care which is highly personalised and continuous. Professional responsibility for patient care then rests with the nurse, who should be held account-able for her actions. Coronary care is ideally suited to primary nursing since patient numbers are few, and the majority of staff are fully qualified. Unfortunately, the practice is not yet widespread. It appears to have been discouraged because many nurses and doctors have felt threatened by such personal care, believing that it might undermine their authority and status. Yet if nursing is to have a positive impact on patients in coronary care it should be individualised, continuous and, hopefully, imaginative.

NURSING THEORIES AND MODELS

Nursing theories and conceptual models may provide a useful and necessary frame-work for the nursing process (Riehl and Roy, 1980; Fawcett, 1984). They have not been designed merely as an academic exercise, but as a sincere attempt to provide the nurse with something that has practical application, so that care planning can be critically analysed, which hopefully will improve the care she gives to her patients. Roy (1984) lists the essential requirement of a model for nursing practice as containing:

- A description of the person receiving care
- A statement of the goal of nursing
- A definition of health
- A specified environment
- A delineation of nursing activities

Some of these models have clear relevance for nursing practice in coronary care, such as the Roy Adaptation Model (1984), and the Orem Self-Care Model (1980). In the United Kingdom, Roper et al, (1980) have described a model which incorporates many of the concepts inherent in Orem's model and Henderson's (1960) conceptual framework. This model certainly provides a useful and more comprehensible framework for practice. Interest in nursing models is growing, with books by Kershaw and Salvage (1986), Pearson and Vaughan (1986) and Wright (1986) attesting to this.

The nursing process can be utilised to implement practice based upon any selected model.

THE NURSING PROCESS

The nursing process serves as a framework for decision making and delivering nursing care, and must be viewed as a thinking exercise and not as a paper exercise. It is depen-dent on the nurse's knowledge and understanding of people, health and nursing. It should also be a dynamic and flexible process so that nursing management can adapt to frequent or rapid changes in the patient's condition. Within coronary care, the nursing process often needs to be completed in a short time and may not, in some instances, be fully documented in an emergency. The nursing process may be considered as a systematic, rational problem-preventing and problem-solving process with four main phases (Ashworth, 1985).

● *Assessment:* appropriate information is collected and an assessment is made
● *Planning:* a plan of action is decided
● *Implementation:* the plan of action is implemented
● *Evaluation:* the results of these actions are evaluated

These phases may overlap and usually form a cyclical process which leads to reassessment, further planning and re-evaluation.

The nurse must be able to elicit subjective and objective data from the patient (and his relatives) to formulate clinical nursing judgments and appropriate plans of care. The outcome of any intervention must then be evaluated. Assessment is based upon all available information, and should establish a nursing diagnosis for which the nurse can prescribe and implement care and evaluate its effect in terms of measurable outcomes.

Assessment

Assessment is probably the most important phase of the entire nursing process. It entails the collection and interpretation of information which is usually factual, but to some extent may be based upon the nurse's impression of the patient. Once information has been gathered, nursing problems should be identified and checked with the patient (*validation*) wherever possible. Nursing assessment therefore permits the nurse to define problems which the patient and his family may have in coping with illness and restoring health.

There are certain basic human needs which take priority over others (Maslow, 1970). The most basic needs are physiological, aimed at self-preservation. However, other important needs are security, belonging and self-esteem. Daily living activities (Henderson 1960; Roper et al, 1980) form part of these human needs and patients may be assessed in terms of their ability to carry out these day-to-day activities.

Compilation of data

Data are compiled through observation, interviewing and physical examination, plus any pertinent laboratory results. Skills are required to assess a patient properly, especially the ability to communicate and observe.

In the UK, unlike North America, it is uncommon for nurses to undertake a detailed physical examination of the patient other than by general observation. Whilst physical examination is usually carried out by the attending physician, an appreciation of the techniques involved and what information may be gained is helpful. Often some signs can be elicited by the nursing staff, and physical finding and examination are therefore discussed further in chapter 4.

Obtaining a clinical history

The history provides subjective information relative to the severity of the illness and how it affects the patient. The nurse must have the interviewing skills necessary to elicit the relevant information. The influence of the nurse, often the first person whom the patient sees upon entering hospital, is paramount. A quick initial assessment usually gives significant clues to his general condition. A calm and efficient approach to patient and family may markedly reduce anxiety and stress. Reassurance, explanation and comfort are required, as well as an ability to anticipate what will be needed.

History-taking improves with experience. The best technique is to allow the patient to relate his problems spontaneously in a calm, unhurried manner. Information should be recorded as soon as it is obtained to minimise omission and distortion of facts. The patient should be comfortable, as relaxed as possible and in an environment free from distraction. Privacy at the bedside is essential, and the nurse should ensure that this is maintained. She should be sensitive and considerate, especially as regards the amount of questioning and discussion the patient can tolerate, particularly if the patient is anxious or in pain. Whilst eliciting the history, the nurse should observe the patient's general appearance, manner of speaking, breathing pattern and evidence of agitation, pain or distress. She should use verbal and non-verbal communication skills, but must ensure that she is making the right inferences from non-verbal cues. Particular care should be shown towards persons who are elderly, confused or have a poor memory and may be unable to provide a reliable history. Help from the patient's relatives or friends should be sought.

History-taking is a continuing accumulation of information throughout the hospital stay. In making an assessment, information may be supplemented by facts gathered from the family, past and existing medical notes and nursing or social reports.

There should be a specific format for obtaining and recording the information the patient gives to establish a complete and accurate database. It is sensible to use a systematic method of evaluation with the following components:

- Personal details
- Presenting complaint (PC)
- History of present condition (HPC)
- Previous medical history (PMH)
- Activity level
- Family history (FH)
- Psychosocial history

Personal details

The database should include the full name of the patient (including what he prefers to be called), sex, age (including date of birth), race, nationality and religion. The marital status and next of kin, with addresses and telephone numbers, are also needed.

His precise occupation should be noted. (What does he actually do? Does it involve physical or emotional stress? If retired, what was his work?)

The source of referral to hospital is important (e.g. family doctor or another specialist) for providing feedback about the admission at a later date.

Presenting complaint

The chief complaint (or the patient's conception of the problem) should be noted. It is normal to write down the exact words he chooses, which can often give valuable insight into the patient's idea of why he has been admitted.

A series of questions can be used to elicit information about the patient's view of the problem (Kleinman et al, 1978):

● What brings you here?
● What do you think has caused your problem?
● Why do you think it started when it did?
● What do you think this illness does to you?
● How severe is your illness?
● What kind of treatment do you think you should receive?
● What important result do you expect from treatment?
● What are the chief problems your illness has caused you?
● What do you fear most about this illness?

The patient should be allowed to describe his own problems and expectations with little or no direction from the interviewer.

History of present condition

This should begin with an elaboration of the chief complaint and provide a detailed history of the present problem from time of onset to the present. Does the patient relate his present problem to his life-style, failure to comply with drug regimens or delay in seeking help?

The history provides subjective information on the severity of the illness and its effect on the patient's life. Relevant information includes:

● Day, time and manner of onset of the problem
● Presence or absence of cardiac risk factors
● Drugs (it should be remembered that side-effects may be responsible for some current complaints)
● Diet
● Physical activity (functional capacities and limitations in day-to-day living)

When information is sought about symptoms that are induced by effort, it is important to determine whether the patient performs the necessary activity sufficient to induce them. Symptoms should be described according to specific factors:

● Site: origin and radiation
● Quality: properties of the symptom ('tight', 'stabbing', etc.)
● Quantity: extent, severity, frequency, duration and intensity
● Chronology: time of onset and sequence of events
● Setting: situation, time, active or resting, emotionally upset or relaxed
● Predisposing, aggravating or alleviating factors: changes with position, temperature, deep breathing or medication (e.g. nitrates or analgesics)
● Associated symptoms: e.g. sweating, nausea

A review of the body systems, particularly the cardiovascular system, may be appropriate here. Symptoms and signs of heart disease that can be obtained from the history and general observation include chest pain, dyspnoea, palpitations, oedema, cyanosis and syncope. All of these are discussed in chapter 4.

Previous medical history

This may or may not be relevant to the present problem. Information about previous illnesses, hospital admissions, treatment, allergies and current medication should be recorded in detail. The reason why the patient is receiving medication and his compliance should also be assessed and recorded.

Activity level

This is a description of the patient's daily level of activity. It should include information on the following:

● Diet: normal habits, calorie intake and any supplements used
● Sleep habits: hours per day, sleep patterns and any sedations or sleep-promoting routines used
● Bowel habit: normal pattern, use of aperients
● Hygiene practices: bath or shower
● Other activities: work, leisure, sexual activity

Family history

This provides an overall picture of the patient's family health, with special regard to first-degree relatives. This should include details of any serious illnesses requiring hospital admission, any operations, with ages and causes of death if applicable. The presence of any familial diseases should be noted or suspected in the light of this information, for example, familial hypercholesterolaemia, diabetes mellitus, hypertension and coronary heart disease.

Psychosocial history

This should include information on the following areas (McGurn, 1981).

1. *Coping mechanisms of the patient and the family:* the changes that the patient's illness imposes and the responses the patient and his family are making to them.

2. *Interpersonal relationships:* the strength and types of relationship the patient has with his family and friends, and whether these will help the patient cope with his illness.

3. *Life-style:* how the patient likes to spend his time and money, and whether his illness will affect this.

4. *Support systems:* the support that may be available from the family, work, friends and neighbours, both while in hospital and when the patient goes home.

5. *Family/community assets:* positive attributes and assets of the family, friends and his work.

It can be seen that proper assessment is not just simply a matter of noting a few facts. The technique of nursing assessment is at an early stage of development and should continue to develop, so that changes in concept, knowledge and direction can emerge from experience and evaluation (Bowman and Thompson, 1986). Flexibility is certainly required with regard to the depth of initial assessment of a patient with acute myocardial infarction.

Nursing diagnosis

When assessment has been completed and interpreted, a nursing diagnosis should be formulated (Gordon, 1982). Nursing diagnosis is a relatively new concept in the UK, but is an integral component of nursing in the USA (Guzzetta and Dossey, 1983). It should be a summary of the problem the patient has experienced or might experience as a result of his illness. It should be written clearly and concisely and include all the factors relating to that problem.

Thus, a full statement of a nursing diagnosis should include identification of the following (Hunt and Marks-Maran, 1986):

- The patient's problem (e.g. pain)
- Aetiology, if known (e.g. ischaemic heart disease)
- Signs and symptoms in relation to the problem (e.g. tachycardia, sweating, grimacing, pallor, in pain)

An example of a nursing diagnosis in relation to an acute myocardial infarction might be:

- 'Retrosternal chest pain caused by ischaemic heart disease. The patient has a tachycardia, is sweating, grimacing, looks pale and says he is in pain'.

Planning

A plan of care should be developed, designed to meet the patient's actual and potential health needs. It involves:

- Establishing aims (or expected outcomes) of care for each problem
- Selecting and documenting the nursing intervention to achieve these goals
- Setting priorities of action

Objectives should be stated in measurable or observable terms, so that achievement can be checked. If possible and appropriate, these goals should be agreed with the patient and his family. A timetable for each agreed point may be useful to motivate the patient. Nursing actions should be realistic, precise, understandable, appropriate and acceptable (Ashworth, 1985).

For the whole planning process to be accomplished, it is evident that time is required. Effective planning is often hindered by pressure of time, unclear purposes and expectations of planning or a failure to delegate responsibility for nursing intervention (Mayers, 1978).

Core care plans

Because of a high turnover of patients in areas such as coronary care, detailed individual care plans are often difficult to organise and complete. A relatively recent development has been the core or emergency care plan (Martin and Glasper, 1986; Glasper et al, 1987). These brief care plans may have a useful role within such areas as coronary care. They are often based heavily on the medical diagnosis and the nurse should be aware of the risk of depersonalised care (Bowman and Thompson, 1987).

The coronary care plan

Planning a care plan for patients on the coronary care unit needs to take into account the following (McGurn, 1981).

1. *Reduction of stress*   The reduction of noxious physical (e.g. temperature, pain) and sensory (e.g. noise, lighting, intrusion) stimuli is desirable. Specific sources should be identified in the assessment plan.

2. *Preservation of routines*   Care should be planned so that the patient's routines are preserved as far as possible. In coronary care, patients' eating, toileting and resting habits are often dramatically changed, sometimes resulting in disorientation and physical complications.

3. *Prevention of non-compliance*   Complex dietary and drug regimens will result in non-compliance, as will failure to explain the reasons for interventions. The nurse needs to ensure that the patient listens to, understands and retains information.

4. *Control of pain*   The nurse must ensure that her patient is free from pain. In coronary care, this often means the liberal use of analgesics and anxiolytic agents such as diamorphine, diazepam and nitrates.

5. *Provision of adequate rest*   Needless disturbance of patients should be avoided, with provision of rest periods. Patients on high-dependency units are often seriously and needlessly deprived of sleep.

6. *Education of the patient*   The nurse should ensure that the patient understands what is happening, and encourage him to take responsibility for his own health.

Although these six areas are important in the care of the coronary patient, they are often inadequately planned and carried out (McGurn, 1981). These and other related topics are discussed in detail in chapters 7 and 8.

Summary of care plans

There are many types of format for recording data, defining problems and outlining goals and intervention strategies. Although different units or wards may have their own care plans it is desirable to have some degree of standardisation to facilitate the transfer of patients between wards, units and hospitals if required. The care plan is the major tool for communicating instructions and providing a permanent and legal record. Entries should be written concisely, legibly and systematically, avoiding jargon and abbreviations to minimise ambiguity about care. The care plan should be kept up to date and made flexible to meet patients' changing needs.

Implementation

Implementation is putting the nursing care plan into action. Care is usually carried out, supervised and co-ordinated by the primary nurse, sometimes assisted by the patient's family, as well as other nurses and members of the health care team. Specific nursing interventions may need delegating to other members of the nursing team if appropriate.

Nursing implementation of the care plan for patients on coronary care should primarily be aimed at preserving the patient's life and meeting the patient's basic needs. Other priorities are then secondary, and the extent and type of nursing intervention required to provide effective care for the coronary patient may vary considerably. It may encompass the administration of cardiopulmonary resuscitation at one time, and encouraging the patient to eat a healthy diet at another. Both of these are central to the patient's welfare.

Evaluation

Critical evaluation can lead to improved assessment and planning and thus more effective intervention, and greater accountability. Evaluation should:

● Determine whether the objectives have been met
● Provide information for reassessment of patients' needs
● Discover which nursing actions are most consistently effective in solving a particular nursing problem

References

Ashworth P (1985) The nursing process and high dependency nursing. In: *High Dependency Nursing Care,* eds. O'Brien D and Alexander S, pp. 6–29. Edinburgh: Churchill Livingstone.
Bowman G S and Thompson D R (1986) Curbing routine and ritual. *Nursing Times, 82:* 43–45.
Bowman G S and Thompson D R (1987) Core care plans go critical. *Nursing Times, 83:* 70.
Fawcett J (1984) *Analysis and Evaluation of Conceptual Models of Nursing.* Philadelphia: F A Davis.
Glasper A, Martin L and Stonehouse J (1987) Core care plans. *Nursing Times, 83:* 55–57.
Gordon M (1982) *Nursing Diagnosis: Process and Application.* New York: McGraw-Hill.
Guzzetta C E and Dossey B M (1983) Nursing diagnosis: framework, process and problems. *Heart and Lung,* 12: 281–291.
Henderson V (1960) *Basic Principles of Nursing Care.* Geneva: ICN.
Hunt J M and Marks-Maran D J (1986) *Nursing Care Plans: The Process of Nursing at Work.* Chichester: John Wiley & Sons.
Kershaw B and Salvage J (1986) *Models for Nursing.* Chichester: John Wiley & Sons.
Kleinman A, Eisenberg L and Good B (1978) Culture, illness and care. *Annals of Internal Medicine,* 88: 251–258.
McFarlane J (1980) *Essays on Nursing.* London: King's Fund.

McGurn W C (1981) The nursing process applied to people with cardiac problems. In: *People With Cardiac Problems: Nursing Concepts,* ed. McGurn W C, pp. 145–221. Philadelphia: J B Lippincott.

Manthey M (1970) Primary nursing: a return to the concept of 'my nurse' and 'my patient'. *Nursing Forum,* **9:** 65–83.

Manthey M (1980) *The Practice of Primary Nursing.* Boston: Blackwell.

Martin L and Glasper A (1986) Core care plans: nursing models and nursing process in action. *Nursing Practice,* **1:** 268–273.

Maslow A (1970) *Motivation and Personality.* New York: Harper and Row.

Mayers M G (1978) *A Systematic Approach to the Nursing Care Plan.* New York: Appleton-Century-Crofts.

Orem D (1980) *Nursing: Concepts of Practice.* New York: McGraw-Hill.

Pearson A and Vaughan B (1986), *Nursing Models for Practice.* London: Heinemann.

Riehl J R and Roy C (1980) *Conceptual Nursing Models for Nursing Practice.* New York: Appleton-Century-Crofts.

Roper N, Logan W W and Tierney A J (1980) *The Elements of Nursing.* Edinburgh: Churchill Livingstone.

Roy C (1984) *Introduction to Nursing—an Adaptation Model.* 2nd edn. Englewood Cliffs, New Jersey: Prentice-Hall.

Wright SG (1986) *Building a Model for Nursing.* London: Edward Arnold.

7

The Management of Acute Myocardial Infarction

In Western countries, myocardial infarction is responsible for between a third and a half of all deaths, and a half to three-quarters of all cardiac deaths. In England and Wales, this means about 150 000 deaths per annum. Patients are probably best managed on coronary care units rather than in general medical wards, since the chances of resuscitation are two to three times higher on specialist units. Indeed in-patient mortality fell by about 10 per cent following the introduction of such units in the 1960s. Mortality rates are still falling, with in-hospital mortality rates of about 10 to 15 per cent in patients under the age of 70 years. The fall in cardiac mortality was initially due to the prompt recognition and treatment of potentially fatal dysrhythmias, but more recently it has been due mainly to improved therapy for cardiogenic shock and heart failure (Goldman and Cook, 1984).

Management of acute myocardial infarction is initially aimed at relieving the immediate symptoms, with rapid haemodynamic stabilisation. The next priority is prompt treatment of any ensuing complications.

PRE-HOSPITAL MANAGEMENT

The first presentation of myocardial infarction may be sudden death. Up to one-half of all coronary deaths occur in the first hour following the onset of symptoms of myocardial ischaemia (table 7.1), and most are due to ventricular fibrillation. As this acute rhythm disturbance can be effectively treated, the care of patients in the first hour is of vital importance. Of course, not all sudden cardiac deaths are necessarily due to dysrhythmia, and infarction of a critical area of myocardium may be responsible, as may myocarditis, aortic stenosis or aortic dissection. Warning symptoms are

Table 7.1. Time between onset of coronary symptoms and death.

Time (h)	Male (%)	Female (%)
< 0.5	35	44
0.5–1	5	5
1–2	5	2
2–3	6	7
4–24	15	12
> 24	34	30

Table 7.2. Premonitory symptoms in 100 sequential cases of myocardial infarction at Leicester General Hospital.

Symptoms*	Percentage
Angina: New	11
Old	17
Chest pain	26
Emotional stress	19
Dyspnoea	13
Lethargy	10
Palpitations	4
None	46

*Note that some symptoms were multiple

common, although their significance frequently goes unrecognised by the patient or by those from whom he may seek advice (table 7.2).

There are two points to note about these findings. First, nearly half of these cases had no warning of impending myocardial infarction. Second, in the majority of those who did experience a warning symptom, it was usually chest pain, although this was not always typically anginal. It is the sole prodromal symptom in 75 per cent of patients, and is usually recurrent. Pain may be felt in the arms (especially in the distribution of the ulnar nerve) or the back, and is frequently attributed to indigestion. It may be present at rest, during exercise or accompanying emotional tension.

Only 40 per cent of acute coronary deaths occur in hospitals (Goldman and Cook, 1984); another 40 per cent occur in the home; and the remainder in public places such as at work (6 per cent) or in the street.

Studies in Seattle, USA, have shown that bystander initiated resuscitation can halve the number of these immediate deaths, and over half of patients who are resuscitated survive to live a normal life (Crampton et al, 1975). 'Coronary ambulances' (Pantridge and Adgey, 1969) are now frequently employed to carry trained staff with equipment for resuscitation, haemodynamic stabilisation and rhythm monitoring to the patient with minimal delay. Initially, these ambulances were manned by medical practitioners and specialist nursing staff, but now paramedical personnel have been trained and provide primary emergency care in many areas (Briggs et al, 1976). The most important part of their training is the rapid use of cardiac defibrillation which has had a major impact on the reduction of out-of-hospital coronary mortality (Eisenberg et al, 1980). These services, however, cannot function satisfactorily unless there has been community education in the recognition of the possible presenting symptomatology of myocardial infarction, with basic training in cardiopulmonary resuscitation, allowing emergency services to reach the patient (Thompson et al, 1979). The effectiveness of such a combined system has been shown in many cities around the world including Brighton, Belfast, Seattle and Melbourne. In these areas pre-hospital care may have decreased the overall observed coronary mortality rate by as much as 14 per cent (Crampton et al, 1975, Goldman and Cook, 1984).

Apart from the role of effective resuscitation, there are other first-line measures which these ambulance services can provide. The insertion of intravenous cannulae and administration of analgesics and oxygen are helpful, and there is evidence from Belfast that the early correction of autonomic imbalance can reduce peri-infarction mortality, and lead to a reduction in the number of patients developing cardiogenic shock (Pantridge and Adgey, 1969; Webb, Adgey and Pantridge, 1972). Parasympathetic overactivity in the first hour following infarction is marked by bradycardia with hypotension, and will respond to treatment with atropine. It is present in about 50 per cent of coronary patients, especially those where the inferior surface of the heart has been involved. Sympathetic overactivity, marked by tachycardia and hypertension, is found in about one-third of cases of myocardial infarction, and here small doses of a short-acting beta-adrenergic blocking agent will improve the haemodynamic status.

There is some controversy about whether or not lignocaine should be given prophylactically to prevent malignant tachydysrhythmias during transportation to hospital or in the immediate peri-infarction period. Intravenous therapy is preferred, since intramuscular drugs are variably absorbed, and may lead to elevation of the muscle enzyme creatinine phosphokinase (CPK) frequently used in the diagnosis of myocardial infarction. Although lignocaine will certainly reduce the frequency of dysrhythmias in high-risk patients (Lie et al, 1974), the value over and above that of prompt resuscitation is minimal (Kertes and Hunt, 1984).

There are several (usually unavoidable) delays between the onset of symptoms and admission to the coronary care unit (Simon et al, 1972). This may occur:

● Between the onset of symptoms and the call for help
● Between the call for assistance and the arrival of medical help
● During transport to hospital
● Within the hospital

It is well recognised that many patients postpone seeking medical attention after the onset of symptoms, and this has been our experience (table 7.3). Where they occur, prodromal symptoms are experienced by 50 per cent of patients up to a week before myocardial infarction, and many can predate symptoms up to a month before the attack. The advice of the patient's family is frequently sought before any contact is made with a medical practitioner, and further time is wasted in waiting for the emergency physician to visit, formulate a diagnosis, arrange hospital admission and organise transport. Travel time to hospital is usually brief, but hold-ups in admission,

Table 7.3. Time between onset of coronary symptoms and call for medical help in 200 patients admitted to coronary care* with and without previous myocardial infarction (MI).

Time (h)	Previous MI	No previous MI
< 0.5	28	20
0.5–1	18	15
1–3	42	27
3–24	5	9
> 24	7	29
Total	100	100

*Leicester General Hospital

radiography or casualty departments can occur. Delays of up to six hours are not infrequent from the onset of symptoms to the arrival in the coronary care unit, and it is obvious that by this time the immediate danger period is over. The role of coronary care units would therefore seem to be limited (Pentecost, 1980), and there has been much debate about whether these patients would be better off kept quietly at home, without being rushed around at a time when they are probably at greatest danger.

THE HOSPITAL VERSUS HOME CONTROVERSY

Conflicting advice about the best place to manage acute myocardial infarction has led to great uncertainty within the medical profession, especially among general practitioners, with whom the decision often lies. There have been three studies attempting to clarify the position.

The Bristol coronary survey (Mather et al, 1971) found that patients treated at home and those treated in hospital did equally well. However, from a total of 1203 coronary patients, a selected group of only 343 were ramdomised to hospital or home care. This 24 per cent chosen for ramdomisation were probably destined to do well anyway, since the more seriously ill patients had already been admitted to hospital.

The Teesside coronary surveys (Colling et al, 1976; Dellipiani et al, 1977) showed that patients treated at home did better, especially if over the age of 65 years. However, patients were not randomly allocated, and we do not know how those doctors involved made the decision to transfer patients to hospital. What was interesting about this survey is that of the 1938 patients sustaining myocardial infarction, only 57 per cent survived long enough to be included in the study.

The final major study in the UK was the Nottingham coronary survey (Hill et al, 1978). This study tried to identify the prognosis in patients treated at home after high-risk patients had been transferred to hospital. A quarter of the cases of myocardial infarction were assessed as being at high risk of complications, and transferred immediately to coronary care. A hospital team stayed with the remaining (76 per cent) patients for two hours, after which the patients were randomly allocated to either hospital or home care. There was no difference in mortality between these two groups (11 per cent vs 13 per cent) although the high-risk group seemed to have been correctly identified (mortality 26 per cent). Whether admission to hospital minimises this mortality is not known.

These studies would suggest that if there is going to be a prolonged delay, or if the patient has presented some time after the onset of chest pain, there will be no difference in mortality of patients treated at home or in hospital. Provided the diagnosis has been established, or is beyond doubt, management at home should be considered if there are no complications, particularly for elderly patients or those living at a distance from the hospital. Home management does of course mean that the general practitioner is committed to frequent visits in the first 48 to 72 hours, which is not always possible in busy practices.

Table 7.4. Analysis of a year's admissions to the coronary care unit at Leicester General Hospital (1985).

Diagnosis	Male	Female	Totals	
			Number	Percentage
Myocardial infarction	267	93	360	37.3
Other cardiac	259	143	402	41.6
Non-cardiac	129	75	204	21.1

Total admissions: 966 patients

MANAGEMENT IN HOSPITAL

There has been a move away from the concept of coronary care units being only for cases of suspected or established myocardial infarction, and they should be available to any condition that merits cardiovascular monitoring facilities, such as dysrhythmia, aortic dissection or major pulmonary emboli. A review of admissions to the Leicester General Hospital unit in 1985 revealed that only 37 per cent of admissions were found to have suffered an acute myocardial infarction (table 7.4). However, a further 21 per cent had ischaemic pain without infarction, and a further 19 per cent of admissions had symptoms that could be described as primarily cardiac in origin. Hence the term Cardiac Intensive Care Unit (CICU) may be more applicable.

Direct admission policies must exist if early cardiac mortality is to be minimised. However, it must be appreciated that if such a policy exists there may be many false alarms, and possible unnecessary admissions to these specialist units. However, our experience (table 7.5) shows that the majority of cases are correctly directed to the cardiac intensive care unit (80 per cent), although only half of these will actually be acute coronaries. A concise and rapid clinical appraisal to assess the likelihood of myocardial infarction and need for hospitalisation is therefore required. An early positive diagnosis is also very helpful, so that any immediate complication which may need urgent treatment can be anticipated.

Of equal importance is the appreciation of the psychological stress placed upon the patient who has been rushed into hospital, usually via an emergency ambulance, to be delivered to the high-technology world of the coronary care unit. Verbal and tactile communication is important and the patient's confidence must be obtained and further developed by careful explanation at all stages.

Immediate management on the unit

There are several areas which need immediate consideration following admission to the coronary care unit. The original approach of watchful waiting over coronary patients has given way to active intervention, with the development of therapies intended to prevent potentially lethal complications and to limit or reduce the extent of the myocardial damage. The role of coronary thrombolysis is so enormously

Table 7.5. Final diagnosis of patients admitted to the coronary care unit.

Diagnosis	Number (% total admissions)
Primarily cardiac	
Myocardial infarction	385 (40)
Angina	204 (21)
Dysrhythmias	98 (10)
Left ventricular failure	55 (6)
Pericarditis	20 (2)
Pulmonary embolism	10 (1)
Aortic dissection	4 (0.5)
Total	776 (80%)
Primarily non-cardiac	
Chest pain of unknown cause	38 (4)
Chest infection	21 (2)
Reflux oesophagitis	46 (5)
Musculoskeletal pain	39 (4)
Other: anxiety, vasovagal episodes, peptic ulceration, biliary colic, pancreatitis, pneumothorax, carcinoma of lung, anaemia, gastrointestinal haemorrhage, cerebrovascular accident, constipation, cervical spondylitis, asthma	46 (5)
Total	190 (20%)

important in this respect that it has been considered separately (chapter 9). The usual period spent by patients on the unit is about 24 to 48 hours, although longer admissions will be needed for those patients with extensive myocardial infarction, severe heart failure or recurrent serious dysrhythmias. About half of the coronary admissions will have an uncomplicated course, and probably need little intensive care (Mulley et al, 1980).

Examination of the patient

The physical appearance and clinical findings in patients suffering from acute myocardial infarction are extremely variable and alter with time and the presence of any coexistent complications. However, it is not uncommon to find no physical abnormalities at all. The initial cardiovascular signs may not only be transient, but may be replaced by other important findings both within and outside the cardiovascular system which develop in the peri-infarction period.

Initial findings

The general appearance of the coronary patient is dependent upon the physical and psychological impact that the illness has upon the particular individual. Hence, although some patients will appear quiet and anxious, others may appear excessively agitated and restless. The situation will be eased or worsened if the patient has had a previous hospital admission (or myocardial infarction), depending upon his clinical and social course within hospital.

Autonomic imbalance or impaired left ventricular function may result in nausea, vomiting, sweating, peripheral vasoconstriction and varying degrees of dyspnoea. The patient will therefore typically be cool, clammy, in pain and frightened.

Pulse and blood pressure

Variation in pulse rate and blood pressure usually depend on the amount of pain, degree of left ventricular dysfunction and area of myocardial necrosis, but may be influenced by the extent of autonomic imbalance (Webb et al, 1972). Inferior and true posterior myocardial infarctions are usually associated with parasympathetic over-activity (bradycardia, hypotension and atrioventricular heart block), whilst anterior and lateral infarctions are associated with sympathetic overactivity (tachycardia and hypertension).

Pulse irregularities may indicate the presence of a dysrhythmia or conduction defect which will usually require electrocardiography for full elucidation.

The jugular venous pressure

The jugular venous pressure (JVP) is usually normal unless there is pre-existing con-gestive cardiac failure or pulmonary disease, or there has been right ventricular infarc-tion (see below). The pressure waveform may, however, be useful in detecting dysrhythmias. For example, cannon waves may be seen in complete heart block, or irregular 'a' waves in ventricular tachycardia.

The heart sounds

The first heart sound at the apex is often diminished and muffled as a result of left ventricular dysfunction, and reversed splitting of the second sound is not uncommon, probably reflecting conduction or mechanical abnormalities of the ischaemic left ventricle.

Fourth heart sounds are nearly always present (Hill et al, 1969), so that their absence makes myocardial infarction an unlikely diagnosis. However, auscultation of these low-pitched sounds is frequently difficult in patients who are obese or have hyperinflated chests, such as those with emphysema. Auscultation over the carotid or subclavian vessels may then reveal the presence of these sounds.

Third heart sounds are less common, and usually reflect left ventricular failure. As such, the presence of this added sound is associated with poor prognosis (Riley et al, 1973).

Cardiac murmurs

The murmur of mitral incompetence is present in about half of all patients in the early stages of myocardial infarction, and is due either to papillary muscle dysfunction, or to dilatation of the mitral ring in association with left ventricular failure (Heikkila, 1967). Other murmurs may indicate pre-existing valvular disease, which may or may not have predisposed the individual to myocardial infarction. For example, aortic valve disease may cause myocardial infarction in the presence of little or no coronary atherosclerosis.

Heparin locks

Initial management should start with insertion of an intravenous line to allow administration of an analgesic and an anti-emetic by injection. Intramuscular routes are inadequate, since drug absorption from vasoconstricted muscle capillary beds in the 'shut-down' patient is erratic. The majority of patients do not need intravenous fluids (which are usually contraindicated) but an emergency intravenous access is necessary in case of cardiac arrest. The routine use of an intravenous port has simplified prolonged venous catheterisation. A Venflon-type catheter can be used, which is inserted under sterile conditions into a peripheral (forearm) vein, and immediately flushed with sterile normal saline. The use of topical antiseptics such as Betadine does not reduce the risk of cannula-related infection, and cleaning the skin with an alcohol swab (Steret) is sufficient (Thompson et al, 1983, 1989). This has the added advantage of removing skin oils, and allowing the cannula to be fixed more securely to the skin with Elastoplast or similar adhesive tape. The cannula needs to be flushed 8 to 12 hourly with normal saline, and before and after every intravenous drug. The use of a heparin solution does not prolong the drip site patency, or reduce infection (Jowett et al, 1986).

Electrocardiographic monotoring

Careful monitoring of cardiac rhythm and the prompt treatment of dysrhythmias have sharply reduced hospital deaths from myocardial infarction (Norris, 1982). Following admission, immediate connection to a suitable cardiac monitor is required (Jowett et al, 1985). If the patient is being transferred via the accident and emergency department, a portable monitor must accompany the patient to the coronary care unit. Chest electrodes should preferably be kept away from areas used for cardiac auscultation or defibrillation (see chapter 5).

Analgesia

The provision of adequate pain relief at the earliest opportunity is of major importance, and should be given by nursing staff on their own initiative. Initial drug therapy should aim at relieving pain and anxiety which may stimulate catecholamine release, leading to a lowered threshold for dysrhythmias, an increase in myocardial work, and provocation of coronary arterial spasm (Lown et al, 1977).

The ideal drug should be effective, short acting and have no deleterious effect on cardiovascular haemodynamics. Intravenous opiates are the drugs of choice, and are usually very well tolerated following myocardial infarction. Morphine will not significantly affect ventricular filling pressures (Lappas et al, 1975), although atropine should be given if there is evidence of parasympathetic overactivity (marked by bradycardia and hypotension) to prevent extreme falls in blood pressure. The commonest side-effects of opiate therapy are nausea and vomiting, which can be reduced by simultaneous administration of an anti-emetic such as prochlorperazine (Stemetil) or metoclopramide (Maxolon). Comparison of the various opiate preparations suggests that diamorphine provides the earliest complete analgesic action with no more side-effects than other similar preparations (Scott and Orr, 1969).

Opiates must be used with care in patients with chronic bronchitis or cor pulmonale. Respiration is depressed by direct action upon the respiratory centre leading to a fall in respiratory rate and tidal volume. There is a reduction in the arterial Po_2, with focal atelectasis and small ventilation/perfusion defects developing in the lungs (Gazes and Gaddy, 1979). Respiratory side-effects occur within minutes of administration of the drug, and may last up to six hours. Opiates should therefore be administered in small, frequent doses, and nalorphine is a useful antagonist to have at hand if in doubt. A less well considered complication of opiate therapy is that of reduced gastric and intestinal motility. Apart from leading to constipation, the oral absorption of important drugs (such as diuretics and antidysrhythmic agents) may be impaired. Persistent anxiety may require treatment with diazepam (Valium), which is an effective anxiolytic agent and has other benefits in that it probably improves left ventricular function by reducing systemic and left ventricular filling pressures (Cote et al, 1976). Another major advantage which may result from the relief of anxiety is the reduced secretion of catecholamines, with a consequent reduced incidence of serious dysrhythmias (Melsom et al, 1976).

Oxygen

Patients with acute myocardial infarction are commonly hypoxaemic, most marked in those with left ventricular failure and cardiogenic shock (Editorial, *British Medical Journal*, 1976). Its severity parallels the clinical condition of the patient, and generally correlates with the degree of left ventricular dysfunction. The reason for hypoxaemia is unknown, but probably results from the interaction of several factors acting simultaneously. Amongst these are pulmonary oedema, pulmonary ventilation/perfusion defects and a slowing of peripheral circulation. Hypoxaemia may increase the size of the infarction (Radvany et al, 1975), and oxygen therapy would therefore seem to be advantageous. Despite a possible associated rise in mean peripheral resistance (afterload), and consequent reduction in cardiac output (McNicol and Kirby, 1972), it is now common practice for low-flow oxygen to be administered to most patients for 24 to 48 hours (100 per cent oxygen at 2 to 4 l/min), on the basis that improved myocardial oxygenation outweighs the theoretical risks of peripheral vasoconstriction. Oxygen therapy is of particular value in patients with left ventricular failure, and is of great psychological value. Even in the absence of heart failure, experimental studies suggest that there will be benefits in oxygen delivery to the ischaemic peri-infarction area with reduction in infarct size (Maroko et al, 1975). Nasal cannulae are preferred to face masks, which spend most of their time oxygenating the skin of the forehead (table 7.6). Care should be observed in patients with coexistent chronic airways disease, and the concentration of inspired oxygen should be altered according to arterial blood gas estimation. In patients with severe heart failure and cardiogenic shock, positive end expiratory pressure ventilation (PEEP) has been used to increase oxygen transport

Table 7.6. Oxygen masks, flow rates and approximate concentrations of delivered oxygen.

Mask oxygen flow (litres/min)	Edinburgh (%)	MC (%)	Nasal cannulae (%)	Hudson (%)
1	25–30	—	25–30	—
2	30–35	30–50	30–35	25–38
4	35–40	40–70	32–40	35–45
6	—	55–75	—	50–60
8	—	60–75	—	55–65
10	—	65–80	—	60–75

to ischaemic tissues, but its use is limited by the accompanying dramatic fall in cardiac output as a consequence of reduced venous return, inhibited by raised intrathoracic pressures.

Arterial hypoxaemia may last for up to three weeks following uncomplicated myocardial infarction, and longer if there has been significant heart failure or shock.

Blood samples

Blood samples should routinely be taken as soon after admission as possible. Samples may be taken via the intravenous cannula if necessary, but haemolysis often occurs if suction is too great. This will lead to incorrect blood counts, and an artificially raised serum potassium on biochemical analysis. In addition, clotting studies may be invalidated if heparin has been used to anticoagulate the intravenous port.

1. *Full blood count*   This may detect anaemia or polycythaemia. The white cell count (WBC) and erythrocyte sedemendation rate (ESR) are initially normal, but rise in response to muscle necrosis. The leucocytosis peaks at about 15 000 cell/mm^3 after two to four days, and higher levels suggest complications, such as infection or pericarditis. The ESR often remains elevated for two to three weeks.

2. *Urea and electrolytes*   These are needed to assess renal function, and for potassium levels. This is particularly important in patients on digoxin or diuretics.

3. *Baseline cardiac enzymes*

4. *Random serum lipid levels*   Early assessment will give an indication of pre-existing hyperlipidaemia (Ryder et al, 1984). If missed on admission, formal assessment will not be possible for about three months.

5. *Blood glucose level*   The venous blood glucose concentration is of prognostic importance (Burden et al, 1978). Those with admission sugars less than 7 mmol/l usually have uncomplicated courses, whereas those over 9 mmol/l are much more likely to have complicated stays in hospital. Hyperglycaemia may be precipitated by the stress of the illness, or may even pre-exist (see below).

Hyperglycaemia and diabetes

Although hyperglycaemia is common in coronary care admissions, so-called 'stress' hyperglycaemia of greater than 10 mmol/l on admission to the unit probably represents pre-existing diabetes mellitus (Husband et al, 1983). The peri-infarction mortality in diabetics is higher than in non-diabetics (Soler et al, 1974), and hence these patients will need special care. High admission blood sugars are frequent in those developing cardiogenic shock, or needing temporary cardiac pacing (Jowett et al, 1989). Oswald et al (1984) estimate that 5 to 6 per cent of coronary admissions are pre-existing undiagnosed diabetics.

Chest radiograph

An anteroposterior (portable) chest film is usually taken on admission. This initial film serves to exclude other causes of chest pain, such as aortic aneurysm, pneumonia and pneumothorax. However, assessment of pulmonary hypertension is not always easy. A normal film excludes significant heart failure, but an abnormal film does not mean that pulmonary pressures have not returned to normal. This is because there may be a 12-hour lag between haemodynamic dysfunction and radiographic appearances of cardiac failure. There may also be a degree of non-cardiac pulmonary oedema, caused by reduced plasma oncotic pressure (serum albumin levels fall in acute myocardial infarction) and aggregation of leucocytes. Radiographic findings also take much longer to resolve (up to four days) following haemodynamic stabilisation (Kostuk et al, 1973).

Review of drugs

All drug therapy being taken on admission needs reviewing. Many medications can be stopped, and should only be reinstituted if specifically required. This will prevent adverse drug actions or interactions. Beta-adrenergic blocking agents should be continued unless there are specific contraindications, such as excessive bradycardia, hypotension or heart failure. Sudden withdrawal of these agents may be accompanied by further chest pain, dysrhythmias or extension of the original area of myocardial infarction.

Hypertension

Many patients with myocardial infarction are found to be hypertensive on admission to coronary care. This may represent pre-existing hypertension, or be a response to the stress of infarction with sympathetic overactivity (Webb et al, 1972). Coronary mortality is higher in hypertensive than normotensive patients, and should therefore be promptly treated (Beck and Hochrein, 1974). If the blood pressure does not settle after relief of pain and anxiety, active treatment should be commenced. This should be considered as urgent when ischaemic pain continues or there is heart failure. Short-acting beta-adrenergic blocking agents (such as metoprolol) are useful for the management of sympathetic overactivity in the early stages of infarction, but caution is required.

Tachycardia and hypertension may represent a cardiovascular response to left ventricular failure, rather than being indicative of pure sympathetic overactivity. Incipient left ventricular failure is more likely in the presence of tachypnoea, a wide pulse pressure and a loud first heart sound (Gunnar et al, 1979), and vasodilator therapy is then a better therapeutic choice.

Anticoagulants

The use of anticoagulants in acute myocardial infarction is controversial, but should be of benefit in:

- Preventing deep vein thrombosis and pulmonary emboli
- Preventing mural thrombi and peripheral embolisation
- Possible limitation of infarct size

The first major investigation of anticoagulant therapy in acute myocardial infarction (Wright et al, 1948) indicated a large reduction in both mortality and thromboembolic complications. However, this trial was carried out at a time when length of bedrest and immobilisation differed markedly from our practice today, and typically involved many weeks in bed. Since that time various studies have shown conflicting results (Gifford and Feinstein, 1969), although it does seem that thromboembolic complications can be reduced by anticoagulant therapy, and should be considered for all patients in the peri-infarction period. The number of patients requiring full anticoagulation are probably few (Ribner and Frishman, 1977), and, for the majority, low-dose heparin therapy is considered sufficient (Goldberg et al, 1984). The efficacy of low-dose heparin therapy was originally demonstrated in patients following surgery (Kakkar et al, 1972). When applied to the coronary patient (Fratantoni and Wessler, 1975) it gave significant benefit, particularly in patients with heart failure.

One recommended practice is for low-dose heparin to be given to all patients who do not have active peptic ulceration or bleeding diatheses and who have not undergone recent ocular surgery. It is continued from admission until the patient is actively ambulant. It has become clear that low-dose therapy is effective only as a prophylactic measure, and has no effect on established thrombus.

Full-dose anticoagulant therapy (heparin followed by warfarin) is given to those considered to be at increased risk of thromboembolic complications. The following are possible indications for full anticoagulation:

- Active thromboembolic phenomena
- Prolonged cardiac failure
- Atrial fibrillation
- Left ventricular aneurysm
- Cardiogenic shock
- Severe obesity
- Patients unable to ambulate

The duration of therapy is not clearly defined, but three months should be adequate in most cases (Genton and Turpie, 1983).

CONFIRMING THE DIAGNOSIS OF MYOCARDIAL INFARCTION

Confirming the diagnosis of myocardial infarction is important for deciding appropriate management of the patient, including where and how he would best be treated, and for assessing prognosis. The coronary care unit is not just for treatment, but has a clear role in establishing the cause of chest pain.

The bedside diagnosis of myocardial infarction is often very difficult. The main aids to the clinical history are the ECG and serum cardiac enzymes. Classically, if two of these are suggestive, myocardial infarction is usually considered definite (Rowley and Hampton, 1981). However, the history is frequently difficult to obtain from a patient who is shocked or in pain, and obtaining an account from the patient's relatives, although often helpful, may confuse the initial clinical impression. Electrocardiographic changes may take time to develop, and enzyme level results may not only take some time to return from the laboratory but may also be non-specific. A high index of suspicion is therefore required when first seeing the patient.

Recently, radionuclide imaging has provided a useful adjunct to the diagnosis of myocardial infarction when the former three diagnostic methods are inadequate. As yet, it is not in routine use.

Clinical history

Although great importance is attached to the clinical history, no two clinicians will always elicit the same account of the present illness. This of course may reflect the skill that any one physician may have in extracting relevant information, but patients have an annoying habit of altering their story each time they recount the details. Often they will tell the doctor what they think he ought to know rather than what he wants to know. Furthermore, obtaining essential information in the acute phase of the illness, when the patient is in pain and feeling faint or nauseated, is not ideal. Often the position becomes clearer when the patient has been settled with analgesics and anti-emetics. Taking a history from patients on coronary care is often much easier; somebody somewhere must have thought the history was suggestive of myocardial infarction.

Serum cardiac enzymes

Following myocardial infarction the levels of some of the myocardial enzymes will rise, and estimation of their serum levels is often of diagnostic importance. They may not only be able to confirm the diagnosis of myocardial infarction (even in the absence of electrocardiographic evidence), but the degree of their elevation may give some indication of the size of the myocardial infarction. Enzyme release is thought to reflect irreversible cell damage (i.e. infarction), and the increased serum concentrations are due to abnormal release from the damaged myocardial cells. The most commonly measured cardiac enzymes are creatinine phosphokinase (CPK), lactate dehydrogenase (LDH) and glutamic oxaloacetic transaminase (SGOT). The timing of their release and peaks in relation to chest pain are also of importance (figure 7.1).

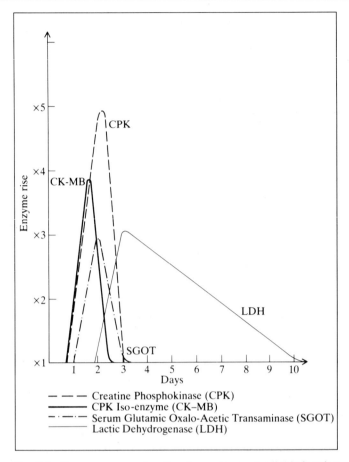

Fig. 7.1   Serum enzyme elevation in acute myocardial infarction

These enzymes are not cardiospecific, and may be released from other tissues in response to different stimuli or illnesses (table 7.7). Isoenzymes of LDH and CPK may be used as cardiospecific enzymes, but assays are usually not available in most district general hospitals. The routine measurement of cardiospecific isoenzymes could improve the speed and accuracy of diagnosis of myocardial infarction (Roberts, 1984).

Creatinine phosphokinase

CPK is found in high concentrations in both skeletal and cardiac muscle, as well as the brain. Its estimation is the most sensitive single enzyme assay for detecting acute infarction (positive in over 90 per cent of cases). Serum levels rise within four to eight hours following myocardial infarction, peak at 24 hours, and return to normal after about five days.

CPK is composed of two subunits, M (muscle) and B (brain), which can be linked together as MM, BB or MB. The last is of greatest diagnostic importance, since it is virtually only found in the human heart. This does not of course mean that it is

Table 7.7. Other possible causes of enzyme elevation.

SGOT	Pulmonary embolism Hepatic congestion Liver disease Shock Trauma (including surgery or cardioversion) Gall bladder disease Drugs (steroids, cholestatic agents and the pill)
LDH	Heart failure Liver disease Renal failure Myocarditis Pulmonary embolism Muscle disease or injury (including severe exercise and intramuscular injections)
CPK	Muscle disease or injury (surgery, intramuscular injections, after defibrillation) Stroke Haemorrhage Following sustained tachycardias

only liberated during infarction of the myocardial cells. Cardiac damage and consequent enzyme release can occur following defibrillation and cardiac surgery (or other trauma) as well as in some myopathies. After acute myocardial infarction, CK-MB levels rise rapidly to reach a peak at 24 hours, and disappear again by about 72 hours.

Lactic dehydrogenase

LDH is found widely throughout the body tissues, especially the liver, as well as skeletal and cardiac muscle. It is elevated in over 85 per cent of cases of myocardial infarction, with elevation starting within 24 to 48 hours, peaking at three to six days and returning to normal over one to two weeks.

Normal LDH is composed of five chemically distinct isoenzymes. There are high concentrations of LDH1 in cardiac tissue, so that release leads to a change in the LDH1:total LDH ratio.

Glutamic oxaloacetic transaminase

The heart is the major source of SGOT, and elevation of this enzyme is found in over 70 per cent of cases of myocardial infarction. Levels start to rise in the serum after 8 to 12 hours, peaking towards the end of the second day, and remaining elevated for about five days.

The ECG in myocardial infarction

There is no single ECG change in myocardial ischaemia and infarction. The findings are dependent upon the duration of the ischaemic insult and the part of the heart affected. The initial ECG is often normal, and even abnormalities are not helpful if they do not change with time. The standard for interpretation of electrocardiograms is the Minnesota code, but this places emphasis on a single ECG rather than an ECG series. It is the daily (often subtle) electrocardiographic changes which follow an

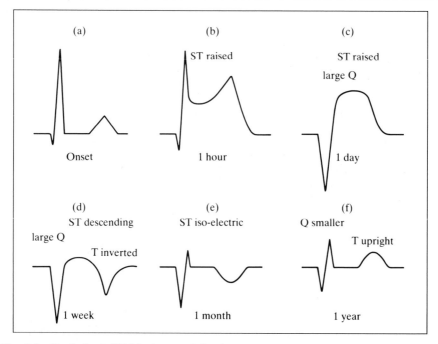

Fig. 7.2   Evolution of ECG changes following acute transmural myocardial infarction
(a)   ECG may be normal or show non-specific changes
(b)   development of Q wave and concave ST segment elevation
(c)   fully developed Q wave and convex ST elevation
(d)   ST segment descends and T wave inverts
(e)   ST segment now isoelectric; T wave often still inverted
(f)   Q wave permanent but smaller. In 10% of patients the ECG is normal

episode of prolonged chest pain that are of value in the diagnosis of myocardial infarction, especially when viewed with the knowledge of the clinical history and changes in serum enzyme levels. Typically, a standard 12-lead ECG is taken on admission and then daily for three days. Early ECG changes (at less than five hours) in patients who are haemodynamically stable and not on beta-adrenergic blocking agents are a reliable indicator of eventual myocardial infarction, and may even be able to predict those at risk from complications (Yusef et al, 1984).

In transmural myocardial infarction, there is typically an evolving sequence of ST–T changes with Q wave formation (figure 7.2). If the ischaemic insult has been insufficient to cause actual infarction, either ST depression or ST elevation (Prinzmetal changes) may be seen. Infarction limited to the inner part of the ventricular wall (subendocardial infarction) interferes with repolarisation (though not depolarisation) leading to ST depression and deep symmetrical T wave inversion (figure 7.3).

Acute transmural myocardial infarction

The hallmark of transmural myocardial infarction is the Q wave. By definition, this is the initial negative (downward) deflection of the QRS complex. Normally there are

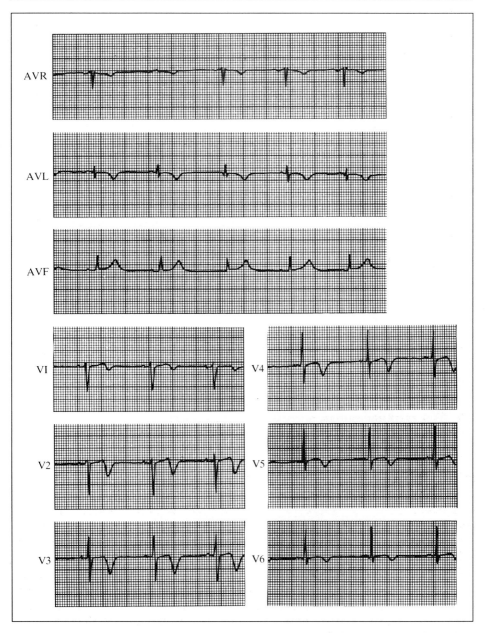

Fig. 7.3   ECG: subendocardial myocardial infarction

small ('septal') Q waves in the left ventricular leads caused by depolarisation of the septum from left to right. Q waves greater than 0.04 second (one small square on standard ECG recording paper) in duration and greater than 2 mm in depth are pathological, and imply infarction. The ventricles are depolarised from the inside outwards, and hence if an electrode were placed inside the heart it would record a large negative deflection, with the impulse travelling from within out. Myocardial necrosis produces an electrical 'window' in the ventricle, so that an overlying recording skin electrode will record a cavity potential, as if the electrode was inside the heart, i.e. a large Q wave.

The Q wave in standard lead III should only be considered abnormal if it exceeds 0.03 second, and if it is accompanied by Q waves in leads II and aVF. The 'normal' Q wave in lead III usually diminishes or disappears on deep inspiration, but a pathological Q wave will remain. Q waves may be produced by any process that forms a myocardial window and, as described above, are usually due to myocardial necrosis or fibrosis. However, other conditions may lead to damage or replacement of myocardial tissue, including myocarditis, cardiomyopathies, amyloidosis and cardiac tumours.

Determining the site of infarction

Infarction Q waves will appear within the first 24 to 48 hours in those leads facing the area of necrosis. Determination of the site of the infarction may be made by correlating the ECG findings with knowledge of the coronary circulation. However, individual differences in the normal coronary vasculature vary widely from person to person, so that it is only possible to make generalisations.

The three major coronary vessels (table 7.8) are:

- The right coronary artery (RCA)
- The left anterior descending artery (LAD)
- The left circumflex artery (LCx)

Table 7.8.   Major coronary arteries and structures supplied by each.

Right coronary artery (RCA)
  right atrium
  right ventricle
  inferior left ventricle
  sino-atrial node
  atrioventricular node
  posterior interventricular septum

Left anterior descending (LAD) coronary artery
  anterior wall of left ventricle
  anterior interventricular septum
  apex of left ventricle
  bundle of His and bundle branches

Left circumflex (LCX) coronary artery
  left atrium
  lateral and posterior left ventricle
  posterior interventricular septum

The RCA supplies the right atrium, the right ventricle and the inferior left ventricle. Blood is also conveyed to the sino-atrial node, the atrioventricular node and the posterior portion of the ventricular septum. Hence, occlusion of the RCA can produce infarction of the inferior and posterior left ventricle and, sometimes, the right atrium and ventricle. Ischaemia of the nodes can produce bradycardia and heart block (figure 7.4).

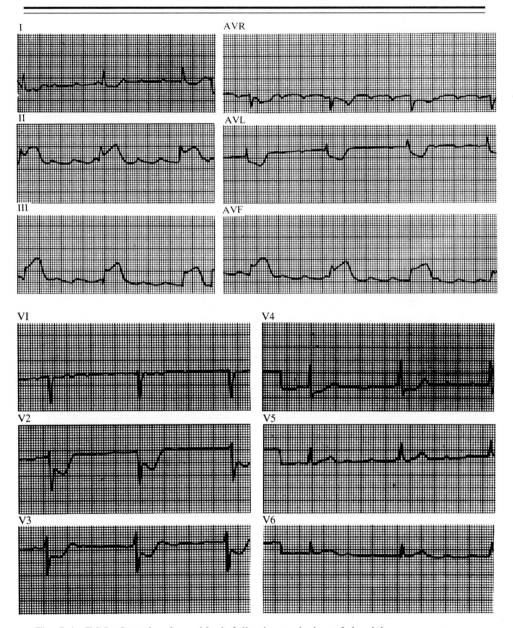

Fig. 7.4 ECG: Complete heart block following occlusion of the right coronary artery.

The left coronary artery ('left main stem') divides into its two main branches: the left anterior descending and the left circumflex. The former supplies the anterior left ventricular wall, the apex and the interventricular septum. There are septal perforating branches which additionally supply blood to the bundle of His and bundle branches. Occlusion of the LAD leads to infarction of the left ventricle, the apex and the septum. The LCx supplies the remainder of the left ventricle and sometimes the posterior part of the septum. In some people, it additionally supplies the sino-atrial

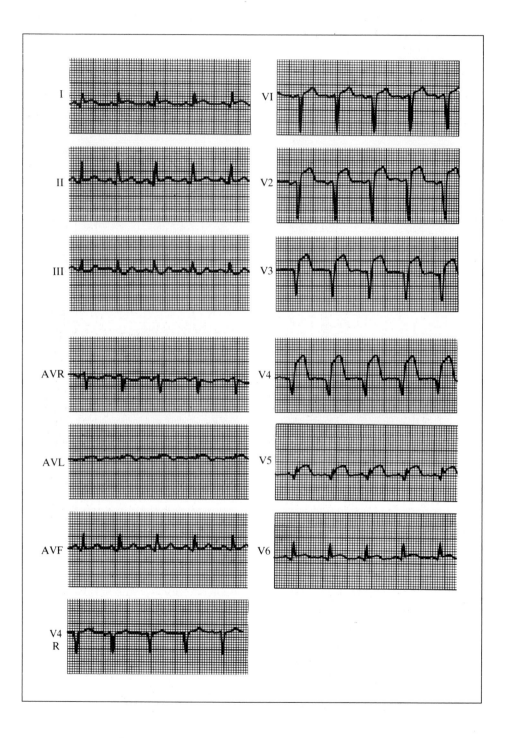

Fig. 7.5 ECG: acute anterior myocardial infarction

and atrioventricular nodes. Occlusion of the LCx leads to lateral infarction, some-times associated with conduction problems.

Common ECG patterns of infarction

The following ECG patterns of infarction can be seen on the standard 12-lead ECG.

1. Anterior infarctions (figure 7.5) give rise to changes in leads V1–4 (anteroseptal), standard leads I and aVL, V4–6 (anteriorlateral).

2. Inferior (diaphragmatic) infarcts are shown in the inferior leads II, III and aVF. (figure 7.6).

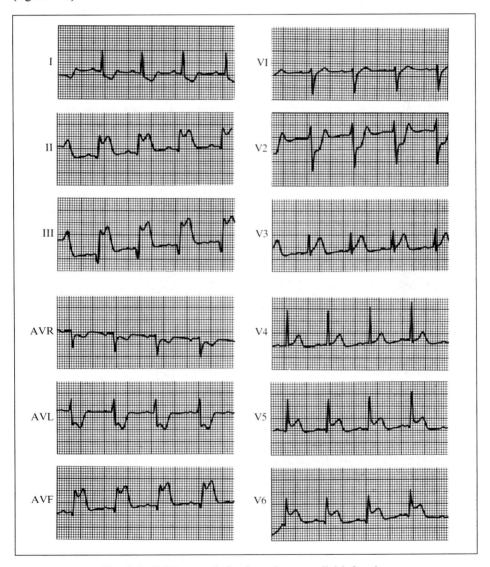

Fig. 7.6 ECG: acute inferolateral myocardial infarction

3. High lateral infarcts may only be seen in leads I and aVL.

4. Apical infarction can be seen in leads V5 and V6.

5. True posterior infarcts do not produce Q waves in the standard 12-lead ECG, since no lead directly overlies the area of necrosis. Instead, the diagnosis must be implied on the basis of reciprocal R waves in leads opposite the area – usually chest leads V1–V3 (figure 7.4).

Further leads may be required to locate infarcts at unusual sites. For example, V7 and V8 (placed further round the chest) are useful for diagnosing lateral infarcts, and leads in the second and third intercostal spaces may locate high lateral infarcts (Marriott, 1983).

Obviously, myocardial infarction does not have strict boundaries, and may be affected by anatomical differences in collateral coronary circulation. Hence, changes do not always appear in classical leads.

In the time following infarction, the Q waves may regress or even disappear. This may be because the scar contracts away from the surface electrode, or because small intraventricular conduction pathways are established in relation to the infarct (Goldberger, 1979).

ST segment and T wave changes

The earliest ECG sign of acute transmural myocardial ischaemia is elevation of the ST segment, the so-called 'current of injury'. This is sometimes accompanied by very tall *hyperacute* T waves. The ST segments are usually convex upwards, although occasionally they are concave or flattened. These acute ST–T wave changes resolve within hours or days to leave inverted T waves. ST segment depression is often seen in leads facing away from the affected area reflecting 'reciprocal' electrical changes. However, it is possible that these changes may indicate ischaemic myocardial tissue away from the infarction site, and could give a clue to the presence of atherosclerotic disease in other coronary vessels.

The ST–T wave changes usually resolve over the following weeks, although T wave inversion may last for an indefinite time. Persistent ST elevation in the chest leads often indicates formation of a ventricular aneurysm.

Right ventricular and atrial infarction

Isolated or additional infarction of the atria or right ventricle is probably more common than realised (Wartman and Hellerstein, 1948) and is difficult to recognise clinically. About one-third to one-half of patients with inferior infarction sustain some damage to the right ventricle, and isolated right ventricular infarction is found in up to 5 to 10 per cent of autopsies (Rodrigues et al, 1986). Right ventricular infarction generally appears as an inferior infarct with changes in standard leads II, III and aVF (Cohn et al, 1974). Lead V4R, however, and also sometimes V5R and V6R, may show ST–T wave changes, with ST elevation of greater than 1 mm. Although change in lead V4R is a useful diagnostic pointer (Klein et al, 1983), false positive recordings may occur in inferior myocardial infarction, left bundle branch block and pericarditis. Atrial infarction is found in about 10 per cent of cases of myocardial infarction, and occurs more commonly on the right. The ECG often shows altered P wave morphology and deviation of the PR segment. Atrial dysrhythmias are a common complication (Liu et al, 1961).

Subendocardial myocardial infarction

The subendocardial portion of the ventricular myocardium is especially prone to ischaemia because its blood supply in impeded by the high intraventricular pressure. In subendocardial myocardial infarction Q waves do not usually appear on the ECG since the damage is not transmural, although they probably will appear if more than 50 per cent of the wall thickness is involved. Infarction is therefore inferred from ST–T wave changes. These are not like those seen in angina or on exercise stress testing, and ST depression may become permanent, and associated with deep symmetrical T wave inversion (see figure 7.3 above).

ECG changes that mimic myocardial infarction (pseudo-infarction)

Reference has already been made to non-pathological Q wave changes in myocarditis or with myocardial infiltrates which may be misdiagnosed as myocardial infarction. Transient Q wave formation may also follow metabolic insult (especially hyperkalaemia or hypoglycaemia), and may even appear in non-infarction ischaemia (Goldberger, 1979).

Left bundle branch block produces loss of precordial R wave progression and inferior Q waves because of abnormal right-to-left septal depolarisation. There is also secondary ST depression with T wave inversion.

Left ventricular hypertrophy also frequently produces poor R wave progression in leads V1 to V3, and QR waves are seen in right ventricular hypertrophy or strain. The S1,Q3,T3 pattern classically described in acute pulmonary embolism is associated with non-infarction Q waves in standard leads III and aVF.

QS complexes occasionally occur in V1 and V2 as a normal variant in tall, thin individuals because of positional changes of the electrodes relative to the heart. Patients with chest deformities (e.g. pectus excavatum) often display poor R wave progression across the chest leads. High ST take-off is frequently seen in the young adult, especially in the septal leads, and ST changes can also be produced by changes in posture, hyperventilation, hypokalaemia and hyperkalaemia. Peaked T waves are characteristic of hyperkalaemia.

T wave changes are very common, and inversion may be normal in leads V1 and V2 (and V3 in negroes). Concave ST elevation with widespread T wave inversion occurs with pericarditis, but it should be noted that reciprocal ST depression does not occur (compare with myocardial infarction).

Very deep inverted T waves are sometimes found after intracerebral bleeds, probably due to altered autonomic tone, and should not be confused with the changes of subendocardial infarction. Similar T wave changes are often seen after tachydysrhythmias, or Stokes–Adams attacks.

DIAGNOSTIC CATEGORIES ON DISCHARGE FROM CCU

It should be possible to categorise patients within coronary care into one of six groups which will help with deciding on therapy and later management on discharge to the general medical wards.

1. Definite myocardial infarction
   ● good clinical history
   ● sequential ST–T wave changes ± Q wave appearance on the ECG
   ● a two-fold rise in serum cardiac enzymes

2. Probable myocardial infarction
   ● good clinical history
   ● diagnostic sequential ECG changes **or**
   ● a two-fold rise in cardiac enzymes

3. Possible myocardial infarction
   ● good clinical history
   ● abnormal (but non-diagnostic) ECG
   ● a small rise in cardiac enzymes

4. Angina
   ● ischaemic chest pain
   ● no ECG/enzyme changes

5. Other definite differential diagnoses (pericarditis, pulmonary embolus, pneumonia, etc.)

6. Chest pain of unknown cause – a diagnosis by exclusion

NUCLEAR IMAGING IN ACUTE MYOCARDIAL INFARCTION

In most cases of myocardial infarction there is adequate diagnostic evidence of myocardial infarction from the history, ECG and cardiac enzymes. However, occasionally the ECG may be difficult to interpret (e.g. in bundle branch block), and nuclear imaging may then complement enzyme studies. Radionuclide scanning techniques have been used to demonstrate areas of myocardial necrosis since the early 1960s, and are particularly useful in those patients who are strongly believed to have suffered myocardial infarction, but have no definitive electrocardiographic or enzyme evidence. Other specific benefits include:

1. Localisation of a myocardial infarction in the presence of:
   a. Left bundle branch block
   b. Subendocardial necrosis

2. Diagnosis of right ventricular infarction

3. Detection of new areas of infarction close to old infarcts or areas of fibrosis

4. Diagnosis of perioperative myocardial infarction. Infarction following cardiac surgery is difficult to diagnose since enzyme studies are unreliable and ECG changes are non-specific (Raabe et al, 1980). Imaging can often be of great help, provided a preoperative scan has been obtained for comparison

Radiolabelled agents identify and delineate areas of myocardial infarction, either by being preferentially taken up by damaged or necrosed myocardium (*hot spot* detection), or by demonstration of areas of hypoperfusion (*cold spot* detection). Technetium-99m is most commonly used for the former and thallium-201 for the latter. Hot spot detection has several advantages over the cold spot technique. Technetium-99m phosphates are inexpensive and easily prepared, the information obtained is easily interpreted and old areas of necrosis usually do not take up tracer. Unfortunately, although positive scans may be recordable at only four hours after the myocardial infarction, radiolabel may not be taken up for a period of up to 48 hours. False positive results may be found after cardioversion, in unstable angina and in the presence of left ventricular aneurysms. Technetium-99m scanning is of particular value in right ventricular infarction (Rodrigues et al, 1986). It can be combined with thallium scanning to separate areas of old and new myocardial infarction.

Table 7.9. Comparative values of hot and cold spot nuclear scanning.

Feature	Thallium-201	Technetium-99m
Diagnosis in first 6 hours	Excellent	Moderate
Diagnosis after 6 hours	Variable	Good
Diagnosis of right ventricular infarction	No help	Useful
Estimation of infarct size	Underestimates	Overestimates
Differentiation of old/new infarctions	Not helpful	Useful
Serial scans possible	No	Yes

The major advantage of thallium-201 cold spot scans is that they are nearly always positive in the first six hours, but are less reliable thereafter (table 7.9). Diagnosis of myocardial infarction may therefore be made in advance of standard laboratory tests. The advantages of cold spot scanning are limited by the high numbers of abnormal scans in patients without myocardial infarction. Reversible defects may be found in patients with coronary artery spasm or crescendo angina, and fixed defects in the presence of myocardial infiltrates or old infarction.

IMPORTANT PHYSICAL FINDINGS IN THE POST-INFARCTION PATIENT

Fever

A low-grade fever frequently follows myocardial infarction in the first three days, and is more common with large areas of myocardial damage. Other causes, such as deep vein thrombosis and infections, should be excluded, especially if the pyrexia exceeds 38 °C. Chest and urinary tract infections are common, and bacteraemia may be caused by intravenous cannulae, pacing wires or urinary catheters. Drugs may occasionally be the cause of late or unusual fevers.

Respiratory findings

Pulmonary embolism

Thromboembolic phenomena have become less frequent since the introduction of low-dose heparin therapy, and the trend towards early mobilisation. The diagnosis must be considered in any patient with chest pain associated with dyspnoea, tachycardia and fever. Physical examination is frequently unhelpful, unless there is pulmonary infarction. It is probably better to treat on suspicion rather than to rely on hard diagnostic criteria.

Chest infections

Chest infections are common, especially in the elderly, the obese and smokers. Pulmonary congestion and frank left ventricular failure predispose to infection, and administration of opiates is associated with small areas of atelectasis and ventilation/perfusion abnormalities in the lungs. Aspiration pneumonias may follow cardiopulmonary resuscitation.

Pneumothorax

This complication may follow central venous catheterisation, temporary cardiac pacing or cardiopulmonary resuscitation. It does not usually need treating, but should be anticipated and drainage carried out if required.

Gastrointestinal tract

Gastric dilatation may sometimes result from nasal administration of oxygen, leading to discomfort, nausea or vomiting.

Constipation and occasional paralytic ileus may result from bedrest, or atropine or opiate therapy. Straining at stool must be avoided to prevent excessive vagal stimulation from the Valsalva manoeuvre.

Gastro-oesophageal reflux is commonly a coexistent cause of precordial chest pain. Even evidence of oesophagitis at endoscopy does not exclude the diagnosis of myocardial infarction. Stress ulceration of the oesophagus, the stomach or duodenum may occur, sometimes presenting as gastrointestinal haemorrhage. This latter complication may be occult, and initially manifest as tachycardia, hypotension and shock in a previously stable patient. An erroneous diagnosis of cardiac failure or cardiogenic shock may lead to the inadvisable administration of diuretics.

Urinary tract

Urinary problems may result from drug therapy or bladder catheterisation. Atropine and opiates may precipitate urinary retention, especially in the elderly male, which is often exaggerated by a sudden diuretic response to frusemide or bumetanide. Catheterisation may be necessary, although is not without risk of introducing infection and excess vagal stimulation.

Acute renal failure may result from prolonged hypotension or renal arterial embolisation from left ventricular mural thrombi.

Nervous system

Alterations in mental state are common on intensive care units, where there may be anxiety or even hostility arising as a response to psychological stress. Decreased cerebral perfusion may give rise to psychiatric symptoms, and is predisposed by pre-existing cerebrovascular disease and drugs. Hypoxaemia and deteriorating left ventricular function will exaggerate these effects. Narcotics and anxiolytic drugs will alter perception, and lignocaine may produce hallucinations and seizures. Neurological findings commonly follow cardiac arrest, although most are transient. Mural thrombi may give rise to cerebral embolisation and stroke.

Table 7.10.   Some causes of lactic acidosis.

Due to impaired tissue oxygenation	Other causes
Myocardial infarction	Diabetes mellitus
Left ventricular failure	Renal failure
Pulmonary embolism	Liver disease
Shock	Drugs:
Sepsis	biguanides
Pancreatitis	alcohol
	cyanide (sodium nitroprusside)
	aspirin

Metabolic problems

Diabetes or gout may be precipitated by myocardial infarction, or by drugs (e.g. thiazide diuretics). The blood glucose concentration should be checked routinely on admission, and monitored if elevated. Dehydration should be avoided by careful monitoring of diuretic therapy. Lactic acidosis is the most common cause of metabolic acidosis in clinical medicine. Whilst it usually develops in situations where tissue perfusion is inadequate, it may also occur where oxygenation is not obviously impaired (table 7.10). Acidosis results because of hypoxia in the tissues, and the accumulation of organic acids, particularly lactic acid. The clinical picture is usually dominated by shock, which should be vigorously treated with oxygen and inotropic support. Although treatment with bicarbonate would seem to be indicated, in patients with myocardial infarction this is limited by possible fluid overload.

References

Beck A O and Hochrein H (1974) Clinical course and prognosis of myocardial infarction in hypertensives. *Deutsche Medizinische Wochenschrift,* **99:** 815–820.

Briggs R S, Brown P M, Crabb M E, Cox T J, Ead H W, Hawkes R A, Jequier P W, Southall D P, Grainger R, Williams J H and Chamberlain D A (1976) The Brighton resuscitation ambulances: a continuing experiment in pre-hospital care by ambulance staff. *British Medical Journal,* **2:** 1161–1165.

Burden A C, Kupfer R, Davies M K and Pohl J E F (1978) Blood sugar and prognosis of myocardial infarction. *Lancet,* **i:** 820–821.

Cohn J N, Guiha N H, Broden M I and Limas C J (1974) Right ventricular infarction – clinical and haemodynamic features. *American Journal of Cardiology,* **33:** 209–214.

Colling W A, Dellipiani A W, Donaldson R J and McCormack P (1976) Teesside coronary survey: an epidemiological study of acute attacks of myocardial infarction. *British Medical Journal,* **2:** 1169–1172.

Cote P, Campeau L and Bourassa M G (1976) Therapeutic implications of diazepam in patients with elevated left ventricular filling pressure. *American Heart Journal,* **91:** 747–751.

Crampton R S, Aldrich R F, Gascho J A, Miles J R and Stillerman R (1975) Reduction of pre-hospital, ambulance and community coronary death rates by the community-wide emergency cardiac care system. *American Journal of Medicine,* **58:** 151–165.

Dellipiani A W, Colling W A, Donaldson R J and McCormack P (1977) Teesside coronary survey: fatality and comparative severity of patients treated at home, in the hospital ward and the coronary care unit after myocardial infarction. *British Heart Journal,* **39:** 1172–1178.

Editorial (1976) Oxygen in myocardial infarction. *British Medical Journal,* **i:** 731.

Eisenberg M S, Copass M K, Hallstrom A P, Blake B, Bergner L, Short F A and Cobb L A (1980) Treatment of out-of-hospital cardiac arrests with rapid defibrillation by emergency cardiac technicians. *New England Journal of Medicine,* **302:** 1379–1383.

Fratantoni J and Wessler S (1975) *Prophylactic Therapy of Deep Vein Thrombosis and Pulmonary Emboli.* DHEW Publication No. (NIH) 76–866.

Gazes P C and Gaddy J E (1979) Bedside management of acute myocardial infarction. *American Heart Journal,* **97:** 782–796.

Genton M D and Turpie A G G (1983) Anticoagulant therapy following acute myocardial infarction. *Modern Concepts in Cardiovascular Disease,* **52:** 49–51.

Gifford R H and Feinstein A R (1969) A critique of methodology in studies of anticoagulant therapy for myocardial infarction. *New England Journal of Medicine,* **280:** 351–357.

Goldberg R J, Gore J M and Dalen J E (1984) The role of anticoagulant therapy in acute myocardial infarction. *American Heart Journal,* **108:** 1387–1393.

Goldberger A L (1979) *Myocardial Infarction: Electrocardiographic Differential Diagnosis.* St Louis: C V Mosby.

Goldman L and Cook E F (1984) The decline in ischaemic heart disease mortality rates. *Annals of Internal Medicine,* **101:** 825–836.

Gunnar R M, Loeb H S, Scanlon P J, Moran J F, Johnson S A and Pifarre R (1979) Management of acute myocardial infarction and accelerating angina. *Progress in Cardiovascular Diseases,* **22:** 1–30.

Heikkila J (1967) Mitral incompetence complicating acute myocardial infarction. *British Heart Journal,* **29:** 162–169.

Hill J C, O'Rourke R A, Lewis R P and McGranahan G M (1969) The diagnostic value of the atrial gallup in acute myocardial infarction. *American Heart Journal,* **78:** 194–201.

Hill J D, Hampton J R and Mitchell J R A (1978) A randomised trial of home versus hospital management for acute myocardial infarction. *Lancet* **i:** 837–841.

Husband D J, Alberti K G and Julian D G (1983) 'Stress' hyperglycaemia during acute myocardial infarction: an indicator of pre-existing diabetes? *Lancet,* **ii:** 179–181.

Jowett N I, Thompson D R and Bailey S W (1985) Electrocardiographic monitoring. I: static monitoring. *Intensive Care Nursing,* **2:** 71–76.

Jowett N I, Thompson D R and Pohl J E F (1989) Temporary transvenous endocardial pacing: six years' experience on one coronary care unit. *Postgraduate Medical Journal,* in press.

Jowett N I, Stephens J M, Thompson D R and Sutton T W (1986) Do indwelling cannulae on coronary care need a heparin flush? *Intensive Care Nursing*, **2**, 16-19.

Kakkar V V, Corrigan T, Spindler J, Flute P T, Fossard D P and Crellin R Q (1972) Efficacy of low doses of heparin in prevention of deep vein thrombosis after major surgery. *Lancet*, **ii:** 101-106.

Kertes P and Hunt D (1984) Prophylaxis of primary ventricular fibrillation in acute myocardial infarction: the case against lignocaine. *British Heart Journal*, **52:** 241-247.

Klein H O, Tordjman T, Ninio R, Sareli P, Oren V, Lang R, Gesen J, Pauzner C, Di Segni E, David D and Kaplinski E (1983) The early recognition of right ventricular infarction: diagnostic accuracy of the V4R lead. *Circulation*, **67:** 558-565.

Kostuk W, Barr J W, Simon A L and Ross J (1973) Correlation between the chest film and hemodynamics in acute myocardial infarction. *Circulation*, **48:** 624-632.

Lappas D G, Geha D, Fischer J E, Lever M B and Lowenstein E (1975) Filling pressures of the heart and pulmonary circulation of the patient with coronary artery disease after large intravenous doses of morphine. *Anesthesiology*, **42:** 153-159.

Lie K I, Wellens H J, Van Capelle F J and Durrer D (1974) Lidocaine in the prevention of primary ventricular fibrillation: a double blind, randomised study of 212 consecutive patients. *New England Journal of Medicine*, **291:** 1324-1326.

Liu C K, Greenspan G and Piccirillo R T (1961) Atrial infarction of the heart. *Circulation*, **23:** 331.

Lown B, Verrier R L and Rabinowitz S H (1977) Neural and psychological mechanisms and the problem of sudden cardiac death. *American Journal of Cardiology*, **39:** 890-902.

McNichol M W and Kirby B J (1972) Oxygen therapy in myocardial infarction. In: *Textbook of Coronary Care*, eds. Melzer L E and Dunning A J. Amsterdam: Excerpta Medica.

Maroko P R, Radvany P and Braunwald E (1975) Reduction in infarct size by oxygen inhalation following acute coronary occlusion. *Circulation*, **52:** 360-368.

Marriott H J L (1983) *Practical Electrocardiography*. Baltimore: Williams and Wilkins.

Mather H G, Pearson N G and Read K L (1971) Acute myocardial infarction - home and hospital treatment. *British Medical Journal*, **3:** 334-338.

Melsom M, Andreassen P, Melsom H, Hansen T, Grendahl H and Hillestad L K (1976) Diazepam in acute myocardial infarction. Clinical effects and effect on catecholamines, free fatty acids and cortisol. *British Heart Journal*, **38:** 804-810.

Mulley A G, Thibault G E, Hughes R A, Barnett G O, Reder V A and Sherman E L (1980) The course of patients with suspected myocardial infarction. The identification of low risk patients for early transfer from intensive care. *New England Journal of Medicine*, **302:** 943-948.

Norris R M (1982) *Myocardial Infarction*. Edinburgh: Churchill Livingstone.

Oswald G A, Corcoran S and Yudkin J S (1984) Prevalence and risks of hyperglycaemia and undiagnosed diabetes in patients with acute myocardial infarction. *Lancet*, **i:** 1265-1267.

Pantridge J F and Adgey A A J (1969) Pre-hospital coronary care: the mobile coronary care unit. *American Journal of Cardiology*, **24:** 666-673.

Pentecost B (1980) The limitations of coronary care. In: *The Medical Annual*, eds. Bradley Scott R and Fraser J. Bristol: John Wright.

Raabe D S, Morise A, Sbarbaro J A and Gundel W D (1980) Diagnostic criteria for acute myocardial infarction in patients undergoing coronary artery bypass surgery. *Circulation*, **62:** 869-877.

Radvany P, Maroko P R and Braunwald E (1975) Effects of hypoxaemia on the extent of myocardial necrosis after experimental coronary occlusion. *American Journal of Cardiology*, **35:** 795-800.

Ribner H S and Frishman W H (1977) Anticoagulation in myocardial infarction: new approaches to an old problem. *Cardiovascular Medicine*, **2:** 787.

Riley C P, Russell R O and Rackly C E (1973) Left ventricular gallop sound and acute myocardial infarction. *American Heart Journal*, **86:** 598-602.

Roberts R (1984) The two out of three criteria for the diagnosis of infarction: is it passé? *Chest*, **86:** 511-513.

Rodrigues E A, Dewhurst N G, Smart L M, Hannan W J and Muir A L (1986) Diagnosis and prognosis of right ventricular infarction. *British Heart Journal*, **56:** 19-26.

Rowley J M and Hampton J R (1981) Diagnostic criteria for myocardial infarction. *British Journal of Hospital Medicine,* **18**: 253-258.

Ryder R E J, Hayes T M, Mulligan I P, Kingswood J and Williams S (1984) How soon after myocardial infarction should plasma lipids be assessed? *British Medical Journal,* **289**: 1651-1653.

Scott M E and Orr R (1969) Effects of diamorphine, methadone, morphine and pentazocine in patients with suspected acute myocardial infarction. *Lancet,* **i**: 1065-1067.

Simon A B, Feinleib M and Thompson H K (1972) Components of delay in the pre-hospital phase of acute myocardial infarction. *American Journal of Cardiology,* **30**: 476-482.

Soler N G, Pentecost B L, Bennett M A, Fitzgerald M G, Lamb P and Malins J M (1974) Coronary care for myocardial infarction in diabetics. *Lancet,* **i**: 475-477.

Thompson D R, Jones G R and Sutton T W (1983) A trial of povidone-iodine ointment for the prevention of cannula thrombophlebitis. *Journal of Hospital Infection,* **4**: 285-289.

Thompson D R, Jowett N I, Folwell A M and Sutton T W (1989) A trial of providone-iodine antiseptic solution for the prevention of cannula-related thrombophlebitis. *Journal of Intravenous Nursing.* In Press.

Thompson R C, Hallstrom A P and Cobb L A (1979) Bystander-initiated CPR in the management of ventricular fibrillation. *Annals of Internal Medicine,* **90**: 737-740.

Wartman W B and Hellerstein H K (1948) The incidence of heart disease in 2000 consecutive autopsies. *Annals of Internal Medicine,* **28**: 41.

Webb S W, Adgey A A J and Pantridge J F (1972) Autonomic disturbances at the onset of acute myocardial infarction. *British Medical Journal* **3**: 89-92.

Wright I S, Marple C D and Beck D F (1948) Report of the committee for the evaluation of anticoagulants in the treatment of coronary thrombosis with myocardial infarction. *American Heart Journal.* **36**: 801-815.

Yusef S, Pearson M, Sterry H, Parish S, Ramsdale D, Ross P and Sleight P (1984) The entry ECG in the early diagnosis and prognostic stratification of patients with suspected acute myocardial infarction. *European Heart Journal.* **5**: 690-696.

8

Nursing Management of Acute Myocardial Infarction

Nursing management of acute myocardial infarction is designed to help the patient overcome various physical and psychological insults. Therapeutic goals are broadly designed to promote healing of the damaged myocardium, prevent complications (such as dysrhythmias, heart failure and shock), and facilitate the patient's rapid return to normal health and life-style.

Meeting the basic needs of the patient, such as comfort, rest, sleep and elimination, forms an essential component of nursing intervention. Some of these needs will require attention immediately, whereas others will be required in later days. The nurse should be aware of what will be required, and should be able to anticipate problems, rather than waiting for them to occur.

Patients in hospital, especially those on high-dependency units, are bound to be under a great deal of stress and anxiety, both during their hospital stay and (usually) after discharge. There will be uncertainty about their surroundings, fear of what has happened to them, and worry about lack of control over what may occur in the following days. The situation may be exacerbated by lack of information, pain, discomfort or inability to obtain adequate rest.

The acute illness brings changes for the patient and family in terms of usual patterns of living which, although hopefully only short term, may persist after discharge from hospital. Acute myocardial infarction, in particular, poses major threats to the patient, usually because of the suddeness of the illness (often with no warning), and because of the connotations that heart disease carries. Fear of sudden death is the immediate worry, usually followed by a realisation that the patient may become disabled for the rest of his days. Apart from these changes in self-image, there are also feelings of loss in terms of status within the family unit, working environment and social circle. The secure knowledge of a regular financial income, the ability to care for the family and continuing full physical fitness are no longer present.

The responses that individual patients make to these threats include emotional crisis, defence mechanisms and coping behaviours. The patient's personal beliefs, attitudes, responsibilities, values and experiences will all influence how he or she will perceive and respond to the infarct. In the unfamiliar and frightening environment of the coronary care unit, the nurse needs to establish a close rapport with the patient and family in order to be effective in reducing anxiety and fear, promoting the resolution of losses, encouraging adjustment to change, and planning together for complete recovery and successful rehabilitation. This will include detailed explanations about the significance of the illness, the nature of coronary heart disease, and the goals of treatment, including the part that the coronary care unit plays. The personnel involved in the provision of care will need introducing, and the roles of these people and the surrounding equipment should be fully explained. The encouragement of independence and the fostering of a realistic but optimistic outlook are of great importance. Such interventions should involve the nurse in providing care in an individualised and flexible fashion rather than the traditional rigid task-orientated system. The coronary care unit is an ideal setting for the nurse, patient and family to meet and discuss progress and future management. Care plans should be based upon an assessment completed within the initial hours of admisson, so that priorities of care can then be established early and modified as the patient improves.

It can thus be seen that nursing intervention involves many challenges in the management of acute myocardial infarction, and a considerate and sensitive approach to the patient and his family is required to permit full evaluation of present and potential problems, and to establish an overall plan of care which will hopefully overcome them.

COMMUNICATION

● There are few, if any, places where patients, their visitors and staff are more in need of good communication, and few where there are more potential or actual impediments to it. (Ashworth, 1984b)

For nursing intervention to be effective, communication between the nurse, the patient, his family and other personnel involved in his care has to be effective. Communication can take many forms – structured or informal, verbal or non-verbal – and tends to be a continuous process in situations where individuals are working within the same environment. Thus, much of nursing management will be directly or indirectly concerned with communication at some level. Contact at the bedside whilst performing physical and technical tasks forms an important part of such communication between nurses and patients, and the nurse is in a unique position in being at the bedside for most of the time. She will therefore be regarded as a prime source of communication (Cassem et al, 1970; Adler, 1976).

There is some evidence that the quality of communication that patients on coronary care receive can influence the speed of recovery and feeling of well-being (Foster, 1974; Garrity and Klein, 1975), and it is a shame that communication skills have not always been seen as a legitimate part of nursing work (Ashworth, 1980).

There are various reasons why nurse–patient communication is often inadequate in coronary care. These include the short duration of the patient's stay on the unit, the severity of his condition and, often, the nurse's preoccupation with handling technical rather than personal requirements. In her review of staff–patient communication in coronary care, Ashworth (1984a) sees the aims of communication as being:

1. For the patient to perceive the nurse as:
   ● friendly
   ● helpful
   ● competent
   ● reliable

2. For the nurse to recognise patients':
- individuality
- perceived needs
- other needs

Coronary care patients are often brought suddenly into the unfamiliar environment of hospital. They change from a position of being in control of their lives to one of having to accept the submissive role of a patient. Effective communication can really only be achieved if the patient is allowed to retain his individuality. The nurse should work with the patient to effect positive adaptation and coping mechanisms by education and counselling. Liaison with the patient and his family is required to ensure that they are aware of the objectives of the cardiac unit and understand the various procedures and treatments. A realistic outlook for the future based on knowledge and understanding may then be achieved. It is important for communication to be clear and comprehensible, using language familiar to the patient (at whatever level) and avoiding the use of jargon. Simple explanations need to be reiterated, since retention of verbal information in medical matters is seldom for long. An atmosphere of optimism should be encouraged by reassuring patients that survival and recovery are fully anticipated.

Cardiac nurses themselves need to be able to demonstrate credibility in their role as communicators. Communication is a two-way process, and there is a need to interact with the patient, adapting the approach to meet changing needs. 'Primary nursing' is the ideal method of maximising nurse–patient contact and increases the likelihood of getting to know the patient as an individual rather than a bed number. The nurse should be able to listen to the patient in a calm, unhurried, sympathetic manner and be genuinely interested in what the patient is saying.

Reassurance is a term frequently used in nursing, often without clarification or evaluation. Broad promises such as, 'Don't worry, everything will be OK' serve little purpose if the patient lacks a basic understanding of his condition and may serve to lessen the nurse's credibility. The majority of patients can be placed at ease during their stay on coronary care provided the right approach is used, even if many may be clinically anxious or depressed.

Some patients may not possess the necessary skills to be able to communicate successfully. They may be too ill or anxious to present themselves as they would wish; they may be physically or mentally handicapped; or they may lack the knowledge and understanding to be able to make realistic decisions regarding their future. This may equally apply to the relatives, who can find the hospital environment imposing. Nurses have an important role to play as advocates to the patient and his relatives, basing advice on experience, knowledge of the illness and the individual patient. As well as structured planned communication to convey specific points, there is also day-to-day conversation, interaction and non-verbal communication. Human contact is possibly more important in a technical environment such as coronary care than on the general medical ward. Patients are likely to appreciate knowing that a nurse is near at hand, especially if they are bedridden, when communication is perhaps the only way that some patients can influence their environment and routine.

In the highly technical and invasive atmosphere of coronary care, there is sometimes a need to stand back and think carefully about what is the best treatment or strategy for the patient. Allowing a critically ill patient to die with peace and dignity is not a failure and may be a better course of action than prolonging life with multiple therapies which mislead the relatives into thinking there is hope. Discussing such subjects openly in a constructive fashion with medical colleagues, in a detached and unemotional manner, involves a sensitive and professional approach, which is necessary, but seldom easy.

Three main approaches have been suggested (Ashworth, 1984a) which might improve nurse–patient communication on coronary care.

1. Planned education to develop communication knowledge and skills

2. Selective scientific reading, and the use of relevant research-based nursing practice information

3. Further research into staff–patient communication

Smooth and effective communication between nurses and other personnel is likely to result in better nurse–patient communication. There is, perhaps, a need to change the emphasis of priorities on intensive care units away from the technical aspects towards the physical and emotional requirements of patients in our care.

ASSESSMENT OF PAIN

● Pain is whatever the experiencing person says it is, existing whenever he says it does. (McCaffery, 1979)

Pain is a complex and personal experience, and it is usually the nursing staff in hospital who are near at hand when the patient experiences pain. It is they who are frequently responsible for its evaluation and for providing relief. In the context of coronary care units, this should be on their own initiative, and it is therefore important that they have formed a proper assessment of the pain the patient is suffering. Inappropriate analgesia is dangerous. It may mask alternative diagnosis or produce cardiac and respiratory depression.

It is clear that the word 'pain' may apply to a variety of qualities, although it is still frequently considered in regard to a single attribute: the intensity of the experience. This, of course, ignores the qualitative dimensions of the pain experienced (table 8.1), but it is nevertheless a useful indication. Moreover, it lends itself to numerical or graphic measurement for research purposes, by using a visual analogue scale (VAS) or a 'pain ruler' (Scott and Huskisson, 1976; Bourbonnais, 1981). Such methods are especially useful for the assessment of acute pain, such as that which commonly accompanies acute myocardial infarction. They are sensitive and reliable indicators for pain evaluation, as well as being easy to use by both the person experiencing the pain and the observer (Huskisson, 1974; Revill et al, 1976).

The relief of pain is a major part of patient care, and is essential for patient comfort and well-being. A careful and detailed assessment of the pain a patient is experiencing is essential if effective relief is to be provided in the minimum of time, and will be more effective if the nurse establishes a rapport with the patient. The assessment should include the patient's own description of the pain and an observation of his

Table 8.1. Words used to describe the quality of pain (Melzack, 1975).

Words describing the sensory qualities of the pain experienced
in terms of:
  ● time (e.g. constant)
  ● space (e.g. radiating)
  ● pressure (e.g. compressing)
  ● temperature (e.g. hot)

Words describing the affective qualities of pain in terms of:
  ● tension (e.g. tiring)
  ● fear (e.g. terrifying)
  ● autonomic properties (e.g. nausea)

Words describing the subjective overall intensity, for example:
  ● excruciating pain

---

reaction to it. It is not always possible to make this evaluation on admission to coronary care if the patient is critically ill, but later on it will be important to determine whether the pain the patient is still suffering is ischaemic pain or pericarditic pain, or is just due to anxiety. Each of these will have different specific antidotes (such as aspirin or indomethacin for pericarditis, diazepam for anxiety) although the disinterested may simply choose to obliterate all possibilities with a large dose of diamorphine. The nurse and doctor must appreciate that the patient is the authority on his own pain. Above all, the patient must be believed; all pain is real, and calling pain imaginary does not make any difference.

In addition to the traditional provision of analgesia with drug therapy, there is a wide range of pain-relieving strategies that can be instituted by the nurse.

● Ensuring peace and comfort
● Careful positioning of the patient
● Reassurance
● Protection from stressful situations
● Limitation of unnecessary activity
● Promotion of sleep

If the patient fully understands the pain and its cause, it may then become less distressing. Coping strategies such as therapeutic touch, relaxation techniques and distraction are useful if they are performed by a skilled nurse. There are other useful methods for the relief of acute pain, which may be used alone or in conjunction with drugs. These include guided imagery, hypnosis and transcutaneous electric nerve stimulation (TENS) and have been discussed elsewhere (Peric-Knowlton, 1984; Wells, 1984).

The nurse needs to be aware of the limitations, as well as the benefits, of the non-pharmacological interventions available. Whereas a small study by Bourbonnais and MacKay (1981) showed that over half the nursing interventions used for the relief of chest pain were ineffective, an approach based upon a holistic approach to the patient resulted in a high degree of pain relief prior to the administration of medication, and greater pain relief than medication alone (Diers et al, 1972).

COMFORT

● 'High tech' medicine should surely require more, not less, hands-on-care from nurses. (Wilson-Barnett, 1984)

The promotion of relaxation and comfort is an essential and fundamental component of nursing. Unfortunately, such skills tend to be overlooked on coronary care units. Careful positioning of the patient, reassurance and the presence of a caring nurse assumes a high priority to ensure complete comfort (Wilson-Barnett, 1984). Careful bed-making, regulation of light, temperature and noise, and the provision of hot milky drinks in the evening may seem mundane and obvious, but are often delegated to the most junior nurse as a low priority in the 'high-tech' environment of coronary care. The inability to get comfortable is a major reason for poor sleep (Jones et al, 1979). This is often due to poor hospital beds, with their hard mattresses covered in plastic causing the patient to feel uncomfortable, hot and sweaty. It may be more beneficial for the patient if he sits in a supportive chair instead of lying in bed. However, it is no use providing such fundamental measures if the patient is in pain. Pain relief should assume the highest priority.

Patient discomfort may be compounded by invasive techniques, such as intravenous cannulation, and the frequent disturbances that occur when routine observations are made or recorded. Invasive monitoring devices and intravenous lines often result in the general enforced immobilisation of the patient which carries with it the attendant risk of pressure sores. Thus, frequent changing of the patient's position in bed and the use of pressure-relieving devices are important in reducing discomfort. Consideration should be given to the siting of intravenous cannulae, and the use of nasal cannulae rather than oxygen masks.

Rest has to be both physical and mental and can be achieved by a variety of factors including:

● Adequate pain relief
● Promotion of relaxation, comfort and sleep
● Ensuring that noise is kept at a low level
● Control of temperature, light and humidity
● Planned rest periods during the day

A warm, stimulating environment should be encouraged, where patients feel they can relax and chat with fellow patients, staff and relatives.

BED REST AND ACTIVITY

Bed rest is usual, but recent trends are towards early mobilisation, with slower schedules being reserved for those with complications. Hospitalisation and enforced bed rest can produce their own problems, such as constipation, bone resorption, thromboembolism, pulmonary atelectasis, pressure sores and urinary retention. It is therefore important that patients mobilise as soon as possible, particularly the elderly who fare worse from complications due to enforced rest than they would otherwise do as a result of myocardial infarction alone. Active and passive leg movements should be encouraged and early chest physiotherapy is advisable, especially in smokers. Rotation of the shoulders is also advisable to prevent 'frozen' shoulders and the shoulder–hand syndrome (Editorial, *Lancet,* 1974).

Although the coronary care unit should theoretically be the ideal environment for resting, in practice it rarely is because of the non-stop activity in and around the patients. Amongst its many other benefits, the purpose of rest following myocardial infarction is to decrease the myocardial demand for oxygen, and limit myocardial work. Inactivity is a major problem in that it serves as a source of frustration and boredom. It is therefore important to stress to the patient the need for temporary limitation, but to reassure him that bed rest is only temporary and is in his own best interest. Enforced bed rest will only have adverse effects on someone who is normally active, by making him perceive himself as more seriously ill. Relaxation, deep breathing, and active and passive leg exercises are useful in reducing boredom and mood changes, as well as the risk of physical complications of bed rest. Such activities will boost patients' morale by making them feel that they are playing an active part in the recovery process.

It is preferable that the patient sits upright in bed rather than lying flat because the latter requires more myocardial work to pump blood through the excess pool of tissue fluid in the lungs (Guyton, 1981). Thus, uncomplicated infarct patients should sit out as early as possible (Long, 1980). Some patients may feel reluctant or hesitant to resume activity, whereas others are over-zealous.

There is no reason why most patients cannot wash, eat and shave themselves. In fact, it is likely that there is danger of more stress resulting from not being allowed to do such activities than the actual performance of them. Patients may require some assistance from the nurse if they are severely restricted by equipment such as short monitor cables, intravenous infusions, pacemaker units, etc., or if they are feeling weak or are generally too ill. The nurse should, in any case, offer to assist as some patients may feel unable to ask. If the patient is bedbound, the nurse needs to ensure that he has everything he needs within easy reach.

EARLY AMBULATION

Only 25 years ago, patients with acute myocardial infarction were kept on strict bed rest for two months, with all activities performed by attending nursing staff. Hospitalisation often lasted for three to four months, with limited mobilisation over the following year. The concern was that early mobilisation would lead to dysrhythmia, heart failure, rupture of the heart or formation of a left ventricular aneurysm. The period of strict rest was based upon pathological studies which indicated that six weeks were required for a firm scar to form from the necrotic myocardium (Mallory et al, 1939). However, it soon became apparent that this form of therapy led to increased incidence of thromboembolic disorders, chest infections and musculoskeletal disorders. Alteration in vasomotor reflexes and hypovolaemia also occurs with prolonged bed rest, leading to tachycardia, hypotension and unsteadiness on standing. The highly controversial approach to early mobilisation in the early 1960s (Cain et al, 1961) was regarded as reckless and dangerous: uncomplicated infarct patients were allowed out of bed after only 15 days.

The emphasis today is on early mobilisation and discharge, especially for those who have an uncomplicated hospital course (Chaturvedi et al, 1974; Gelson et al, 1976; McNeer et al, 1978). This type of approach minimises physical and psychological disability, and reduces the risk of thromboembolism. There is no doubt that peri-infarction mortality is higher in patients who have had complications (Norris et al, 1974), such as:

● Prolonged or recurrent chest pain
● Left ventricular failure
● Cardiogenic shock
● Significant dysrhythmia (e.g. ventricular tachycardia or fibrillation)
● Heart block
● Severe pericarditis
● Extensive infarcts
● Complicating disease (e.g. diabetes)

Early mobilisation should certainly be delayed in these patients, even when the underlying complication has been corrected. However, most of these potential high-risk cases may be identified in the first 24 hours following admision, and provisional selection for early discharge made within 48 hours (Lau et al, 1980).

Nursing should reflect the current pattern of care for coronary patients, which has been characterised by an increase in physical activity soon after infarction and has led to a decrease in imposed invalidism and an earlier discharge from hospital. Patients with an uncomplicated infarct are kept in bed for a maximum of 24 to 48 hours only. Indeed, in some units, patients are encouraged to sit out on the day of admission provided they are free of pain and significant dysrhythmia (Sloman, 1981). Certainly, gradual but early mobilisation should encourage patients to walk around the ward by the end of a few days. It is important that an individualised approach takes preference over a strict regimen.

When the patient resumes activity it is helpful if the nurse knows the normal activity levels and habits of the patient. This should have been ascertained during the nursing assessment. A plan can then be developed by the nurse and patient to provide a framework as to what level of activity he can realistically be expected to achieve by a specific time. This will need to be a tentative plan, and it is important to stress that only guidelines and not strict regimens can be formulated, because each patient will be different in his abilities. An ideal method for quantifying the energy spent under-taking various activities is the *metabolic equivalents system* (METS). One MET is equal to the resting oxygen uptake of approximately 3.5 ml/kg/min. The average male can attain a level of 12 METs, and an uncomplicated post-infarct patient can probably achieve no more than 9 METs.

The stress that various activities have on the body can be assessed by observing heart rate and rhythm, respiratory rate and blood pressure. However, these should be monitored in an informal manner to avoid unduly worrying the patient. The development of symptoms such as chest pain, shortness of breath, palpitations or faintness are indications to cease activity. The patient should be made aware of this, and encouraged to inform the nurse if such symptoms should occur.

In uncomplicated cases, patients should be encouraged to climb one or two flights of stairs before they are discharged home. They will need to be advised about what they will be able to do at home, including information on eating, drinking and driving. A realistic appraisal of the prospect of a full recovery and early return to work is essential. Further detailed guidlines concerning these are dealt with in chapter 13 ('Rehabilitation').

SLEEP

● Sleep is the golden chain that ties health and our bodies together. (Thomas Dekker)

The function of sleep is unknown. It is thought to be a period of bodily and brain restitution (Adam and Oswald, 1984), although Meddis (1977) challenges the idea that sleep is necessary at all, believing that sleep is an instinct which merely serves as a means of segregating periods of inactivity and activity.

Sleep may be roughly divided into two broad stages;

● *Non-REM* (rapid eye movement) or orthodox sleep
● *REM* or paradoxical sleep

Non-REM sleep is characterised by lowering of the blood pressure, heart and respiratory rates, whilst REM sleep is characterised by the opposite and is strongly correlated with dreaming.

Many people experience onset or worsening of an illness during the night. Cardiovascular events often occur with a high frequency during sleep, and especially during REM sleep. Patients with nocturnal angina are more likely to suffer their attacks during periods of REM sleep (King et al, 1973), and there is also an increase in the frequency of premature ventricular contractions (Rosenblatt et al, 1973). The onset of symptoms of acute myocardial infarction is more frequent in bed, especially just after falling asleep and on waking (Thompson et al, 1985).

It is clear that coronary patients experience marked sleep disturbances in hospital, particularly in specialised units (Broughton and Baron, 1978). Additionally, much of this sleep is desynchronised, and therefore less effective. The reasons for this poor sleep are many. Sleep may be affected by several factors, including age, noise, temperature, comfort, pain and anxiety (Webster and Thompson, 1986). Noise is a major problem in specialised units (Hilton, 1976), mainly due to electromechanical equipment, staff movement and conversation. Bentley et al (1977) found that noise levels in three hospital areas, including an intensive care unit, were about 25–40 dB higher than limits internationally recommended (30 dB at night, 40 dB during the evening, 45 dB during the daytime).

Patients will be able to sleep better if they are comfortable, free from pain and in a quiet and peaceful environment. The promotion of comfort and relaxation are important, as discussed in the previous section, with control of environmental factors (e.g. reduced noise, regulated room temperature and dimmed lights). Pain relief is of course essential. Unnecessary nursing or medical observations or interventions disrupt the continuity and efficiency of patients' sleep, and essential procedures should be organised in a fashion that ensures that patients are only minimally disturbed. With current advanced technology, multichannel monitoring facilities make many routine observations easy to perform without waking the patient.

Nursing assessment should incorporate information about the patient's usual sleeping habits and patterns, information such as quality and quantity of normal sleep, and the identification of any routines that the patient feels will enhance his ability to sleep. Hot milky drinks such as Ovaltine and Horlicks often form part of the night-time ritual and have been shown to improve sleep significantly (Brezinova and Oswald, 1972). The use of a sleep questionnaire (such as the St Mary's Hospital Sleep Questionnaire, Ellis et al, 1981) is a useful adjunct in the assessment of sleeping habits.

DIET

Although diet is not usually considered in the early stages following myocardial infarction, there are many reasons why adjustments may need to be made. In the early hours following admission, nausea and vomiting are common, and there is a higher risk of cardiorespiratory arrest which may lead to bronchial aspiration of gastric contents. A liquid diet is therefore probably best given initially until a normal diet can be instituted. Caffeine should be avoided because of its possible dysrhythmic effect, and salt should be avoided because of its deleterious effect on cardiac failure. In order to assist the healing process, adequate and appropriate nutrition is essential. The nurse should possess some of the knowledge and necessary skills to assess and advise on the nutritional requirements of the patient. Nurses, by the very nature of their close involvement with the patient and his family, are ideally placed, yet all too often they seem to ignore their responsibility in this area, prematurely enlisting the help of a usually overworked dietitian. A careful assessment of the patient's usual eating habits and life-style is essential. Many patients will have preconceived ideas obtained from their relatives and the media about good dietary habits. Nurses play a major role in nutrition education, and often have to perform the notoriously difficult task of persuading the patient to consider a change in dietary habits. The major difficulty is not in giving the advice to patients and their relatives, but in achieving appropriate behavioural responses which should be in their own interests.

Many misconceptions regarding diet litter the popular press and even the fringe scientific literature. The problem is compounded by conflicting and unsubstantiated information and advice given by friends, relatives or health professionals, particularly with regard to coronary heart disease.

Other considerations in relation to diet include the following.

1. Patients on coronary care units feel nauseated or not hungry. Nourishing drinks and small snacks at times other than established meal times may be more appreciated.

2. Ethnic minorities will require special consideration, and relatives need to be consulted as they can offer valuable advice and assistance by bringing in their own meals.

3. Although some patients may require parenteral or nasogastric feeding, these methods should not be undertaken lightly. Not only are they likely to be stressful to the patient, but they may be associated with metabolic disturbance and infection.

4. Fluid restriction may be warranted if the patient is in heart failure. Such patients will require thoughtful mouth care, including mouth washes, and sips of cold or iced water. Confiscating the water jug is not sufficient; the patient should be informed of what is being done and why. A notice concerning fluid restriction is needed above the bed to remind others that fluids are being monitored, and the patient will be able to prevent the tea-lady filling him up with fluid if he is aware of what the fluid restriction is trying to achieve.

Nurses should be aware that they are serving as role models in providing credibility to any health education. It is difficult to convince patients of such change if the nurse herself is overweight or smokes.

ELIMINATION

Prolonged bed rest or general physical inactivity should be avoided as this inhibits gastrointestinal motility and leads to constipation. The faeces may additionally become hardened because of increased water resorption or use of diuretics. The constipated patient will strain at stool, with excessive isometric work which leads to vagal stimulation. This is likely to produce bradycardia or heart block, and may severely compromise venous return, with dramatic falls in cardiac output. A 'bedpan' vasovagal collapse may result, but staff should be aware that patients with acute pulmonary emboli often call for a bedpan as a terminal event. Similar vasovagal effects may result with the use of a bedpan, upon which most patients seem to strain, whether constipated or not. They are most uncomfortable and stressful contraptions, which probably need banning. Using a bedside commode is easier, more comfortable and places the patient in a more familiar position for defaecation (Winslow, et al 1984). In fact, there appears to be little scientific evidence to support the use of a bedpan in preference to the commode. Laxatives may be warranted to prevent excessive straining at stool, and may be helped by careful attention to the fluid and fibre content of the diet. The patient needs to be reassured that many patients have altered bowel habit following admission to hospital. This may simply be due to different dietary habits, or enforced bed rest, but certain drugs can alter normal elimination habits. For instance, opiates cause constipation and broad spectrum antibiotics may cause diarrhoea. Additionally, many patients feel extremely embarrassed about using a commode or urinal in the vicinity of others. This in itself may give rise to constipation or retention. They are more likely to feel at ease in a private room or cubicle than in the middle of an open-plan area, even if they do have the benefit of partially-closed curtains through which different faces keep appearing. Perhaps more patients should be permitted to use a toilet at an earlier stage.

Careful recording of fluid balance is essential for patients on diuretic therapy. Daily weighing of the patient may be more accurate than a fluid balance chart for assessment in congestive cardiac failure. The patient should be warned of the resulting increase in quantity and frequency of urine. Consideration regarding the timing of diuretic administration should be given so that the patient is minimally disturbed during the night. Bumetanide (Burinex) is probably a shorter acting loop diuretic than frusemide (Lasix), and will limit the duration of diuresis.

HYGIENE

Bathing and hygiene

Many patients admitted to coronary care have been unprepared for admission because of the sudden onset of symptoms and may feel acutely embarrassed and uncomfortable, particularly if they are sweating, have vomited or are partly naked. Patients are likely to be feeling too unwell in the immediate stages to look after themselves and, although the nurse will need to assist acutely, she should avoid encouraging the patient to become dependent on her help. The psychological aspects of bathing and hygiene are important. For example, patients feel better after a shower or bath, and appreciate simple things such being offered hand-washing facilities after using the commode without having to ask.

Oral hygiene

Mouth toilet should be offered to all patients, especially those who wear dentures, are on fluid restriction or have been vomiting. Patients with dentures are often very embarrassed about cleaning them in the presence of others, and should be afforded the necessary privacy and facilities.

Use of the bath and shower

It appears that coronary patients move more slowly and deliberately than normal when bathing in order to conserve energy (Winslow et al, 1985). Patients may prefer to shower if it has been their normal domestic routine, particularly during the later stages of their stay in hospital. However, oxygen consumption of coronary patients is higher in patients who shower than in those who use a bath (Johnston et al, 1981), and this should be taken into consideration. The isometric activity required by some patients to get out of a bath may result in a steep rise in arterial blood pressure which increases myocardial work. Hence, before a patient is first bathed the nurse needs to evaluate any potential difficulties. If the patient is weak, obese or generally likely to have difficulties, bathing is probably contraindicated.

EMOTIONAL DISTURBANCES

Emotional disturbances after infarction may adversely influence subsequent mortality, speed of rehabilitation and ability to return to work. The manner in which a patient adapts emotionally to having sustained a myocardial infarction will be determined to a large extent by his premorbid personality (Byrne and Whyte, 1980; Totman, 1979). Emotional disturbances are extremely common in patients admitted to coronary care. Anxiety is, not surprisingly, very common, especially in women, and many patients are depressed, agitated or even openly hostile (Hackett et al, 1968; Cay et al, 1972). Many complain of difficulty in concentrating, and nearly half of the patients will have difficulty with sleep. If anxiety is unrelieved, depression usually supervenes, and both may persist for long periods of time in many patients (Cay et al, 1973).

The nurse is often the first and ideal person to identify the emotional disturbances that may affect the patient in hospital. She needs to be able to recognise verbal and non-verbal cues to emotional distress, and understand the basic mechanisms that the patient is using to cope. The profound emotional distress that often accompanies acute myocardial infarction can adversely affect the recovery process. For instance, severe anxiety during the initial phase of the illness results in an increased heart rate, blood pressure, and myocardial oxygen demand. These cardiac effects, mediated through the sympathetic nervous system, may lead to life-threatening complications, including dysrhythmias, heart failure, pulmonary embolism and extension of the infarct. Moreover, the patient's emotional adjustment during the period on coronary care significantly influences rehabilitation and long-term survival.

Three of the commonest acute emotional responses following acute myocardial infarction are fear, dependency and disorientation. These may later be replaced by anxiety and depression.

Fear

The patient's immediate reaction is usually fear, not only of death, but also of the threat the illness poses to his life-style (Cay, 1982). This fear can be reduced by an explanation of the purpose of coronary care, the monitoring equipment and the high nurse–patient ratio. Patients need to be warned of and informed about routine observations, investigations and drug administration. Knowing the names of staff and the ease of summoning them increases their security. In general, the unit environment should become more reassuring than frightening to the patient, and later his family too.

Dependency

This can be reduced by encouraging the resumption of usual activities as soon as possible in an attempt to minimise the sense of damage and helplessness. Involving the patient in planning his own care helps to increase feelings of self-worth and independence. Involving the spouse or other family members is a useful adjunct.

Disorientation

Disorientation, together with social isolation, can be reduced by the provision of a suitable environment which includes calendars, clocks, radios, televisions, newspapers and windows with a view of the outside world. The additional comforts and provision of items such as personal photographs indicate extra thoughtfulness.

Anxiety

Anxiety is a normal but complex human phenomenon which is difficult to define exactly. Mild anxiety is part of normal everyday life but, in excess, it impairs physical and mental performance. Empirically, anxiety is used to describe an unpleasant emotional state, although it is also used to describe differences in anxiety-proneness as a personal characteristic.

Various studies have reported raised anxiety levels in coronary patients. Dellipiani et al (1976) compared patients admitted to a coronary care unit in Edinburgh, and patients in the Teesside coronary survey, who were treated at home, on a coronary care unit or on general medical wards. The pattern of anxiety was similar in both groups regardless of where they were treated, although throughout the study period the Teesside patients were more anxious. Their level of anxiety was high early in the illness, fell rapidly and rose again towards the end of their stay in hospital. Anxiety soon after admission to coronary care units is no higher than for patients admitted as emergencies to general medical wards (Vetter et al 1977).

Anxiety is certainly the most common initial response to acute myocardial infarction. The main source is the prospect of sudden death, and the signs of anxiety are more likely to be noticed during the initial phase of the illness, when recurrent symptoms such as chest pain or shortness of breath develop, or when special procedures such as the insertion of a temporary pacemaker or cardioversion are required. A less obvious symptom that evokes anxiety is the feeling of weakness and complete exhaustion. Patients who have normally been fit and strong, but are now feeling weak as a consequence of an infarct, may experience extreme anxiety and frustration. Anxiety about transfer to the ward and discharge home is likely to be particularly high if the patient is discharged abruptly with little or no warning.

Anxiety can be identified subjectively and objectively. Subjectively, patients will appear tense, apprehensive and restless. They may have a sustained tachycardia, sweat freely and constantly seek reassurance. Care must be taken not to mistake these symptoms for heart failure. Objectively, anxiety can be measured in a variety of ways, including physiological and biochemical indices, such as blood pressure, heart rate, and plasma or urinary catecholamine levels. However, in cardiac patients such methods are more likely to reflect the physical than the psychological state. Questionnaires such as the Spielberger State-Trait Anxiety Inventory (Spielberger et al, 1970), the Cattell 8-Parallel-Form Anxiety Battery (Scheier and Cattell, 1960), or visual analogue scales may prove more practical and quick to use.

Once anxiety has been assessed, intervention can be more specifically tailored to the patient's needs. The patient with a mild level of anxiety is usually alert and able to absorb information and solve problems, even though he may be restless and irritable. In contrast, the patient with a very high level of anxiety is often terrified and much too distressed to perceive and communicate normally.

A reduction of anxiety can usually be achieved in the majority of patients by considerate, attentive and competent nurses who can be a major source of reassurance. Close and consistent nurse–patient contact increases the patient's feelings of security. Relaxation techniques which involve progressive muscle relaxation may be effective in minimising undue stress.

Depression

Depression is common in coronary patients, and will often follow anxiety, especially if the latter is untreated. This is particularly so after a second myocardial infarction (Cay et al, 1972). It is a reactive rather than endogenous depression, and seldom assumes psychotic status. It is an understandable response to myocardial infarction because of the implied loss of health, loss of earning capacity, impairment of physical activity and diminution of general status within family and society. It is important that depression is recognised and dealt with promptly because it may interfere with the recovery process. Patients who are depressed make the poorest long-term recovery as measured by their ability to return to work and resume sexual activity. They may experience sadness, disinterest, sleep disturbances and loss of appetite. In the acute phase, depression usually appears on the third to fifth day, when the patient is at an emotional low ebb. Denial is the commonest coping mechanism and can often be recognised by statements the patient makes. There may be refusal to acknowledge that he has suffered a heart attack and is becoming depressed as a consequence. Denial is usually a temporary phenomenon, and may serve to protect the patient from further psychological deterioration. Gradual acceptance of the illness and active participation in recovery usually follows. However, denial is dangerous to the patient when its presence allows him to engage in some form of behaviour that threatens his welfare, for example by trying to take too much exercise too soon. The nurse needs to examine to what extent denial is interfering with the treatment and endangering the patient.

Depression is often accompanied by anxiety. Some patients may be irritable, oversensitive or prone to bouts of tearfulness. Others may experience feelings of hopelessness and helplessness which results in them forming a generally pessimistic outlook. A full assessment of the patient's situation is required to ascertain whether the depression is part of the normal process of adapting to illness or whether it is related to other events. It may be helpful for the nurse to sit quietly with the patient and attempt to determine the major worries. Many of his fears may be quite realistic, and are likely to prove difficult to resolve or alleviate. Some concerns may be unfounded and, once these are identified, the nurse can help correct any misconceptions that the patient may hold. Having someone to talk with, or to hold or cry with, may enable the patient to organise his thinking and help positively to reassess his future. An optimistic but realistic outlook which conveys hope and gives him energy and enthusiasm is usually what is required. Probably the best antidote is early mobilisation to counter the physical and psychological problems associated with immobility. The sooner the patient is back on his feet the sooner will feelings of self-worth and self-esteem return. The nurse will need to avoid overprotection or the encouragement of dependency.

Anger and hostility

Once patients are aware of the fact that they have had a heart attack (and what this may imply), it is possible that their reaction may be one of anger, hostility or both. There is much emphasis and media coverage today on healthy living, and patients who consider that they have taken special care of their health may feel cheated that this has happened to them. Anger occurs in response to frustration, threat or injury. It may be expressed actively or passively or may be self-directed. Active expressions of anger include sarcasm, criticism, irritability and argument. Passively, it may be expressed through non-compliance, boredom, withdrawal or forgetfulness. Self-directed anger is manifested as depression, self-depreciation, accident proneness and somatic symptoms such as headaches and dizziness.

It is often difficult to remain objective, especially when the patient is critical of the care he is receiving or of the personnel who provide it. The attending medical staff and others may feel powerless or may experience anger themselves. They need to try to help the patient clarify his ideas and feelings, and explain constructive ways of dealing with such feelings. A consistent approach should be adopted towards the patient, and staff should not allow themselves to be played off against each other.

THE REACTION OF THE FAMILY

Hospital is a frightening place for the majority of the general public, especially cardiac intensive care and high-dependency units with their very titles suggestive of danger and bodily assault. The family will have more time to sit and think about the implications of these titles, and may actually fear the coronary care unit more than the patient who is usually too busy being ill. Relatives often feel that their loved one has been taken away and isolated from them. They frequently feel helpless, frightened and unnecessarily excluded from close involvement with their loved one. All members of the family (but especially the spouse) fear that the patient may die, and there may be many recriminations and feeling of guilt if there have been recent family arguments or upsets. Friction or tension within the family unit prior to myocardial infarction is mentioned by about 20 per cent of patients (Solomon et al, 1969) and this may be unresolved if the patient dies, causing untold guilt in the future.

Professional support from nurses and doctors is sadly lacking where the family is concerned (Skelton and Dominian, 1973), and that which they do get is often inadequate or inappropriate (Hentinen, 1983; Thompson and Cordle, 1988). Nursing intervention is aimed at assessing and supporting the family's coping mechanisms by providing information and reassurance and involving other appropriate professional help and opinion. Family members may view the patient's illness as a loss; they may feel they have lost the security of having certain needs consistently and reliably met, especially economic and emotional security. They are therefore likely to need information, reassurance and support, but often feel reluctant to seek out staff and indicate their concerns. Many feel that by doing so they may be in the way, stopping important work, or that they may cause friction with the staff, resulting in a deterioration of their relative's care. It is therefore important for the coronary care staff to take the initiative in making and maintaining contact with the family, especially the spouse, who is more likely to benefit from involvement in the care of her partner. She can also provide a unique service by giving insight into her partner's preferences, dislikes and frame of mind, and by generally supporting the partner in recovery. Unnecessary distress may be prevented by including the spouse in discharge planning and preparing the family for the patient's homecoming. Anticipation of any difficulties will facilitate a smooth and continuous transition from hospital to home.

The reaction of the spouse to the illness is likely to be influenced by a number of factors, not least of which will be the general state of the marriage (Skelton and Dominian, 1973). She will need to be warned that she is likely to experience emotional and physical responses to her husband's illness, such as fatigue, anxiety, depression, difficulty in sleeping, weight loss and sexual difficulties. These are expected stress reactions to the patient's return home. The spouse will often feel that if she shows concern, she may be accused of being overprotective, and if she does not she may be regarded as callous and unsympathetic.

Once the patient returns home family members are often afraid to express their true feelings to the patient in case they induce another heart attack. Such cautious suppression of feelings inhibits frank and easy communication within the family and often results in a general atmosphere of tension. Both partners and their families should be invited to follow-up visits to continue education and to provide an opportunity to discuss their problems and receive advice about possible resolution. Groups for the partners of post-infarction patients may be beneficial in offering support, providing information, and encouraging changes in life-style. These will be discussed in chapters 13 and 14.

TRANSFER FROM THE CORONARY CARE UNIT

Although transfer to the ward may be interpreted by the patient as evidence of improvement, it may sometimes be viewed as an indication of lack of care or rejection. Anxiety and even fear about transfer are not uncommon, and these are likely to be compounded if the patient is transferred abruptly or during the night. Such negative reactions can be reduced by careful preparation and explanation at the time of transfer. Anxiety levels in patients who receive structured pre-transfer teaching are significantly less than in those who do not (Toth, 1980). A pre-transfer teaching programme should therefore be incorporated into the training of coronary care personnel, and become a routine in the management of acute myocardial infarction. The incidence of cardiovascular complications is reduced in patients who are prepared for transfer from the unit, especially if cared for by the same nurses and doctors throughout their stay in hospital (Klein, et al, 1968). There is also evidence that family support during the transfer phase can reduce associated cardiovascular morbidity and patient stress (Schwarz and Brenner, 1979). Pre-discharge management can be further improved upon if the patient's nurse follows the patient from the coronary care unit to the ward, to serve as a liaison between the patient and the ward staff.

It is important to warn the patient and family that after transfer there is usually a marked change in daily routine, with greatly reduced nursing and medical attention and possible changes in medication, diet and activity. Although it may be thought that the majority of coronary patients would be concerned about no longer being closely monitored, this does not seem to be the case (Thompson et al, 1986). Most assume that they must have virtually recovered, since they no longer have monitoring equipment, cannulae or high nurse–patient ratios. Perhaps worse still, ward staff may perceive the patient in the same light, and there is a real danger that the post-coronary patient will be left alone to 'self-care' in the belief that he requires minimal nursing contact. It is vital that, during handover from the unit to the ward, a full explanation of what has happened to the patient, and what is required in terms of care and treatment, is given. A fully documented up-to-date care plan, with suggested plan of further management and expected outcome is highly desirable. Ideally, such a handover should involve the patient, who can clarify any points and make a valid contribution.

Preparing patients for transfer from coronary care forms an important part of nursing management, and requires more attention than it frequently is afforded. There is certainly a need for a systematic evaluation of this process. An inventory has been developed to evaluate changes in the patient's condition as a result of transfer to a general ward at the time the patient is presumably out of danger (Minkley et al, 1979). This myocardial infarct stress-of-transfer inventory (MISTI) is an important aid to measuring the effectiveness of nursing intervention, and should perhaps be included in all coronary care courses.

References

Adam K and Oswald I (1984) Sleeps helps healing. *British Medical Journal,* **289:** 1400–1401.
Adler D (1976) Critical care nursing. *Nursing Mirror,* **143:** 54–55.
Ashworth P M (1980) *Care to Communicate. An Investigation into Problems of Communication between Patients and Nurses in Intensive Therapy Units. RCN Research Series.* London: Royal College of Nursing.
Ashworth P M (1984a) Staff–patient communication in coronary care units. *Journal of Advanced Nursing,* **9:** 35–42.
Ashworth P M (1984b) Communication in an intensive care unit. In: *Communication,* ed. Faulkner A, pp. 94–112. Edinburgh: Churchill Livingstone.
Bentley S, Murphy F and Dudley H (1977) Perceived noise in surgical wards and an intensive care area: an objective analysis. *British Medical Journal,* **ii:** 1503–1506.
Bourbonnais F (1981) Pain assessment: development of a tool for the nurse and the patient. *Journal of Advanced Nursing,* **6:** 277–282.
Bourbonnais F and MacKay R C (1981) The influence of nursing interventions on chest pain. *Nursing Papers,* **13:** 38–48.
Brezinova V and Oswald I (1972) Sleep after bedtime beverage. *British Medical Journal,* **ii:** 431–433.
Broughton R and Baron R (1978) Sleep patterns in the ICU and on the ward after acute myocardial infarction. *Electroencephalography and Clinical Neurophysiology,* **45:** 348–360.
Byrne D G and Whyte H M (1980) Life events and myocardial infarction revisited. The role of measures of individual impact. *Psychosomatic Medicine,* **42:** 1–10.
Cain H D, Frasher W G and Stivelman R (1961) Graded activity program for safe return to self-care after myocardial infarction. *Journal of the American Medical Association,* **171:** 111.
Cassem N H, Hackett T P, Bascom C and Wishnie H (1970) Reactions of coronary patients to the CCU nurse. *American Journal of Nursing,* **70:** 319–325.
Cay E L (1982) Psychological aspects of cardiac rehabilitation. *Hospital Update,* **8:** 161–170.
Cay E L, Vetter N J, Philip A E and Dugard P (1972) Psychological reactions to a coronary care unit. *Journal of Psychosomatic Research,* **16:** 437–447.

Cay E L, Vetter N J, Philip A E and Dugard P (1973) Return to work after a heart attack. *Journal of Psychosomatic Research,* **17:** 231–243.

Chaturvedi N C, Walsh M J, Evans A, Munro P, Boyle D and Barber J M (1974) Selection of patients for early discharge after acute myocardial infarction. *British Heart Journal,* **36:** 533–535.

Dellipiani A W, Cay E L, Philip A E, Vetter N J, Colling W A, Donaldson R J and McCormack P (1976) Anxiety after a heart attack. *British Heart Journal,* **38:** 752–757.

Diers D, Schmidt R L, McBridge M A B and Davis B L (1972) The effect of nursing interaction on patients in pain. *Nursing Research,* **21:** 419–428.

Editorial (1974) Shoulder–hand syndrome. *Lancet,* **i:** 850.

Ellis B W, Johns M W, Lancaster R, Raptopoulos P, Angelopoulos N and Priest R G (1981) The St Mary's Hospital Sleep Questionnaire: a study of reliability. *Sleep,* **4:** 93–97.

Foster S B (1974) An adrenal measure for evaluating nursing effectiveness. *Nursing Research,* **23:** 118–124.

Garrity T F and Klein R F (1975) Emotional responses and clinical severity as early determinants of six-month mortality after myocardial infarction. *Heart and Lung,* **4:** 730–737.

Gelson A D N, Carson P H M, Tucker H H, Phillips R, Clarke M and Oakley G D G (1976) Course of patients discharged early after myocardial infarction. *British Medical Journal,* **i:** 1555–1558.

Guyton A C (1981) *Medical Physiology.* Philadelphia: W B Saunders.

Hackett T P, Cassem N H and Wishnie H A (1968) The coronary care unit, a reappraisal of its psychologic hazards. *New England Journal of Medicine,* **279:** 1365–1370.

Hentinen M (1983) Need for instruction and support of the wives of patients with myocardial infarction. *Journal of Advanced Nursing,* **8:** 519–524.

Hilton B A (1976) Quantity and quality of patients sleep, and sleep disturbing factors in a respiratory intensive care unit. *Journal of Advanced Nursing,* **1:** 453–468.

Huskisson E C (1974) Measurement of pain. *Lancet,* **ii:** 1127–1131.

Johnston B, Watt E W and Fletcher G F (1981) Oxygen consumption and hemodynamic and electrocardiographic responses to bathing in recent post-myocardial infarction patients. *Heart and Lung,* **10:** 666–671.

Jones J, Hoggart B, Withey J, Donaghue K and Ellis B W (1979) What the patients say: a study of reactions to an intensive care unit. *Intensive Care Medicine,* **5:** 89–92.

King M J, Zir L M, Kaltman A J and Fox A C (1973) Variant angina associated with angiographically demonstrated coronary artery spasm in REM sleep. *American Journal of Medical Science,* **265:** 419–422.

Klein R F, Kliner V A, Zipes D P, Troyer W G and Wallace A G (1968) Transfer from a coronary care unit. *Archives of Internal Medicine,* **122:** 104–108.

Lau Y K, Smith J, Morrison S L and Chamberlain D A (1980) Policy for early discharge after acute myocardial infarction. *British Medical Journal,* **i:** 1489–1492.

Long C (1980) *Prevention and Rehabilitation of Ischaemic Heart Disease.* Baltimore: Williams and Wilkins.

McCaffery M (1979) *Nursing Management of the Patient with Pain.* Philadelphia: J B Lippincott.

McNeer J F, Wagner G S, Ginsburg P B, Wallace A C, McCants C B, Contey M J and Rosati R A (1978) Hospital discharge after acute myocardial infarction. *New England Journal of Medicine,* **298:** 229–232.

Mallory G K, White P D and Salcedo-Salgar J (1939) The speed of healing of myocardial infarction: a study of the pathologic anatomy in 72 cases. *American Heart Journal,* **18:** 647.

Meddis R (1977) *The Sleep Instinct.* London: Routledge and Kegan Paul.

Melzack R (1975) The McGill Pain Questionnaire: major properties and scoring methods. *Pain,* **1:** 277–299.

Minkley B, Burrows D, Whrat K, Harper L, Jenkin S A, Minkley W F, Page B, Schramm D E and Wood C (1979) Myocardial infarct stress-of-transfer inventory: development of a research tool. *Nursing Research,* **28:** 4–10.

Norris R M, Caughey D E, Mercer C J and Scott P J (1974) Prognosis after myocardial infarction: six year follow up. *British Heart Journal,* **36:** 786–790.

Oswald G A, Corcoran S and Yudkin J S (1984) Prevalence and risks of hyperglycaemia and undiagnosed diabetes in patients with acute myocardial infarction. *Lancet,* **i:** 1265–1267.

Peric-Knowlton W (1984) The understanding and management of acute pain in adults: the nursing contribution. *International Journal of Nursing Studies,* **21:** 131–143.

Revill S I, Robinson J O, Rosen M and Hogg M I J (1976) The reliability of a linear analogue for evaluating pain. *Anaesthesia,* **31:** 1191–1198.

Rosenblatt G, Hartmann E and Zwilling G R (1973) Cardiac irritability during sleep and dreaming. *Journal of Psychosomatic Research,* **17:** 129–134.

Scheier I H and Cattell R B (1960) *Handbook for the IPAT 8-Parallel-Form Anxiety Battery.* Champaign, Illinois: IPAT.

Schwarz L P and Brenner Z R (1979) Critical care transfer: reducing patient stress through nursing interventions. *Heart and Lung,* **8:** 540–546.

Scott J and Huskisson E C (1976) Graphic representation of pain. *Pain,* **2:** 175–184.

Skelton M and Dominian J (1973) Psychological stress on wives of patients with myocardial infarction. *British Medical Journal,* **ii:** 101–103.

Sloman J G (1981) Management of myocardial infarction. In: *Recent Advances in Cardiology – 8,* eds. Hamer J and Rowlands D J, pp. 29–46. Edinburgh: Churchill Livingstone.

Solomon H A, Edwards A L and Killip T (1969) Prodromata in acute myocardial infarction. *Circulation,* **40:** 463–471.

Spielberger C D, Gorsuch R L and Lushene R (1970) *Manual for the State-Trait Anxiety Inventory (Self-evaluation Questionnaire).* Palo Alto, California: Consulting Psychologists Press.

Thompson D R and Cordle C J (1988) Support of wives of myocardial infarction patients. *Journal of Advanced Nursing,* **13:** 223–228.

Thompson D R, Blandford R L, Sutton T W and Marchant P R (1985) Time of onset of chest pain in acute myocardial infarction. *International Journal of Cardiology,* **7:** 139–146.

Thompson D R, Bailey S W and Webster R A (1986) Patients' views about cardiac monitoring. *Nursing Times Occasional Paper,* **82(9):** 54–55.

Toth J C (1980) Effect of structured preparation for transfer on patient anxiety on leaving coronary care unit. *Nursing Research,* **29:** 28–34.

Totman R (1979) What makes 'life events' stressful? A retrospective study of patients who have suffered a first myocardial infarction. *Journal of Psychosomatic Research,* **23:** 193–200.

Vetter N J, Cay E L, Philip A E and Strange R C (1977) Anxiety on admission to a coronary care unit. *Journal of Psychosomatic Research,* **21:** 73–78.

Webster R A and Thompson D R (1986) Sleep in hospital. *Journal of Advanced Nursing,* **11:** 447–459.

Wells N (1984) Response to acute pain and the nursing implications. *Journal of Advanced Nursing* **9:** 51–58.

Wilson-Barnett J (1984) *Key Functions in Nursing* (Fourth Winifred Raphael Memorial Lecture). London: Royal College of Nursing.

Winslow E H, Lane L D and Gaffney F A (1984) Oxygen consumption and cardiovascular response in patients and normal adults during in-bed and out-of-bed toileting. *Journal of Cardiac Rehabilitation,* **4:** 348–354.

Winslow E H, Lane L D and Gaffney F A (1985) Oxygen uptake and cardiovascular responses in control adults and acute myocardial infarction patients during bathing. *Nursing Research,* **34:** 164–169.

9

Management of Unstable Angina and Limiting the Size of the Infarct

---

UNSTABLE ANGINA

About half of all patients who sustain a myocardial infarction have warning symptoms (Fulton et al, 1972), the commonest of which is worsening angina. This may either occur in a known angina sufferer or in a previously fit patient, and has been termed unstable, crescendo or pre-infarction angina. Despite the latter term not all patients with this syndrome subsequently sustain a myocardial infarct, but its occurrence does highlight a group of patients at increased risk. The mean incidence of myocardial infarction after the onset of unstable angina is about 40 per cent, with a mortality of 17 per cent (Cairns et al, 1976). Recognition of this condition with appropriate therapy may therefore prevent myocardial infarction and its consequent problems.

Definition

Unstable angina describes symptoms in patients (usually males aged between 40 and 60 years) caused by myocardial ischaemia which are:

- Of recent onset (within four weeks)
- Occurring at rest or with minimal activity
- Different from previous anginal pain (in duration or by accompanying symptoms)

Of course, all these findings may occur with myocardial infarction and, indeed, subclinical myocardial infarction ('micro-infarction') probably occurs in patients with unstable angina (Jaffe et al, 1979).

Aetiology

Typical exercise-induced angina results from an imbalance between myocardial oxygen supply and demand, usually because of a fixed stenosis in one or more coronary arteries. Medical therapy is aimed at reducing cardiac work, thus re-establishing the balance between supply and demand. However, in patients with unstable angina there

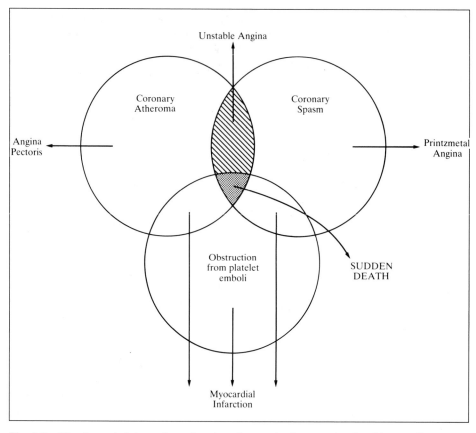

Fig. 9.1 The dynamic interaction of various factors in the genesis of sudden cardiac events

is seldom any demonstrable reason for this imbalance. There appears to be no difference in the severity or distribution of coronary atheroma in patients with stable and unstable angina. It may be that, in angina of recent onset, collateral blood vessels have not had time to form or, alternatively, coronary artery spasm may be the prime initiating factor, leading to a reduction in coronary artery blood flow (Maseri et al, 1978). Waters et al (1983) followed up 100 patients with unstable angina, and found that coronary angiography was normal in 52 per cent of cases, showing the large part that coronary artery spasm plays in unstable angina. Other considerations include the dynamic interaction of atheromatous plaque rupture and haemorrhage, coronary arterial emboli and coronary thrombosis (figure 9.1).

Clinical features

Chest pain is the usual presenting symptom. It is typically anginal in nature, but worse in respect of intensity, duration and accompanying symptoms (e.g. nausea and sweating). Attacks at rest (especially nocturnal) are frequent and are probably caused by coronary artery spasm (Higgins et al, 1976).

Examination may reveal signs of ischaemia, such as dysrhythmias, a third or fourth heart sound, reversed splitting of the second heart sound or transient mitral systolic murmurs. Blood pressure and pulse are normal, but may rise transiently at the onset of pain. If hypotension and pyrexia are present, myocardial infarction has probably already occurred.

Investigations

The electrocardiogram

Between episodes of pain, the 12-lead ECG may be normal although local or generalised changes are frequently present. During pain the ECG shows either ST elevation (25 per cent of cases) or more usually ST depression, reflecting transmural and subendocardial ischaemia respectively (Braunwald, 1978). T wave flattening, peaking and inversion also often occur with pain. Serial ECGs may show both ST elevation and depression (Maseri et al, 1978). The appearance of Q waves usually implies infarction, although even these can be a transient manifestation of ischaemia (Goldberger, 1979). The ischaemic changes in the ECG during pain do not always predict subsequent angiographic findings.

Cardiac enzymes

Increases in enzyme levels usually signify myocardial necrosis. Mild increases (up to 50 per cent) were previously thought to be compatible with the diagnosis of unstable angina if they were unaccompanied by ECG changes. However, it is possible that these enzyme changes represent subclinical 'micro-infarctions', which may be confirmed if the highly sensitive assays for CK-MB are used. It can thus be seen that the spectrum of stable/unstable angina has very indistinct boundaries.

Radionuclide studies

Pyrophosphate scanning can be used to differentiate between areas of acutely infarcted and non-infarcted myocardium. However, pyrophosphate is probably also picked up by areas of critical ischaemia such as may occur in unstable angina. Thallium-201 scintigraphy can be used to outline normal myocardium, highlighting ischaemic areas as cold spots. This will not differentiate between infarcted and non-infarcted myocardium, but may be used to exclude other causes of non-ischaemic rest pain.

ECG stress testing

This is contraindicated unless there have already been normal serial ECG and enzyme investigations and, preferably, a pyrophosphate scan. Cold pressor tests may be used to identify patients with variant (Printzmetal) angina, but these should be delayed until complete stabilisation to avoid precipitating myocardial infarction.

MANAGEMENT

Initial management

Unstable angina is a cardiological emergency and admission to a specialist unit is required for therapy to avert myocardial infarction and any sequelae. In addition, other clinical manifestations of severe myocardial ischaemia (e.g. dysrhythmias or heart failure) need controlling.

It is usually not possible to exclude myocardial infarction on admission, but differentiation may be important because emergency bypass surgery can be carried out in centres where immediate coronary angiography and surgery are available (DeWood et al, 1979; Rahimtoola, 1984).

Initial management does not differ from that given to patients who have sustained a confirmed myocardial infarction, with attention being paid to adequate pain relief and alleviation of anxiety. Oxygen should be given continually via nasal cannulae.

Drug therapy

It is possible to stabilise the majority of patients with medical therapy using combinations of beta-blockers, nitrates and calcium antagonists. Low-dose aspirin (325 mg daily) for three months may be of value. Anticoagulation has generally not been proved to be of value, but full heparinisation may stop pain quickly and completely. The mechanism is not known.

Beta-adrenergic blocking agents

Beta-blockers are the mainstay of therapy for unstable angina, and will control pain initially in about three-quarters of patients. They act predominantly by reducing the heart rate and myocardial oxygen consumption. There is a small theoretical disadvantage of unopposed alpha-adrenergic vasoconstriction precipitating coronary arterial spasm and leading to worsening myocardial ischaemia. However, since most patients will concurrently be treated with nitrates and calcium antagonists (see below), this is rarely a clinical problem. The main practical consideration is therefore the risk of impaired left ventricular function by direct action on the myocardium or secondary to an induced bradycardia. Beta-blocking agents should therefore be given in small and frequent doses to reduce the pulse rate to about 60 beats per minute, and it is probably better to select an agent with a short duration of action as it is not possible to anticipate which patients will react adversely. The shorter-acting agents may also reverse more easily with prenalterol (2 to 5 mg). Prenalterol is a specific beta-1-agonist which increases cardiac output and has been used to treat cardiac failure complicating myocardial infarction. Care is required when giving this drug to avoid precipitating further anginal pain. A cardioselective beta-blocker (e.g. metoprolol) is preferred, since coronary sympathetic vasodilator tone is mediated by the beta-2 receptor; this is particularly important if coronary artery spasm is suspected.

Nitrates

These drugs reduce cardiac work and oxygen consumption by reducing preload and some afterload. Subendocardial blood flow is also improved. However, some of these effects may be offset by an increase in heart rate, so that nitrates are best given with a beta-blocker. They may be given orally or transdermally, although intravenous nitrates are easier to titrate against blood pressure and headaches. The starting dose should be 2–5 μg, increasing to as much as 300 μg per minute depending on systemic blood pressure. The systolic blood pressure should not be allowed to fall below 100 mmHg or coronary perfusion pressures will fall and may precipitate infarction. If hypotension develops at low doses of nitrate therapy, it may be advisable to insert a Swan–Ganz catheter so that unsuspected hypovolaemia is not missed, and to ensure that the patient has an adequate left ventricular filling pressure.

Nitrates are of major value in patients with coronary vasospasm and should be administered to all those who show ST elevation on the ECG when in pain.

Calcium channel blockers

These drugs inhibit calcium influx in myocardial and smooth muscle, producing relaxation. Hence there is a decrease in myocardial contractility (decreasing myocardial work), and a vasodilator action both systemically (reducing afterload) and in the coronary arteries (improving myocardial perfusion). Nifedipine, nicardipine, diltiazem and verapamil are all currently available, but probably do not offer any major therapeutic benefit over the nitrates. Verapamil and diltiazem are particularly useful if there is a fast pulse rate unresponsive to beta-blockade. Nicardipine has the least cardiodepressant activity, which may be an important consideration when prescribing beta-blockers. Nifedipine capsules can be administered sublingually for a rapid onset and short duration of action.

Anticoagulants

Although there has been much controversy, there is good evidence that myocardial infarction is actually caused by coronary thrombosis, so that the risk of infarction may theoretically be reduced with the use of anticoagulants (Roberts, 1974). Early studies found large differences in the subsequent infarction and mortality following treatment, and concluded that withholding anticoagulant treatment was unethical (Wood, 1961). Since non-occlusive thrombi are present in some patients with unstable angina (Holmes et al, 1981), there is a rational basis for acute administration of anticoagulants. However, heparin may lead to thromboxane A2 release. This is a potent coronary vasoconstrictor and additionally causes platelet aggregation, thus theoretically predisposing to myocardial infarction (Lewy et al, 1979). Despite these reports, intravenous heparin often has a swift analgesic action when infused in doses of 25 units/kg/h, and may be effective in preventing myocardial infarction (Telford and Wilson, 1981).

Fibrinolysis is the system whereby inactive plasminogen is converted to the powerful enzyme, plasmin, which digests and solubilises the fibrin skeleton of coronary (and other) thrombi. This is normally activated spontaneously within the body for this precise purpose, but activating the system artificially with streptokinase (Ganz et al, 1984; Davies et al, 1984) has been used with good effect in the very early stages of myocardial infarction. Interest is now being shown in 'fibrin-specific' agents such as urokinase and tissue plasminogen activator.

Aspirin

Unstable angina is associated with enhanced platelet reactivity, increased plasma concentrations of platelet factor 4 and beta-thromboglobulin and release of thromboxane B2 from the coronary sinus. This increased activity may aggravate the degree of coronary obstruction. Administration of aspirin (325 mg/day) will reduce cardiac mortality and should be given unless contraindicated (Petch, 1986).

Intra-aortic balloon counterpulsation

Some centres still advocate the use of counterpulse balloon pumping if other medical therapies have failed. However, there is an appreciable insertion mortality and morbidity, particularly with regard to vascular injury and lower limb ischaemia. Most patients with unstable angina can be controlled for short periods, but they cannot usually be weaned off the balloon pump without rapidly worsening myocardial ischaemia, often associated with cardiogenic shock. As a consequence, once the balloon has been inserted, there is little choice but to proceed to cardiac catheterisation and surgery (either coronary artery bypass grafting or angioplasty).

Later management

The majority of patients with crescendo angina will settle with conservative management in the first 24 hours. Those who do not should be considered for emergency bypass surgery. This must be weighed against the additional morbidity and mortality of coronary angiography performed in the acute phase of unstable angina. Angiography should usually be carried out anyway in most cases as soon as they are stabilised to identify those patients who will benefit from bypass surgery. Those with left main stem disease, triple coronary artery disease and ventricular aneurysms are usually considered for early surgery. Patients with single discrete lesions may be suitable for coronary angioplasty.

Many patients who settle with conservative therapy will suffer pain later, and about one-third will need coronary artery surgery within two years. Thereafter, prognosis is good (the 10 year survival rate is 83 per cent).

ESTIMATION OF INFARCT SIZE

Limiting the extent of myocardial necrosis following acute myocardial infarction has become a major goal in clinical cardiology, because it is the extent of myocardial damage that is the major determinant of survival and long-term well-being. However, experimental support for such strategies (especially in humans) has been held back by the difficulties in estimating infarct size, and hence judging the success of any given therapy.

The precise estimation of infarct size is difficult, but the following techniques have been used.

Ventriculography

Myocardial infarction produces abnormalities of ventricular movement and hence ventriculography (using echocardiography or nuclear angiography) may be able to demonstrate areas of necrotic myocardium. Unfortunately, this method does not differentiate between long-standing scar tissue and acutely non-contracting ischaemic areas that are potentially salvageable.

Cardiac enzymes

The extent of myocardial necrosis may be estimated from the measurement of creatine kinase (CPK) levels, or preferably from its myocardial isoenzyme CK-MB. However, to be accurate, levels probably need to be taken every three to six hours for the first two to three days following infarction, and even then levels may be altered by enzyme release following myocardial reperfusion, or concurrent drug therapy.

The electrocardiogram

The standard 12-lead electrocardiogram can give some indication of the extent of infarction, both from classical infarct changes and from ST depression in leads facing the non-infarcted myocardium. 'Reciprocal depression' has long been regarded as a purely electrical phenomenon reflecting ST elevation on the opposite side of the heart. However, it does not explain why these changes are not always present in cases where there is very marked ST elevation. It is possible that these 'reciprocal' changes reflect remote ischaemia and highlight a group of patients at increased risk of complications because of a greater degree of left ventricular damage (*Lancet*, 1986). Myocardial ECG mapping techniques using multiple electrodes are probably required to maximise any information from this method of study, but even so inferior and posterior infarcts cannot be mapped with any degree of accuracy.

Radioisotopes

Thallium cold spot scanning has been shown to be of value in the assessment of infarction size (see chapter 5). Unfortunately, confusion may arise in the differentiation of old scars, new infarcts or areas of ischaemia. Recently, radiolabelled monoclonal antibodies to cardiac myosin have been introduced for assessing infarct size. If these labelled antibodies are injected within 48 hours of myocardial infarction, they will bind to any myosin exposed by myocardial cell rupture. The result may then be visualised using a conventional gamma-camera. The principal advantage of this technique is the ability to distinguish between myocardial ischaemia and myocardial infarction. As the half-life of the tracer (indium-111) is 2.5 days, serial scans can be used to assess the progress of the infarct. European trials using this techniques are at present under way.

LIMITING THE EXTENT OF INFARCTION

Therapeutic intervention in the course of acute myocardial infarction aims to prevent or limit the extent of myocardial necrosis and preserve normal myocardial performance. This demands early reperfusion of the myocardium at risk. The important zone of potentially salvageable myocardium lies between the irreversibily damaged central core and normal myocardial tissues at the periphery. The size of this 'border zone' will be influenced by the severity and location of the coronary artery stenosis, the patency of other coronary arteries and the presence of collateral vessels. A restoration of the imbalance of oxygen supply and demand within this border zone is required to prevent subsequent necrosis, and may be achieved by:

1. Improving oxygen supply to the injured myocardium by:
   ● Supplemental oxygen therapy
   ● Coronary arterial surgery
   ● Thrombolytic therapy
   ● Reversal of coronary artery spasm

2. Limiting oxygen requirements by:
   ● Mechanical myocardial support
   ● Cardiac depressant drugs to reduce cardiac work
   ● Retarding inflammation at the infarct site

Improving oxygenation

Supplemental oxygen

Most patients with acute myocardial infarction have arterial hypoxaemia. There is some evidence from ST segment mapping that oxygen therapy can reduce myocardial ischaemia. Apart from correcting arterial hypoxaemia, oxygen may also induce vasoconstriction and it is postulated that, by constricting normal coronary arteries, blood is diverted to the affected coronary artery. Certainly, the oxygen gradient between the normal myocardium and border zone myocardium is increased, thus helping myocardial oxygenation.

Coronary artery surgery

Peri-infarction surgery includes coronary angioplasty and coronary artery bypass grafting. Restoration of perfusion will lead to increased oxygenation and should limit infarction size. Widespread application of these techniques is still limited by the resources and expertise required.

Thrombolytic therapy

The majority of patients with acute myocardial infarction have evidence of fresh coronary arterial thrombus formation in association with a fissured atheromatous plaque. The use of streptokinase and other thrombolytic agents is described later, and these drugs may be utilised to increase or re-establish myocardial perfusion. Thrombolysis (especially if performed within two hours of onset of myocardial infarction) may limit infarct size, preserve global and regional left ventricular function and increase survival (Van der Laarse et al, 1986).

Reversal of coronary artery spasm

Coronary artery spasm in the presence of a fixed atheromatous lesion may complicate over one-third of cases of myocardial infarction. Use of nifedipine and nitrates may help to overcome this and aid myocardial reperfusion.

Reduction of oxygen requirements

The major factors that increase myocardial oxygen requirements are heart rate, strength of contractility and left ventricular tension (determined by left ventricular volume, pressure and mass). Reduction in myocardial oxygen requirement may thus be achieved by several methods.

Mechanical myocardial support

Intra-aortic balloon pumping helps reduce left ventricular work by reducing afterload and left ventricular pressure. It also increases coronary artery perfusion. However, although it has been used widely in cardiogenic shock, there is no evidence that it is helpful in uncomplicated myocardial infarction. Furthermore, it is an invasive and expensive procedure with an appreciable morbidity rate.

Cardiac depressant drugs

Beta-adrenergic blocking agents reduce myocardial work by reducing heart rate and contractility. The use of beta-blockers to limit infarct size has been extensively investigated, and results (mostly from animal studies) suggest a beneficial effect (Taylor et al, 1982). Clinical trials have shown that beta-blockers will reduce the degree of ST elevation which correlates with 2-year post-infarct mortality. However, ST elevation does not necessarily correlate with myocardial viability (Hearse et al, 1986), and strategies designed to reduce ST elevation will not necessarily reduce the size of the infarct. Dysrhythmias (including ventricular fibrillation) are reduced by acute parenteral administration of beta-blockers, and prevention of excessive oxygen utilisation by inappropriate tachycardias will reduce oxygen requirements, with subsequent limitation of the size of infarction. Early administration of beta-blockers has been reported to decrease the final infarct size by 15–20 per cent (Herlitz and Hjalmarson, 1986).

Nitrates may be useful in reducing preload, and thus reducing myocardial work and increasing endocardial perfusion. In addition, they reduce left ventricular volume, thus reducing compression on the collateral coronary arteries which may enhance collateral coronary blood supply.

Reducing inflammation

Steroids are thought to protect ischaemic tissue by membrane stabilisation, prevention of lysosomal rupture and reduction of energy requirements. However, their use may delay the healing of the myocardium and predispose to the formation of left ventricular aneurysms.

Non-steroidal anti-inflammatory agents (e.g. aspirin) will reduce inflammation and additionally have an antiplatelet action. The beneficial use of aspirin in unstable angina has been confirmed, and it may be that a combination of reduction of inflammation with prevention of coronary platelet emboli may limit the extent of myocardial necrosis following acute infarction. However, caution is required; indomethacin has been reported to precipitate coronary vasoconstriction and may thus increase the size of the infarct (Friedman et al, 1981). Whether this is clinically important, or even applicable to other non-steroidal anti-inflammatory agents, is not known.

TREATMENT OF CORONARY THROMBOSIS

Whether anticoagulation is of any value in the treatment of acute myocardial infarction would seem to depend upon whether or not myocardial infarction is caused by an acute coronary artery thrombosis. This was widely believed to be the case in the early 1960s when anticoagulation became routine (hence the terms coronary thrombosis and myocardial infarction being used synonymously). The concept of acute coronary thrombosis then became less popular and accordingly fewer patients were anticoagulated. However, the increasing use of coronary angiography has demonstrated that most cases of myocardial infarction are indeed associated with the presence of fresh thrombus in the affected coronary artery (*Lancet*, 1985), usually at the site of a ruptured atheromatous plaque (Davies and Thomas, 1985). Coronary artery thrombus has also been found in many patients suffering sudden cardiac death and as many as 95 per cent of patients dying from acute transmural myocardial infarction (Davies et al, 1976).

The main controversy now surrounds whether acute thrombosis causes the sudden cardiac event or whether it forms as a result of the myocardial infarction. Thrombotic occlusion may occur without resulting in infarction, and subendocardial infarction can follow acute coronary insufficiency without evidence of thrombosis. In the majority of cases of transmural myocardial infarction, complete absence of blood flow in the diseased coronary artery is typical, although spontaneous thrombolysis may take place to a varying degree in about 30 per cent of patients within the first 12 to 24 hours (DeWood et al, 1980). Present evidence suggests that there is a dynamic interaction involving coronary artery spasm, platelet aggregation and a fissured atheromatous plaque (Gold and Leinbach, 1980; Davies and Thomas, 1985). Occlusive thrombi probably originate at the site of an intimal tear and, before the artery becomes occluded, it is likely that small coronary emboli are shed causing multiple small distal occlusions in the area supplied by the coronary vessel ('micro-infarcts'). The tear may either heal and regress or initiate thrombosis leading to complete occlusion. Hence there may be varying consequences ranging from micro-infarcts to full transmural infarction (Stehbens, 1985). This raises the question of whether coronary thrombosis can be treated to re-establish myocardial perfusion, and thus limit the extent of myocardial infarction, or even prevent it (Davies et al, 1984). There is much interest in the possibility of achieving this by thrombolysis.

Coronary thrombolysis

Coronary thrombolysis promises to become one of the most significant advances in the treatment of acute myocardial infarction. Ironically, the observation in the 1930s that streptokinase (a breakdown product of some streptococcus strains) could lyse clotted blood came long before coronary care units, bedside monitors, defibrillators and loop diuretics existed. It was another 25 years before attempts to recanalise the coronary arteries with streptokinase were reported in the treatment of acute myocardial infarction (Fletcher et al, 1958). Although there are many drugs that may be used to break up thrombi, most clinical trials so far have reported the use of streptokinase and urokinase. Intracoronary administration of streptokinase in acute myocardial infarction has been studied in the USA since 1978, and has now become routine practice in some centres. The exceptionally important GISSI study (1987) has shown that early administration of streptokinase can reduce short-term mortality, and long-term results are eagerly awaited. More recently tissue plasminogen activator (tPA), an acylated form of streptokinase (APSAC) and pro-urokinase have been utilised, having been found to be more 'clot-specific' and associated with fewer complications, particularly those due to haemorrhage and allergy. The results of trials using these agents are awaited.

Before therapeutic intervention is carried out with these agents, there are certain considerations including:

● Who should be treated
● How and when to administer the drug
● The choice of thrombolytic agent
● What to do with any residual stenosis

Who should be treated

At present it would seem that thrombolytic agents should be offered to all patients presenting in the early phase of acute myocardial infarction, as well as those with persistent ischaemic pain and ST elevation unresponsive to nitrates. Patients with unstable angina should probably also receive thrombolytic therapy.

The main contraindications to administration are:

● A high risk of bleeding (recent surgery or trauma, stroke, peptic ulceration)
● Uncontrolled hypertension (BP more than 200/120)
● Proliferative diabetic retinopathy

Although early work has suggested that less than 50 per cent of cases of myocardial infarction may be suitable for thrombolysis (Murray et al, 1987; Jagger et al, 1987), this may be because trial protocols are more rigid than criteria that could be applied outside this setting (De Bono, 1987).

Drug administration

Many reports have now shown a reduction in mortality of 15 to 20 per cent in patients treated with thrombolytic agents following acute myocardial infarction (*Lancet*, 1987), and the outcome is better in those treated early. For myocardial salvage to be effective, thrombolysis must be attempted within four hours of onset of chest pain, and probably not later than six hours. Lack of improvement in left ventricular function may result if there is a delay in reperfusion, although any time limit may be prolonged by such factors as the presence of a pre-existing collateral circulation, residual antegrade coronary blood flow and the oxygen requirements of the ischaemic myocardium (Rude et al, 1981; Rogers et al, 1984). As a result, benefit has been noted in some patients when thrombolysis has been delayed for up to 18 hours following the onset of chest pain. Unfortunately, admission to hospital after the start of symptoms may vary widely, and has been reported to be between and 13 and 505 minutes (mean 80 minutes) in the UK, often with a further delay of 70 minutes between arrival at the hospital and transfer to the coronary care unit (*Lancet*, 1987). Ideally an intravenous thrombolytic agent should be given at the patient's home or in the ambulance on the way to hospital.

The route of administration has also been subject to study and controversy (Marder and Francis, 1984). Increasing access to occluded coronary arteries has led to fibrinolytic agents being infused directly at the site of required action. An angiographic catheter is introduced via the femoral artery and nitrates or nifedipine are given to alleviate any coronary artery spasm before thrombolysis is commenced. Because this method of drug administration involves acute coronary catheterisation, widespread acceptance of the use of thrombolysis has not occurred. Systemic administration is of course preferable, and this method of giving thrombolytic agents will probably emerge as the preferred technique because of its simplicity and low risk of provoking dysrhythmias, and because it is applicable to units without facilities for angiography. Furthermore, systemic administration of the drug enables the distal surface of the thrombus to be reached by retrograde coronary flow through collateral blood vessels.

The main problems with thrombolysis are dysrhythmias and bleeding which may be severe in about 5 per cent of cases (Timmis et al, 1982). Fever and allergic reactions are frequent and may be minimised by prior treatment with intravenous chlorpheniramine (10 mg) and hydrocortisone (100 mg). Platelet activity should be considered, and some centres administer aspirin (300 mg) routinely. Short-term beta-blockade may help protect the myocardium during thrombolysis, and could reduce the incidence of reperfusional dysrhythmias. Such dysrhythmias often accompany recanalisation and reperfusion of the ischaemic myocardium. Idioventricular rhythm is the most frequent abnormality, although 10 per cent of cases will develop ventricular tachycardia or fibrillation.

Successful reperfusion of the myocardium is usually accompanied by relief of chest pain, with ST segments on the ECG returning quickly to normal. The ejection fraction increases (Valentine et al, 1986), and global and regional left ventricular function have been shown (by echocardiography and radionuclide ventriculography) to improve, particularly in patients with anterior infarcts and those with their first infarct (Res et al, 1986).

Venepuncture following thrombolysis must be carried out with care to prevent bleeding and bruising. Pacemakers and Swan–Ganz catheters may be better inserted via the antecubital fossa or femoral vein to prevent possible occult bleeding following central catheterisation.

Choice of thrombolytic agent

Plasmin is a protein-splitting enzyme which breaks down the insoluble fibrin network within the thrombus. It is present in the plasma, as its inactive precursor plasminogen. Streptokinase is a metabolic product of the group C beta-haemolytic streptococcus which causes activation of plasminogen leading to lysis of the fibrin within the thrombus. It may be given systemically or directly into the affected coronary artery. Intravenous streptokinase has been used to break up thrombi (with a success rate of about 45 per cent), but intracoronary infusion has been found to be more effective. It is infused into the mouth of the affected artery at a rate of 2000 to 4000 units/min (after a loading dose of 10 000 to 20 000 units) until patency is restored, and then continued for a further one to two hours to ensure complete thrombolysis. This approach will recanalise the infarct-related artery in up to 90 per cent of cases within 30 minutes (Rentrop, 1985), with reduction of pain and resolution of electrocardiographic changes (Rentrop et al, 1981).

Higher doses of streptokinase (500 000 to 1 700 000 units/min) are now being used during peripheral administration. If given for up to an hour, they may be as effective as traditional intracoronary infusion (Taylor et al, 1984). However, new evidence has shown that these high doses of streptokinase can be safely and effectively infused directly into the affected vessel, producing reperfusion in over 90 per cent of cases and limiting the size of infarction (*Lancet*, 1985). Other studies do not confirm such high figures for recanalisation, and only one showed an improvement in left ventricular function (Rentrop, 1985), but these results may reflect the speed of administration. It is probable that the greater the delay in institution of therapy, the less likely it is that left ventricular function will be improved. Although intracoronary streptokinase does achieve a better patency rate than systemic streptokinase, the former route may never become routine (except in specialist units) because of the expertise and equipment required for coronary catheterisation. The extra time needed to arrange transfer of patients to such units may negate the possible benefits. If intracoronary administration of thrombolytic agents does become the method of choice, the systemic route may still have a place in that they may be started before transfer to a centre where angiography is available.

Other agents such as tissue plasminogen activator, anisoylated plasminogen–streptokinase activator complex (APSAC) and pro-urokinase are gaining popularity as their administration may be associated with lower risks of systemic anticoagulation and bleeding.

Urokinase is a product of human renal tubular cells and directly activates the fibrinolytic system. It is more clot-specific and less antigenic than streptokinase and when infused directly into the coronary vasculature (2 000 to 24 000 units/min) yields recanalisation rates of 62 to 94 per cent (Tennant et al, 1984; Yasuno et al, 1984).

Tissue-type plasminogen activator (tPA) is a naturally occurring protein with greater clot specificity than streptokinase and urokinase, and hence should be less likely to activate systemic fibrinolysis. Recent cloning of the tPA gene has provided large quantities of the drug for clinical investigation and early reports are very encouraging. It has been found to be highly fibrin-specific and thus cause fewer bleeding problems. In addition, because it is very potent, it may be given systemically and still restore patency in infarct-related coronary vessels (Verstraete et al, 1985). Since this agent is produced by genetic engineering, the cost is likely to fall in the coming years.

There have been two major trials with tPA in Europe (Verstraete et al, 1985) and America (TIMI Study Group, 1985). The TIMI study showed that infusion of 80 mg tPA over 90 minutes restored patency in 55 per cent of cases compared with only 35 per cent of those treated with streptokinase (1 500 000 units). The European study showed that recanalisation occurred in 61 per cent of cases treated with tPA and only 20 per cent of cases treated with placebo. Re-occlusion, however, may be higher following treatment with tPA (Sherry, 1987) because of its short half-life. It must therefore be given as a prolonged infusion. However, the great advantage of agents with a short half-life is that if haemorrhage occurs treatment can be stopped and its activity will rapidly disappear.

Management following thrombolysis

Once the coronary thrombus has been successfully lysed, the circumstances that caused it usually still prevail, and may lead to re-accumulation of thrombus. Estimates of up to 40 per cent reoccurrence in the first week have been made, and strategies aimed at preventing re-occlusion are therefore required. Following reperfusion, patients should therefore receive antiplatelet therapy (aspirin or dipyridamole) to counter platelet aggregation, and calcium blocking agents (e.g. nifedipine) to prevent coronary artery spasm. Anticoagulation is probably important to prevent recurrent thrombosis, especially when clot-specific agents have been used. Heparin is commonly given for two to three days, followed by warfarin for at least three months (De Bono, 1987). Early coronary angiography will identify those needing coronary angioplasty (PTCA) or coronary artery bypass operations (CABG). Residual atheromatous stenosis may be found after thrombolysis in 80–90 per cent of cases (Serruys et al, 1983). Angioplasty is thus the logical next step, although it is not as yet widely available. Using a combination of intracoronary streptokinase and PTCA, very high rates of reperfusion may be obtained in patients following acute myocardial infarction, leading to improved left ventricular function (Erbel et al, 1986). Re-occlusion rates may also not be so great. Although the hospital mortality associated with this approach is at present high, this figure will certainly fall as units become more adept at managing acute myocardial infarction in this way.

A milestone for myocardial infarction?

The benefits of thrombolysis are already of such magnitude that thousands of lives stand to be saved every year. Use should be routine.

All patients with evidence of acute myocardial infarction, and no important contraindications should receive thrombolytic therapy (irrespective of the patient's age, sex or location of the infarct). A time-window of 4 to 6 hours is desirable, although the major thrombolytic trials suggest they may be effective for up to 24 hours (GISSI Study Group, 1987; ISIS-2, 1988). Why it continues to be effective beyond the vital first few hours is unclear. It is likely that acute coronary occlusion is not always a sudden, but a stuttering event, often marked by episodic chest pain. Since aspirin reduces platelet aggregation which is responsible for progression of the infarct, early administration (at home or in the ambulance) should now be routine. The second international study on infarct survival (ISIS-2) has additionally shown the additive role of aspirin to streptokinase, especially in those admitted after 6 hours. It probably also makes subsequent anti-coagulation unnecessary.

Specific therapy for acute myocardial infarction now exists; it is organisation of care which now needs to be improved (Julian et al, 1988).

References

Braunwald E (1978) Coronary spasm and acute myocardial infarction – new possibility for treatment and prevention. *New England Journal of Medicine,* **299:** 1301–1303.

Cairns J A, Fantus I G and Klassen G A (1976) Unstable angina pectoris. *American Heart Journal,* **92:** 373–386.

Davies G J, Chierchia S and Maseri A (1984) Prevention of myocardial infarction by very early treatment with intracoronary streptokinase. *New England Journal of Medicine,* **311:** 1488–1492.

Davies M J and Thomas A C (1985) Plaque fissuring – the cause of acute myocardial infarction, sudden death and crescendo angina. *British Heart Journal,* **53:** 363–373.

Davies M J, Woolf N and Robertson W B (1976) Pathology of acute myocardial infarction with particular reference to occlusive coronary thrombi. *British Heart Journal,* **38:** 659–664.

De Bono D (1987) Coronary thrombolysis. *British Heart Journal,* **57:** 301–305.

DeWood M A, Spores J, Notske R N, Lang H T, Shields J P, Simpson C S, Rudy L W and Grunwald R (1979) Medical and surgical management of myocardial infarction. *American Journal of Cardiology,* **44:** 1356–1364.

DeWood M A, Spores J, Notske R, Mouser L T, Burroughs R, Golden M S and Lang H T (1980) Prevalence of total coronary occlusion during the early hours of transmural myocardial infarction. *New England Journal of Medicine,* **303:** 897–902.

Erbel R, Pop T, Henrichs K-J, von Olshausen K, Schuster C J, Rupprecht H J, Stevernagel C and Meyer J (1986) Percutaneous transluminal coronary angioplasty after thrombolytic therapy. *Journal of the American College of Cardiology,* **8:** 485–495.

Fletcher A P, Alkjaersig N, Smyrniotis F E and Sherry S (1958) The treatment of patients suffering from early myocardial infarction with massive and prolonged streptokinase therapy. *Transcripts of the Association of American Physicians,* **71:** 287–295.

Fulton M, Lutz W and Donald K W (1972) Natural history of unstable angina. *Lancet,* **i:** 860–865.

Friedman P L, Brown E J, Gunther S, Alexander R W, Barry W H, Mudge G H and Grossman W (1981) Coronary vasoconstrictor effect of indomethacin in patients with coronary artery disease. *New England Journal of Medicine,* **305:** 1171–1175.

Ganz W, Geft I, Shah P K, Lew A S, Rodriguez L, Weiss T, Maddahi J, Berman D S, Charuzi Y and Swan H J C (1984) Intravenous streptokinase in evolving myocardial infarction. *American Journal of Cardiology,* **53:** 1209–1216.

GISSI Study Group (1987) Long-term effects of intravenous thrombolysis in acute myocardial infarction: final report of the GISSI study. *Lancet,* **ii:** 871–874.

Gold H K and Leinbach R C (1980) Coronary obstruction in anterior myocardial infarction: thrombus or spasm? *American Journal of Cardiology,* **45:** 483.

Goldberger A L (1979) *Myocardial Infarction: Electrocardiographic Differential Diagnosis.* St Louis: C V Mosby.

Hearse D J, Yellon D M and Downey J M (1986) Can beta-blockers limit myocardial infarction size? *European Heart Journal,* **7:** 925–930.

Herlitz J and Hjalmarson A (1986) The role of beta-blockade in the limitation of infarct development. *European Heart Journal,* **7:** 916-924.

Higgins C B, Wexler L, Silverman J F and Schroeder J S (1976) Clinical and angiographic features of Prinzmetal's variant angina: documentation of etiological factors. *American Journal of Cardiology,* **37:** 831-839.

Holmes D R, Hartzier G O, Smith H C and Fuster V (1981) Coronary artery thrombosis in patients with unstable angina. *British Heart Journal,* **45:** 411-416.

ISIS-2 (1988) ISIS-2: a randomised trial of intravenous streptokinase, oral aspirin, both or neither among 17,187 cases of suspected myocardial infarction. *Lancet,* **2:** 349-360.

Jaffe A S, Klein M S, Patel B R, Siegel B A and Roberts R (1979) Abnormal technetium-99m pyrophosphate images in unstable angina: ischaemia versus infarction. *American Journal of Cardiology,* **44:** 1035-1039.

Jagger J D, Murray R G, Davies M K, Littler W A and Flint E J (1987) Elegibility for thrombolytic therapy in acute myocardial infarction. *Lancet,* **i:** 34-35.

Julian D G, Pentecost B L & Chamberlain D A (1988) A milestone for myocardial infarction. *British Medical Journal,* **297:** 497-498.

Lancet (1985) Treatment of coronary thrombosis. *Lancet,* **i:** 375-376.

Lancet (1986) Reciprocal changes accompanying acute myocardial infarction. *Lancet,* **ii:** 1370-1371.

Lancet (1987) Thrombolytic therapy for acute myocardial infarction. *Lancet,* **ii:** 138-140.

Lewy R I, Wiener L, Smith J B, Walinsky P and Silver M J (1979) Intravenous heparin initiates in vivo synthesis and release of thromboxane in angina pectoris. *Lancet,* **ii:** 97.

Marder V J and Francis C W (1984) Thrombolytic therapy for acute transmural myocardial infarction: intracoronary versus intravenous. *American Journal of Medicine,* **77:** 921-927.

Maseri A, Severi S, Nes M D, L'Abbate A, Chierchia S and Parodi O (1978) 'Variant' angina: one aspect of a continuous spectrum of vasospastic myocardial ischaemia. *American Journal of Cardiology,* **42:** 1019-1035.

Murray N, Lyons J, Layton C and Balcon R (1987) What proportion of patients with myocardial infarction are suitable for thrombolysis? *British Heart Journal,* **57:** 144-147.

Petch M C (1986) Aspirin for unstable angina? *British Medical Journal,* **293:** 1-2.

Rahimtoola S H (1984) Coronary bypass surgery for unstable angina. *Circulation,* **69:** 842-848.

Rentrop K P (1985) Thrombolytic therapy in patients with acute myocardial infarction. *Circulation,* **71:** 627-631.

Rentrop P, Blanke H, Karch K R, Kostering H, Oster H and Leitz H (1981) Selective intracoronary thrombolysis in acute myocardial infarction and unstable angina pectoris. *Circulation,* **63:** 307-317.

Res J C, Simoons M L, Van der Waal E E, Van Eenige J, Vermeer F, Verheugt F W, Wijns W, Braat S, Remme W J and Serruys P W (1986) Long-term improvement in global left ventricular function after early thrombolytic treatment in acute myocardial infarction. *British Heart Journal,* **56:** 414-421.

Roberts W C (1974) Coronary thrombosis and fatal myocardial ischaemia. *Circulation,* **49:** 1-3.

Rogers W J, Hood W P, Mantle J A, Baxley W A, Kirklin J K, Zorn G L and Nath H P (1984) Return of left ventricular function after reperfusion in patients with myocardial infarction: importance of sub-total stenosis and intact collaterals. *Circulation,* **69:** 338-349.

Rude R E, Muller J E and Braunwald E (1981) Efforts to limit the size of myocardial infarcts. *Annals of Internal Medicine,* **95:** 736-761.

Serruys P W, Wijns W, Van Den Brand M, Ribeiro V, Fiorretti P, Simoon M, Kooijman C J, Reiber J H and Hugenholtz P G (1983) Is transluminal coronary angioplasty mandatory after successful thrombolysis? Quantitative coronary angiographic study. *British Heart Journal,* **50:** 257-265.

Sherry S (1987) Recombinant tissue plasminogen activator: is it the thrombolytic agent of choice for evolving myocardial infarction? *American Journal of Cardiology,* **59:** 984-989.

Stehbens W E (1985) Relationship of coronary artery thrombosis to myocardial infarction. *Lancet,* **ii:** 639-642.

Taylor G J, Mikell F L, Moses H W, Dove J T, Batchelder J E, Thull A, Hassen S, Wellons

H A and Schneider J A (1984) Intravenous versus intra-coronary streptokinase therapy for acute myocardial infarction in community hospitals. *American Journal of Cardiology,* **54:** 256–260.

Taylor S H, Silke B and Lee P S (1982) Intravenous beta-blockade in coronary heart disease. *New England Journal of Medicine,* **306:** 631–635.

Telford A M and Wilson C (1981) A trial of heparin versus atenolol in the prevention of myocardial infarction in the intermediate coronary syndrome. *Lancet,* **i:** 1225–1228.

Tennant S N, Dixon J, Venable T C, Page H L, Roach A, Kaiser A B, Fredriksen R, Tacogue L, Kaplan P and Babu N S (1984) Intra-coronary thrombolysis in patients with acute myocardial infarction: comparison of the efficacy of urokinase with streptokinase. *Circulation,* **69:** 756–760.

TIMI Study Group (1985) The thrombolysis in myocardial infarction (TIMI) study. Phase 1 findings. *New England Journal of Medicine,* **312:** 932–936.

Timmis G C, Gangadharan V, Hauser A M, Rames R G, Westveer D C and Gordon S (1982) Intracoronary streptokinase in clinical practice. *American Heart Journal,* **104:** 925–938.

Valentine R P, Pitts D E, Brooks-Brunn L, Woods J, Nyhuis A, Van Hove E and Schmidt P E (1986) Effect of thrombolysis on left ventricular function during acute myocardial infarction. *American Journal of Cardiology,* **58:** 896–899.

Van der Laarse A, Vermeer F, Hermens W T, Willems G M, de Neef K, Simoons M L, Serruys P W, Res J, Verheugt F W and Krauss X H (1986) Effects of early intra-coronary streptokinase in infarct size estimated from cumulative enzyme release and on enzyme release state: a randomised trial of 533 patients with acute myocardial infarction. *American Heart Journal,* **112:** 672–681.

Verstraete M, Bleifeld B, Brower R W, Charbonnier B, Collen D, de Bono D P, Dunning A J, Lennane R J, Lubsen J and Mathey D G (1985) Double blind randomised trial of intravenous tissue type plasminogen activator versus placebo in acute myocardial infarction. *Lancet,* **ii:** 965–969.

Waters D D, Miller D D, Szlachcic J, Bouchard A, Methe M, Kreeft J and Theroux P (1983) Factors influencing the long-term prognosis of treated patients with variant angina. *Circulation,* **68:** 258–265.

Wood P (1961) Acute and sub-acute coronary insufficiency. *British Medical Journal,* **i:** 1779–1782.

Yasuno M, Saito Y and Ishida M (1984) Effects of percutaneous transluminal angioplasty: intracoronary thrombolysis with urokinase in acute myocardial infarction. *American Journal of Cardiology,* **53:** 1217–1220.

10

Complications of Acute Myocardial Infarction and their Management

There are numerous complications that may arise as a consequence of acute myocardial infarction. The major risk factors are:

● The extent of the present myocardial infarction
● The cumulative loss of functional myocardium if there have been previous infarctions
● The extent and severity of coronary arterial disease

Abnormal electrical activity in ischaemic or necrotic cardiac tissue can precipitate disturbances in cardiac rate, rhythm and conduction ('the dysrhythmias') whilst the loss of left ventricular myocardium leads to pump failure ('heart failure').

Dysrhythmias are the most common complication of myocardial infarction, occurring in about 90 per cent of all cases. Most are caused by re-entry mechanisms or from enhanced automaticity in pacemaker cells (see p. 207). They need treating if there is a deterioration in circulatory function (hypotension, heart failure or syncope) or if the rate is increasing myocardial work such that ischaemia is worsened. Many dysrhythmias can be prevented or abolished by relief of pain and anxiety, correction of hypoxaemia and treatment of heart failure.

Heart failure complicates about a quarter to a half of myocardial infarcts, and arises from the loss of contractility in the damaged myocardium. Myofibril shortening no longer produces a forceful contraction, but allows the injured myocardium to bulge passively outwards during ventricular systole. As a result, the ejection fraction falls and there is a concomitant rise in the left ventricular end-diastolic pressure (LVEDP). A fall in the intra-aortic pressure reduces coronary artery perfusion and this, with arterial hypoxaemia and acidosis, leads to a further reduction in myocardial performance. The development of heart failure is primarily determined by the extent of myocardial necrosis; loss of over 40 per cent of the left ventricular myocardium is associated with cardiogenic shock and a high mortality. Loss of myocardium may be acute or acute-on-chronic, with a cumulative loss of contracting myocardium following more than one ischaemic event.

Cardiogenic shock complicates about 10 per cent of acute myocardial infarcts, and is characterised by hypotension, oliguria and peripheral hypoperfusion. Although it usually occurs as a consequence of extensive myocardial infarction, other underlying causes (e.g. pulmonary embolism, cardiac tamponade or acute mitral incompetence) need excluding since they require specific therapy.

Hypertension may be caused by sympathetic overactivity in the early stages of acute myocardial infarction (Webb et al, 1972), or may have been present beforehand. If the blood pressure remains elevated after pain relief and treatment of cardiac failure, hypotensive therapy should be administered. If sympathetic overactivity is suspected, beta-blockade is the logical approach, although care is needed in case cardiac failure is precipitated. Alternatively a peripheral vasodilator may be effective, and will additionally relieve any associated left ventricular failure. Controlling the blood pressure in the acute phase of myocardial infarction will reduce myocardial oxygen requirements and aid myocardial perfusion, and thus may limit the size of the infarct.

Pericarditis is common (about 20 per cent of cases), and is characterised by precordial pain made worse by inspiration and lying flat. A pericardial friction rub is usually audible, but may be very localised and transient. Treatment with aspirin is usually effective and pain settles within 48 hours.

Dressler's syndrome presents as recurrence of pericardial pain in the first six weeks following myocardial infarction, and is associated with fever, pleurisy and a high ESR. It probably has an autoimmune basis and antibodies to myocardial tissue are sometimes detectable in the serum. Mild cases may be treated with aspirin or indomethacin, but severe cases often require a short course of corticosteroids.

Cardiac arrest complicates about 3 per cent of cases that reach hospital and may be recurrent. Circulatory standstill is usually associated with ventricular fibrillation, asystole or electromechanical dissociation (EMD), although many other dysrhythmias can have serious haemodynamic consequences during the acute phase of myocardial infarction (e.g. supraventricular tachycardia, ventricular tachycardia and complete heart block). Resuscitation methods have recently been modified ('new cardiopulmonary resuscitation') and are described in chapter 11.

RIGHT VENTRICULAR INFARCTION

Although coronary artery disease and subsequent infarction usually result in left ventricular dysfunction, the right ventricle may also be involved, either alone or with the left ventricle (Cohn et al, 1974). Estimates from post-mortem studies suggest an incidence of between 8 and 14 per cent (Wartman and Hellerstein, 1948), but involvement via extension from acute inferior myocardial infarction is very common (Rodrigues et al, 1986). Early recognition is required since sudden and profound haemodynamic effects may develop which can be treated or even averted by intravenous fluids. Despite high right-sided intracardiac pressures, these patients usually need expansion of the intravascular volume to maintain left-sided pressures and cardiac output. Inappropriate treatment with pressor agents (e.g. dopamine) or diuretics may be fatal.

Patients present with right ventricular failure disproportionate to left ventricular failure, and the clinical appearance may suggest cardiac tamponade. The right atrial pressure is elevated to about 20 mmHg and systemic hypotension is common. The neck veins are distended and fail to empty on inspiration (*Kussmaul's sign*). A systolic murmur which increases with inspiration, caused by functional tricuspid regurgitation secondary to right ventricular dilatation, may be heard at the left sternal edge. Electrocardiography is frequently unhelpful, even if the V4R lead is used. Echocardiography will exclude small pericardial effusions (which may not be suspected radiologically) and often shows a dilated right ventricle. Significant right ventricular infarction is best detected and followed by radionuclide ventriculography (Rodrigues et al, 1986). Measurement of intracardiac pressures will support the diagnosis, and is of major value during therapy to optimise cardiac output.

LEFT VENTRICULAR ANEURYSM

Major coronary artery occlusion frequently leads to sudden death, but if the patient survives, destruction of cardiac muscle and subsequent replacement by scar tissue can lead to the formation of a cardiac aneurysm. The incidence of left ventricular aneurysm is between 10 and 15 per cent of patients following acute myocardial infarction. They are more common in the presence of diffuse coronary artery disease, hypertension or where there has been extensive myocardial damage. The site is usually anterolateral (60 per cent), whilst 20 per cent occur in the inferior wall. The apex and septum are sometimes also affected. During ventricular systole, the aneurysm bulges outwards and thus reduces the ejection fraction by passively absorbing the force of myocardial contraction. The aneurysm itself may act as a focus for abnormal electrical activity (often ventricular tachycardia) and also as a site for thrombus formation. Systemic embolisation complicates about 50 per cent of cases. Death in patients with cardiac aneurysms is associated with either a dysrhythmia or systemic embolisation, and it is rare for cardiac rupture to take place through the aneurysm (Alpert and Braunwald, 1984).

Patients are often identified because of refractory left ventricular failure, or because of persistent ST elevation on the electrocardiogram. Diagnosis may be confirmed by a standard chest radiograph, echocardiography or a MUGA scan. The definitive investigation is left ventriculography, which is normally performed with coronary angiography. Surgical excision is often combined with revascularisation procedures (40 per cent) and postoperative mortality is about 7 per cent. The five-year survival is nearly 70 per cent (Keenan et al, 1985).

MURAL THROMBI

Left ventricular mural thrombi may develop over areas of acutely inflamed endocardium following acute myocardial infarction. They may become dislodged (especially if there are paroxysmal dysrhythmias) and lead to peripheral arterial embolisation. A left atrial thrombus often forms when the left atrium is dilated, as in mitral valve disease and left ventricular failure, especially in the presence of atrial fibrillation.

Low-dose heparin therapy may be helpful in the prevention of mural thrombosis but patients with recurrent dysrhythmias, severe heart failure and dyskinetic hearts should be fully anticoagulated with warfarin.

Silent myocardial infarcts with subsequent embolisation may frequently present as a cerebrovascular accident. An electrocardiogram should therefore be carried out in all cases of stroke.

CARDIAC RUPTURE

After dysrhythmias and cardiogenic shock, the commonest cause of death following acute myocardial infarction is cardiac rupture, which complicates about 10 per cent of cases (Mundth, 1972; Alpert and Braunwald, 1984). It usually occurs in the healing stages following infarction (three to five days) and the risk is higher in the presence of hypertension, diffuse coronary artery disease, anticoagulant therapy and extensive infarction. It is more common in women (M : F = 1 : 4), especially the elderly, and with their first infarct.

Rupture of the free wall of the left ventricle

The commonest site for rupture is through the free left ventricular wall. It classically occurs in the first week following infarction, manifesting as chest pain, hypotension, dyspnoea and distended neck veins. Death is rapid and caused by an acute haemopericardium leading to cardiac tamponade. Recurrent chest pain without ECG changes may warn of imminent rupture, and cardiac collapse in the presence of normal complexes on the electrocardiogram is typical (electromechanical dissociation).

Occasionally, these patients may present subacutely with a slowly accumulating haemopericardium giving rise to cardiac tamponade. Others may seem to have developed a left ventricular aneurysm, but the dilatation is in fact a pseudo-aneurysm of a partially contained rupture. The walls are formed by organised clot and fibrous tissue, and may be demonstrated by echocardiography or ventriculography. Differentiation from a true ventricular aneurysm is important, since complete rupture may occur at any time (Vlodaver et al, 1975).

Rupture of the interventricular septum

The interventricular septum is supplied by both the left and the right coronary arteries, but occasionally by the left coronary artery alone. These patients are at risk of septal infarction and subsequent rupture following thrombosis of the left coronary artery. Rupture of the septum affects 2 per cent of cases of acute myocardial infarction, and it is frequently a late complication, occurring in the healing phase. A left-to-right shunt is formed, with blood being forced from the powerful left ventricle into the right ventricle, resulting in a marked fall in cardiac output with pulmonary circuit overload and severe pulmonary oedema. A loud pansystolic murmur is audible at the left sternal edge, with a systolic thrill. Chest pain is usual at the time of rupture, which typically occurs four to five days after the onset of the acute myocardial infarction.

Rupture of the papillary muscles

The papillary muscles are projections of the ventricular endocardium which attach to the tough chordae tendineae which anchor the leaflets of the mitral and tricuspid valves. They may become ischaemic and infarcted like any other part of the ventricular myocardium, and rupture in the healing stages. The posteromedial papillary muscle can rupture as a consequence of inferior myocardial infarction or, more rarely, the anterolateral papillary muscle may rupture following anteroseptal infarction. Acute mitral regurgitation results, with a fall in cardiac output and acute pulmonary oedema. An apical pansystolic murmur develops, which radiates to the axilla. Prognosis is better than for septal rupture, and depends upon the degree of left ventricular dysfunction (Alpert and Braunwald, 1984).

SILENT MYOCARDIAL INFARCTION

Most cases of myocardial infarction are diagnosed as a result of typical signs and symptoms. However, the diagnosis may sometimes pass unrecognised in the acute phase because of atypical symptoms, especially if the patient has not suffered any pain. The sudden onset of cardiac failure without any prior warning is a typical example. Such myocardial infarcts are often only discovered when a routine ECG is performed, and are known as 'silent' myocardial infarcts. Various theories have been advanced to explain why some ischaemic episodes are perceived, whilst others are not. It may be that silent episodes involve smaller areas of the myocardium, or perhaps that the patient's pain threshold is higher. The pain mechanism may be defective, and this particularly applies to patients with diabetes and cardiac neuropathy. Asymptomatic coronary disease may present with silent myocardial infarction, sudden cardiac death or episodes of silent ischaemia on Holter monitoring. Prolonged periods of Holter monitoring have demonstrated that two-thirds of ischaemic episodes may be pain-free, with the ischaemic episodes lasting from a few seconds to many hours. The prevalence of unrecognised myocardial infarction is commoner than might be expected. The Framingham study suggests that about one-third of infarcts may occur this way (Kannel and Abbott, 1984). However, although initial symptoms are absent, 14 per cent of these patients later develop angina, and about 5 per cent die each year following the diagnosis. The 10-year mortality in these patients is higher than that in patients with symptomatic myocardial infarction. It seems likely that, since this group of patients does not receive typical post-infarction advice and intervention, prognosis is worse.

THE DYSRHYTHMIAS

Acute myocardial infarction commonly causes potentially fatal dysrhythmias, and their detection and treatment was the primary reason for the creation of coronary care units. It is probable that both the size and the location of the infarction play an important part in their aetiology. Dysrhythmias need swift and effective therapy if there is circulatory impairment or compromised ischaemic myocardium, or if they predispose to more severe (malignant) dysrhythmias such as ventricular tachycardia or ventricular fibrillation.

Following acute myocardial infarction, patients almost invariably show overactivity of the autonomic nervous system (Webb et al, 1972). Vagal overactivity is particularly common with inferior and posterior myocardial infarction, manifest as a sinus bradycardia, atrioventricular blockade and hypotension. Sympathetic overactivity (tachycardia and transient hypertension) may be present in nearly half of all patients (particularly those with anterior infarction) and lowers the threshold for ventricular fibrillation.

Dysrhythmias may arise by one or more of the following mechanisms:

● Abnormal impulse formation
● Abnormal conduction
● Ectopic activity

The cardiac dysrhythmias may then be classified as in table 10.1.

Table 10.1. A classification of cardiac dysrhythmias.

Abnormal impulse formation and ectopic beats	*Conduction disturbances*

1. At the sino-atrial node
  Sinus arrhythmia
  Sinus bradycardia
  Sinus tachycardia
  Sinus arrest
	1. In the sino-atrial node
	  Sino-atrial block
	
	2. In the atrioventricular node
	  First, second and third-degree AV block

2. In the atria
  Atrial ectopic beats
  Atrial tachycardia
  Atrial flutter
  Atrial fibrillation
  Wandering atrial pacemaker
	3. In the bundles of His
	  Left bundle branch block
	  Right bundle branch block
	  Left anterior and posterior hemiblocks

3. In the atrioventricular node
  Nodal ectopic beats
  Junctional rhythm
  Junctional tachycardia
	4. Others
	  Intra-atrial block
	  Ventricular pre-excitation
	  Atrioventricular dissociation

4. In the ventricles
  Ventricular ectopic beats
  Idioventricular rhythm
  Ventricular tachycardia
  Ventricular fibrillation	

Consequences of cardiac dysrhythmias

Clinical consequences of dysrhythmias arise because of impaired circulation or myocardial oxygenation. Such consequences are extremely variable but are always more pronounced in patients with cardiac disease. The healthy heart can withstand many rhythm disturbances but the diseased heart cannot, and sustained tachycardias may present with circulatory collapse or ischaemic pain. Any circulatory embarrassment is serious following acute myocardial infarction, since it may compromise perfusion in areas of marginally ischaemic myocardium. If these then become infarcted, the cycle may be repeated.

Increases in heart rate are associated with a reduction in diastolic timing. Ventricular filling may therefore be critically reduced with a dramatic fall in cardiac output. Coronary arterial blood flow also takes place during diastole, especially to the left ventricle. A shortened filling time may reduce oxygen supply to the myocardium at a time when demand is high, and this may precipitate angina or even myocardial infarction.

A final consideration is the synchrony of atrioventricular contraction. The acute loss of atrial transport (e.g. at the onset of atrial fibrillation) may severely impair cardiac output if the diseased heart is dependent on atrial systole.

Management of acute dysrhythmias

Asymptomatic disturbances of rhythm are common and were discovered in the early days of ambulatory monitoring. Treatment is not usually required unless they are producing distressing symptoms. However, ventricular dysrhythmias may occasionally give early warning of myocardial ischaemia or cardiomyopathy, and should perhaps be further investigated. Within the coronary care unit, treatment is usually given for those rhythm disturbances that:

1. Are producing or will soon produce haemodynamic decompensation

2. May be a precursor of cardiac arrest

The treatment of acute rhythm disturbances aims to restore normal sinus rhythm and to prevent recurrence. Often establishment of sinus rhythm is not possible (e.g. in chronic atrial fibrillation) and treatment is then designed to slow the ventricular rate and increase cardiac output.

The treatment is usually either electrical or pharmacological. If drugs are used, these should be given intravenously, since absorption by other routes may be slowed because a low cardiac output will impair tissue perfusion.

Wherever possible, attention should be directed towards the precipitating cause. Pain, fear, hypoxia, acidosis and electrolyte imbalance should be considered. Restoration of normal rhythm will be difficult if these factors remain uncorrected.

The bradydysrhythmias

Bradycardia usually occurs either as a result of sino-atrial dysfunction, when the generation of the impulse at the SA node is inhibited, or when conduction through the heart is slowed or blocked (heart block). Bradycardia predisposes to cardiac standstill which may present as Stokes–Adams attacks, during which the patient transiently loses consciousness. Although most often caused by sudden ventricular standstill, these attacks may be associated with short bursts of ventricular tachycardia or fibrillation.

Sinus bradycardia

This is arbitrarily defined as a sinus rhythm slower than 60 beats per minute. It is common in normal individuals especially during sleep and in those who are physically fit. It may complicate hypothyroidism, raised intracranial pressure or infections such as acute rheumatic fever or typhoid fever. Drug therapy with digoxin, beta-blockers, disopyramide and procainamide is also associated with a sinus bradycardia.

It is seen in about one-third of patients following myocardial infarction, especially acute inferior infarction. Bradycardia here may be caused by stimulation of afferent vagal fibres which are more frequent on the inferior surface of the heart. In addition, infarction may lead to increased acetylcholine release from autonomic fibres in the atria and atrioventricular node, making bradycardia more likely. The slowing in heart rate is a protective mechanism which attempts to limit myocardial work by the acutely injured heart. However, it may result in hypotension secondary to a low cardiac output which reduces coronary perfusion. Escape rhythms and ventricular ectopic activity are also more likely, and may predispose to ventricular tachycardia and fibrillation.

Symptoms are usually not present, but sudden bradycardia may cause syncope. No therapy is required unless there are signs of a low cardiac output, when a single dose of atropine (0.3 to 0.6 mg) is usually sufficient to raise the pulse and restore blood pressure to normal. Further doses can be given at two to three minute intervals up to a total dose of 2.4 mg. Sympathomimetic agents such as adrenaline or isoprenaline may be used, but should be administered with care in acute myocardial infarction, since increased myocardial work may result in extension of the infarct size.

Temporary cardiac pacing may then be considered. Atrial pacing is ideal, as it has less of an effect on cardiovascular haemodynamics than does traditional ventricular pacing (since atrial systole is preserved). However, ventricular wires are usually more stable, and should be used preferentially if the sinus bradycardia has complicated anterior myocardial infarction, since sudden, complete atrioventricular block is likely to follow. Temporary pacing to raise the sinus rate will sometimes control ectopic (escape) ventricular activity (ventricular ectopics, ventricular tachycardia) without need to resort to antidysrhythmic agents.

Prenalterol is a selective beta-1 adrenergic agonist which may help reverse beta-blockade. Care is needed during administration since it may increase ectopic ventricular activity.

Sino-atrial block

If the SA node fails to initiate one or more stimuli or there is block of transmission of the impulse into the atria, *sino-atrial block* is said to occur (figure 10.1). The atria and ventricles will not be activated and long pauses may result. The causes of sino-atrial block are the same as for sinus bradycardia. They are particularly common

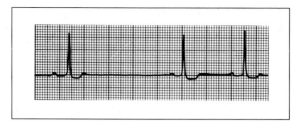

Fig. 10.1   ECG: sino-atrial block

following inferior myocardial infarction, since the right coronary artery supplies the SA node in 50–60 per cent of patients and the branch to the SA node may be affected.

Block at the SA node has been classified in a similar fashion to *atrioventricular block* (i.e. first, second and third degree), although first-degree block cannot be recognised electrically.

Second-degree SA block may be present in two forms.

1. The PP interval becomes progressively shorter until there is a long pause between two beats (*sino-atrial Wenckebach*). This is very similar in appearance to a sinus arrhythmia, from which it must be differentiated.

2. A long pause appears following multiple regular PP cycles. The frequency of the pause may be every three or four beats, although if it occurs every other beat a sinus bradycardia will result from halving of the pulse rate.

Third-degree SA block (*sinus arrest*) is characterised by cardiac standstill for a variable period of time. Escape beats from the atria, the AV node or ventricles often take over control of the heart rhythm (*escape rhythm*).

Dropped beats may be appreciated on feeling the pulse and are sometimes felt by the patient ('my heart keeps stopping'). Syncope may occur with prolonged pauses.

No treatment is required if pauses are short and asymptomatic. If drugs are responsible, they should be stopped or the dose reduced. Atropine, isoprenaline or cardiac pacing is sometimes required, as in sinus bradycardia.

Junctional (nodal) rhythm

If junctional rhythm is present, the atria and ventricles are often stimulated simultaneously by a pacemaker in the AV junctional region (figure 10.2). The stimulus spreads normally into the ventricles, but will pass into the atria in a

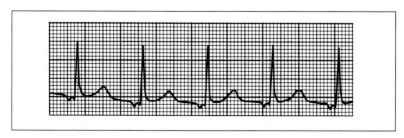

Fig 10.2   ECG: junctional bradycardia, lead aVF. The junctional focus has also activated the atria, as shown by the fact each ventricular complex is preceded by an inverted P wave

retrograde fashion. As a result, the P wave may appear slightly before, after or buried in the QRS complex, depending on the velocity of antegrade and retrograde conduction. The retrograde spread can be recognised by the shape of the P wave which is abnormal and usually inverted (except in lead aVR).

Nodal rhythm is conducted to the ventricles alone if there is retrograde block or interference with retrograde conduction by simultaneous sinus impulses. In both cases, the sinus P wave is dissociated from the junctional QRS complexes (i.e. there is AV dissociation).

Junctional rhythms are usually produced by sinus node depression as described before, but may be a transient normal occurrence. They are often seen in anaesthetised, hypoxic or acidotic patients.

Because the atria and ventricles beat simultaneously, the atria contract against closed mitral and tricuspid valves. Blood is pumped retrogradely into the superior vena cava and neck resulting in the appearance of giant 'v' waves in the venous pulse.

The dysrhythmia is usually short-lived, and no treatment is required apart from stopping any medication that may be depressing the SA node. Isoprenaline or atropine may restore sinus rhythm.

Conduction disturbances

Conduction abnormalities arising within the AV node, bundle of His or bundle branches may result in bradycardia with hypotension and reduced cardiac output. Alternatively, there may be ventricular standstill and death.

Atrioventricular block (heart block)

Heart block exists when conduction from the atria to the ventricles is either slowed or blocked. This condition may be transient, intermittent or permanent. The dysfunction may be classed as first, second and third-degree atrioventricular block.

First-degree AV block

The PR interval varies with age, but does not usually exceed 0.2 second. In first-degree heart block (figure 10.3) the impulse passing through the AV node is delayed resulting in an increase in the PR interval on the ECG. No change in heart rate occurs, and it is primarily an electrocardiographic finding. It complicates up to 14 per cent of acute myocardial infarcts (Alpert and Braunwald, 1984) and is more common with inferior myocardial infarction.

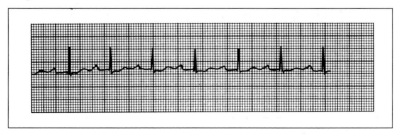

Fig 10.3   ECG: first-degree atrioventricular block

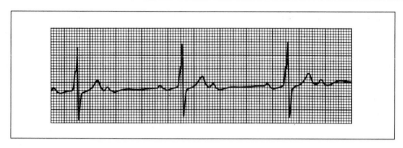

Fig. 10.4   ECG: second-degree atrioventricular block (Mobitz type II), with 2 : 1 AV conduction

Second-degree AV block

This is a partial block which occurs when some atrial impulses fail to reach the ventricles (figure 10.4). This results in so-called 2 : 1, 3 : 1 or 4 : 1 heart block, where the figures show the ratio of atrial to ventricular beats. There are two types of second-degree AV block.

1. *Wenckebach (Mobitz type I)*   This is the commonest form of second-degree heart block (90 per cent). Each successive stimulus from the atria finds it more difficult to pass through the AV junction, reflected as progressive prolongation of the PR interval with each beat. Eventually, the stimulus is unable to pass through to the ventricles and the P wave is not followed by a QRS complex. When the next P wave reaches the AV junction, it is able to pass through normally since the tissues have recovered, and the cycle is then repeated. The frequency of dropped beats varies with the number of beats per cycle which may be numerous or very few.

2. *Mobitz type II*   Here, the AV junction fails to respond to each atrial stimulus and more than one atrial beat is required before the stimulus can pass to the ventricles. The PR interval is constant and the pulse rate is regular. The QRS complex may be widened because simultaneous blockade of the His–Purkinje fibres often coexists.

Third-degree (complete) heart block

This affects about 5 to 10 per cent of patients with acute myocardial infarction, and again is more common with acute inferior myocardial infarction. Atrial stimuli are blocked at the AV junction or below the bundle of His (see figure 10.5). An escape rhythm takes over from within the distal AV node, the His–Purkinje system or ventricles.

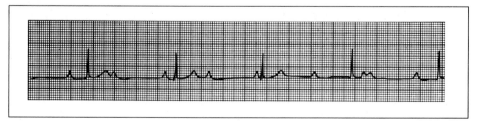

Fig 10.5   ECG: third-degree atrioventricular block

When complete heart block is due a lesion within the AV node, the block develops slowly and is characterised by an escape rhythm of 40 to 60 beats per minute. The QRS complex is narrow as it originates just below the node. Patients with complete heart block originating within the node have a mortality of 20 to 25 per cent.

If complete heart block complicates acute anteroseptal infarction, the block usually originates in the bundle branches which may have undergone necrosis. The onset is usually sudden and the emerging pacemaker is slow (fewer than 45 beats per minute). The wide QRS complexes resemble those of bundle branch block. However, if the pacemaker arises within the AV junction, the QRS may be near normal in configuration. The rate is slow and regular (30 to 60 beats per minute), but may be irregular and fall to very low rates. The faster rates are more commonly seen when the pacemaker arises in the His–Purkinje fibres, and the lower rates are more usual when there is a ventricular origin. Irregularity of the QRS complexes is seen when the origin of the stimulus varies, or when there is transient ventricular standstill or ventricular ectopic beats. P waves appear regularly, but have no fixed relationship to the QRS complexes. When complete heart block complicates acute anteroseptal infarction, the mortality is very high (75 per cent), although this is probably because of associated left ventricular damage, rather than the heart block itself.

Aetiology of heart block

Fibrosis of the AV junction is probably the most common cause of complete heart block, although acute and chronic ischaemia are often the underlying causes, particularly following acute inferior myocardial infarction.

The AV node may also be transiently affected in myocarditis and collagen disorders or by drugs such as digoxin and beta-blockers.

Clinical features

First-degree heart block produces no symptoms, although the intensity of the first heart sound is inversely proportional to the duration of the PR interval. Second-degree heart block is also usually asymptomatic, but may be associated with palpitations due to forceful contractions or dropped beats. Complete heart block may be asymptomatic in the presence of a fast, regular escape rhythm. However, the pulse is usually slow and regular, and the pulse pressure widened; systolic blood pressure is elevated by forceful ventricular ejection due to the high stroke volume, and the diastolic blood pressure falls because the prolonged diastolic period allows the blood pressure to fall by about 50 to 60 mmHg. Cannon waves may be seen occasionally in the jugular vein when the right atrium contracts against a closed tricuspid valve. Stokes–Adams attacks may occur, particularly with acute onset heart block.

Investigations

Acute onset and transient complete heart block complicating acute myocardial infarction will not usually need investigation, but chronic and persistent conduction abnormalities may need further elucidation.

His-bundle electrocardiography may help in locating the site of the block since the normal ECG does not yield much information about electrical activity within the AV junction. His-bundle activity is recorded by an electrode placed in the right ventricle close to the tricuspid valve. The usual technique is to pass a wire from the femoral vein into the right atrium to lodge close to the interventricular septum. Bipolar electrodes from this area show spikes of potential when the atrium depolarises, followed by a smaller 'His' deflection after conduction delay in the AV node. Later, there is the major depolarisation of the ventricles. These three groups of electrical spikes are called:

1. A spikes: caused by depolarisation of the low right atrium

2. H spikes: caused by passage of the impulse through the bundle of His

3. V spikes: caused by the start of ventricular depolarisation close to the recording lead

The intervals between these spikes can be measured, and the site of the block defined.

Treatment

First- and second-degree (Wenckebach) heart block usually need no treatment, although cardiodepressant drugs should be stopped. Mobitz type II carries a bad prognosis by virtue of the high risk of progression to symptomatic complete heart block.

Symptomatic heart block requires insertion of a temporary pacemaker, although an isoprenaline infusion or an atropine bolus can sometimes help as a temporary measure to raise the ventricular rate. Pacemakers are discussed in detail in chapter 12.

Atrioventricular dissociation

This is often confused with complete heart block, and occurs when a ventricular escape rhythm emerges following vagal depression of the sino-atrial node (figure 10.6). The atria and ventricles beat independently, the ventricular rate being the same or slightly faster than the atrial rate. If the ventricles and atria contract simultaneously, the AV node is stimulated at the same time and usually becomes refractory. However, if an atrial contraction reaches it whilst it is non-refractory, it is conducted normally (a *capture beat*).

The rhythm manifests as P waves which bear no relationship to the QRS complexes and, as sinus rhythm is slower than ventricular rhythm, the PP interval is longer than

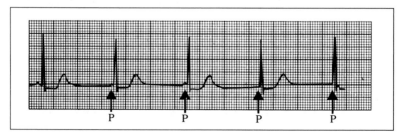

Fig 10.6   ECG: atrioventricular dissociation, with respective atrial and ventricular rates of 49 and 51 per minute. The last two P waves are covered by superimposed QRS waves

the RR interval. As a result, the P waves gradually overtake the QRS complexes, become superimposed upon them, and eventually appear after the QRS complex. When the P wave is far enough beyond the QRS, a sinus beat will 'capture' a QRS, resulting in an early PQRS complex. AV dissociation should therefore always be suspected where the PR interval progressively shortens. The condition is usually benign and may complicate acute infections, myocardial infarction or drug therapy. No treatment is required unless drugs are responsible, when the medication should be withdrawn. Demonstrating atrioventricular dissociation is very important in the diagnosis of ventricular tachycardia (see p. 215).

Intraventricular block

Conduction disturbance may also arise within the ventricles. Bundle branch block may complicate 10–20 per cent of cases with acute myocardial infarction, and is more common with anterior infarction. Right bundle branch block (RBBB, 2 per cent) is associated with the later development of complete heart block. Left anterior hemiblock (LAHB, 4 per cent) is considered benign. Left posterior hemiblock (LPHB, 1 per cent) is usually only seen with very large infarctions, since it has a good blood supply. It is therefore associated with a high mortality, as is left bundle branch block (LBBB). Bifascicular block commonly leads to complete atrioventricular heart block and prophylactic pacing wires are commonly inserted.

Ventricular asystole

Sudden death associated with acute myocardial infarction is usually due to ventricular fibrillation (VF). Even apparent asystole on monitors may in fact be fine VF and, in the clinical setting of acute myocardial infarction, defibrillation may be the first line therapy of choice.

Asystole (figure 10.7) may complicate up to 14 per cent of patients admitted to coronary care, and the prognosis is very bad: the mortality exceeds 90 per cent (Alpert and Braunwald, 1984).

The tachydysrhythmias

Myocardial infarction directly increases sympathetic cardiac stimulation via receptors in the atria and ventricles. There may also be increased plasma concentrations of catecholamines with local release of catecholamines from nerve endings within the

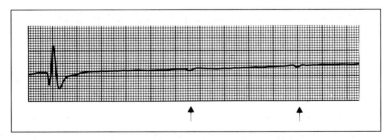

Fig 10.7 ECG: ventricular asystole. The arrows indicate residual atrial complexes

heart. The ischaemic heart is highly vulnerable to the dysrhythmogenic effect of sympathetic stimulation, and resulting tachydysrhythmias may have a deleterious effect upon cardiac function following acute myocardial infarction. These abnormally fast rhythms increase myocardial oxygen requirements, and compromise cardiac output by limiting the time available for coronary perfusion and ventricular filling in diastole. Aggressive management is therefore indicated. Therapy not only involves the use of antidysrhythmic drugs, but also the correction of hypoxaemia, acid–base balance and electrolyte levels.

Mechanism of the tachydysrhythmias

There are two major mechanisms that lead to the production of the dysrhythmias:

● Enhanced automaticity
● Re-entry (circus) movement

Enhanced automaticity

Automatic cells from specialised areas of the myocardium have the property of slow (phase 4) diastolic depolarisation (see chapter 2). When a critical point is reached (the *threshold potential*) an action potential automatically develops. The intrinsic rhythmicity of the heart is thus governed by the speed of phase 4 depolarisation. If there has been an ischaemic (or metabolic) insult to these cells, the speed of phase 4 depolarisation may quicken leading to 'enhanced automaticity'. In other words spontaneous discharge from pacemaker cells will lead to a speeding up of the heart rate.

Re-entry

This mechanism describes the continual circus movement of a single impulse around a normal or abnormal electrical pathway. There must be two interconnecting pathways which under abnormal circumstances function independently (e.g. have different refractory periods when stimulated). This is shown diagrammatically in figure 10.8.

Re-entry can take place within the AV and SA nodes, in the atria and ventricles, and between the atria and ventricles via an accessory pathway (*reciprocating tachycardia*).

Supraventricular tachydysrhythmias

The main supraventricular tachydysrhythmias are atrial tachycardia, atrial flutter and atrial fibrillation. Each may present acutely as a sustained or a paroxysmal dysrhythmia. Treatment is usually directed towards the restoration of sinus rhythm, although in the case of chronic or unstable dysrhythmias, controlling the ventricular rate is the aim of therapy. Other supraventricular causes of fast or irregular heart rhythms are sinus tachycardia and atrial ectopic beats.

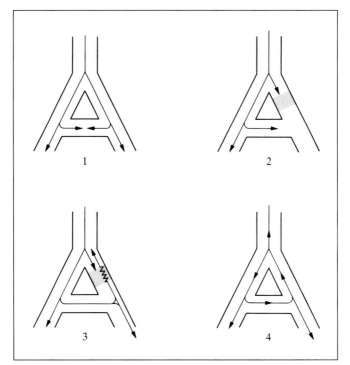

Fig. 10.8   Circus movement during re-entry tachycardia
(1) Normal electrical conduction through a common proximal piece of tissue which splits into
two pathways.
(2) A unidirectional block develops in one limb of tissue (possibly because of a slowing in the
refractory period) and this fails to conduct the impulse. The other pathway conducts normally.
(3) The normal conduction wave is carried round to the proximal side of the block which, if
it has recovered functionally, will transmit the impulse in a retrograde direction.
(4) If the normal limb of tissue has recovered, it can be stimulated by the returning impulse,
and a circus movement about the area of conducting tissue is set up which is self-propagating.
This gives rise to a re-entrant dysrhythmia.

Sinus tachycardia

Sinus tachycardia is arbitrarily defined as a sinus rhythm greater than 100 beats per
minute, and commonly ranges between 100 and 160 beats per minute. At higher heart
rates, the P wave tends to merge with the preceding T wave, and the PR and QT intervals decrease as the heart rate increases.

A sinus tachycardia during exercise is, of course, normal and in young individuals
can sometimes attain a rate of 180 beats per minute. At rest, a sinus tachycardia may
be due to anxiety, fever, drugs or shock. Patients may complain of palpitations – particularly those who are anxious.

A sinus tachycardia is found in one-third of patients with acute myocardial infarction and represents an attempt to maintain cardiac output in the face of a reduced
stroke volume. The tachycardia may be worsened by increased sympathetic drive due
to anxiety, fear and pain. As a sinus tachycardia is a physiological response to heart
damage, it probably does not require therapy following acute myocardial infarction.
However, if the haemodynamic status is such that beta-blockade can be tolerated,

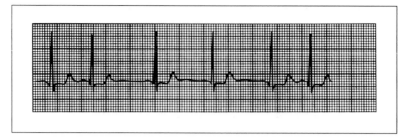

Fig. 10.9   ECG: atrial ectopic beats. Note that the ectopic P waves are slightly different from those of sino-atrial origin

slowing the pulse rate will reduce myocardial work and possibly limit infarct size (Herlitz et al, 1984). Metoprolol is a suitable short-acting beta-blocker, and can be given in doses up to 5 mg (12 mg/min), repeated if required.

The mortality of patients with sinus tachycardia following acute myocardial infarction is higher than for those with sinus bradycardia, and death is usually due to left ventricular failure (Bigger et al, 1977).

Atrial ectopic beats (premature atrial contractions, PACs)

Atrial ectopic beats are very common is both health and disease, and occur when an atrial focus discharges before the sino-atrial pacemaker. They are seen on the ECG as a premature (often abnormally shaped) P wave, usually followed by a normal QRS complex (figure 10.9). An incomplete compensatory pause follows the ectopic beat because the premature impulse depolarises the SA node which must recover before it is able to initiate another sinus beat. The PP interval is therefore only slightly longer than the normal PP interval. Complete compensatory pauses are a feature of ventricular ectopic beats.

Conduction of atrial impulses to the ventricles depends on the recovery status of an AV node. If an atrial ectopic arises near the AV node (seen as an abnormal P wave and a short PR interval) the AV node may be refractory. The impulse is blocked, and no QRS complex follows. Other atrial impulses (normal or shortened PR interval) may find that part of the conducting system below the AV node is refractory (e.g. one of the bundle branches), and then an aberrantly conducted beat is seen. A prolonged PR interval is seen when an atrial ectopic beat encounters a partially refractory AV node, and is thus delayed.

In heart disease, atrial ectopics often precede sustained atrial dysrhythmias. Junctional ectopic beats may also be seen as QRS complexes occurring in the absence of a preceding P wave, with the P wave buried within the QRS complex or even after it.

Atrial ectopic beats are usually asymptomatic and cause no haemodynamic upset. Generally, no therapy is required unless they are frequent or multifocal in origin. In the post-infarct patient, excessive autonomic activity is associated with frequent atrial ectopics and may be abolished by beta-adrenergic blockers or sedation. However, care is required, since frequent atrial ectopic beats may indicate atrial dilatation in early heart failure. Atrial ectopics need therapy if they are seen to be initiating re-entry tachycardias.

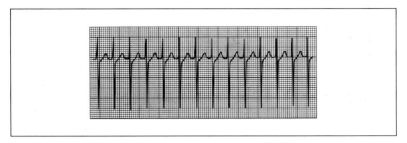

Fig. 10.10 ECG: supraventricular tachycardia

Supraventricular tachycardia

It is sometimes not possible to determine the exact atrial rhythm during tachycardias unless specialised (e.g. oesophageal) leads are used, and the term *supraventricular tachycardia* (SVT) is generally applied to tachydysrhythmias arising above the AV junction (figure 10.10).

Paroxysmal atrial tachycardia

Paroxysmal atrial tachycardia (PAT) is caused by the rapid discharge of an atrial pacemaker at a regular rate of between 160 and 250 beats per minute. The stimulus arises from one or more foci in the atria, and a re-entry mechanism commonly occurs through the AV node (90 per cent). This is either solely within the node (58 per cent) or as a reciprocating tachycardia, where antegrade conduction is through the node with re-entry via an accessory pathway (30 per cent). The P wave will be obscured by the simultaneous QRS complex in the former case and the P wave will occur after the QRS complex in reciprocating tachycardias. Re-entry tachycardias start abruptly, often preceded by an abnormal P wave, whereas ectopic tachycardias usually speed up. The heart rhythm is usually regular unless interspersed by atrial ectopics or if beats are blocked at the AV node. P waves are present and usually abnormally shaped. The QRS complexes may be normal or aberrantly conducted.

Aberrant conduction is the term applied when a widened and abnormal QRS complex is seen following a supraventricular beat, and is caused by transmission to the ventricles by an abnormal conduction pathway. Differentiating ventricular ectopic beats from aberrantly conducted supraventricular beats may be difficult. With aberrant conduction P waves may be seen, and the ectopic is of a right bundle branch block (RBBB) pattern. There is no compensatory pause. In contrast, ventricular ectopics usually show a monophasic or biphasic QRS in V1. P waves are not seen and ectopics are followed by a compensatory pause.

PAT versus sinus tachycardia

During a sinus tachycardia, the heart rate is usually less than 140 beats per minute, and varies with respiration. It does not start or finish abruptly and P waves are normal. 'Sinus' rates of about 150 per minute are on closer inspection usually due

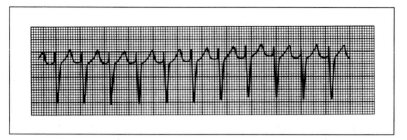

Fig. 10.11   ECG: junctional tachycardia

to atrial flutter with 2 : 1 block. After cessation, post-tachycardia T wave changes may be seen which can be present for days or weeks. These changes do not occur following sinus tachycardias.

PAT with block

Here, the atrial rate is between 150 and 200 beats per minute, and AV block is present (second or third degree). The ventricular response is usually not rapid and causes little upset in cardiac function. Although classically described in relation to digoxin toxicity, this is only the case in about 10 per cent of cases. Serious heart disease is usually present.

Digoxin should be withdrawn and potassium given. Phenytoin and propranolol may be effective. If the dysrhythmia occurs in the absence of digoxin, the drug can be used with good effect.

Junctional (AV nodal) tachycardia

The majority of junctional tachycardias (except for escape rhythms) are paroxysmal, caused by circus movement involving the atrioventricular node (figure 10.11). Hence therapy directed towards the AV node is usually effective.

A non-paroxysmal junctional (*idionodal*) tachycardia can occur. The heart rate is usually less than 130 beats per minute and the onset and termination are not so abrupt.

Treatment of supraventricular tachycardia

Nearly 30 per cent of episodes of SVT occur in normal hearts. They can also complicate thyrotoxicosis, pulmonary disease, acute and chronic myocardial ischaemia and the Wolff–Parkinson–White syndrome. The urgency of treatment depends upon symptoms and, whilst usually well endured, cardiac output falls as the heart rate rises due to the loss of atrial transport. Ischaemic pain may be produced in patients with coronary artery disease. In the peri-infarction period, ventricular work must be limited to prevent extension of the infarct, and prompt therapy should be given.

Carotid sinus massage may terminate atrial tachycardias or increased AV block to allow differentiation of PAT from atrial flutter (figure 10.12). The carotid sinus is located anterior to the sternomastoid muscle at the upper level or just above the thyroid cartilage. The right carotid artery is massaged against the transverse process

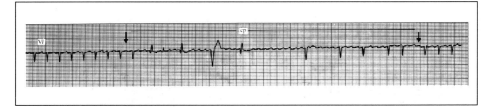

Fig. 10.12 Supraventricular tachycardia slowed by pressure on the carotid sinus (cp = carotid pressure). This has increased block at the atrioventricular node showing that the underlying rhythm is atrial flutter

of the 6th cervical vertebra for 10 to 20 seconds. Massage of the left carotid artery is usually not so successful.

Flutter is never terminated by carotid compression, but it will increase blockade at the AV node, allowing a correct diagnosis of atrial flutter with 2 : 1 block to be differentiated from atrial tachycardia of 150 beats per minute.

Other methods of vagal stimulation are the Valsalva manoeuvre, or glottal stimulation (putting fingers deep in the throat or sucking ice). Eyeball pressure is not recommended since damage to the cornea may result.

The most successful treatment is *d.c. cardioversion*, but this is infrequently used since drug therapy is very effective. Cardioversion is the treatment of choice in the face of rapid haemodynamic deterioration, regardless of prior digitalisation.

There are many drugs that may be employed to restore sinus rhythm. The drug of choice is verapamil. A bolus injection (5 to 10 mg) usually achieves sinus rhythm within two minutes in 90 per cent of cases. It can depress myocardial contractility, and is contraindicated if the patient is taking beta-blockers. Digoxin is also very useful, after which carotid sinus massage can be tried again. Other agents include practolol, disopyramide and amiodarone. Prophylaxis should be considered for repeated and poorly tolerated attacks.

Atrial flutter

Atrial flutter is probably caused by re-entry within the atrial muscle. The atria contract at a rate between 250 and 350 beats per minute, and the ECG shows flutter (F) waves with a sawtooth appearance in the inferior leads (figure 10.13). Leads V1 and

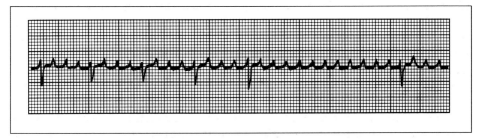

Fig 10.13   ECG: atrial flutter, with varying degrees of atrioventricular block

V2 often appear to show large biphasic P waves. Flutter waves may be obscured by the QRST complexes if the rate is very fast. Although the AV node can respond to atrial rates of about 300 beats per minute, there is usually some degree of AV heart block, often resulting in a ventricular rate of 150 beats per minute (with 2 : 1 block). Higher degrees of blockade usually occur in the presence of drugs or after damage to the conducting system. Vagal stimulation increases AV block and may make the diagnosis more obvious (figure 10.12).

Exercise decreases AV block, and may lead to a doubling of the pulse rate. As a result, the apparently normal patient with a pulse rate of 75 beats per minute may feel faint on exertion when switching from 4 : 1 block to 2 : 1 conduction. During 2 : 1 AV conduction, QRS conduction may be aberrant and appear like ventricular tachycardia on the ECG.

Atrial flutter is usually associated with cardiorespiratory disease or hyperthyroidism. Atrial flutter is unstable and should always be converted to sinus rhythm unless present for years. Cardioversion is the therapy of choice, and generally only low energies are required (25 J). Digoxin converts atrial flutter to atrial fibrillation by increasing the atrial rate. If the digoxin is then stopped, sinus rhythm commonly results, although this may take a few days. Intravenous verapamil increases AV block temporarily, and may produce sinus rhythm in about 20 per cent of cases.

Atrial fibrillation

Paroxysmal or *sustained* atrial fibrillation is one of the most common rhythm disturbances. Amongst the better known underlying causes are ischaemic heart disease, thyrotoxicosis, mitral valve disease, hypertensive heart disease and constrictive pericarditis. *Benign* (or *lone*) atrial fibrillation is that which occurs in the absence of recognisable cardiac disease.

Normal atrial contraction is replaced by a continuous series of irregular fibrillation waves which are ineffective for atrial emptying, and functionally the atria remain in diastole. As such, the presence of atrial fibrillation makes the heart less efficient since atrial systole accounts for 5 to 10 per cent of cardiac output (Matsuda et al, 1983). There is incomplete filling of the ventricles leading to a reduction in stroke volume.

Although the presence of atrial fibrillation makes the heart less efficient, the most important consequence is that of thromboembolism, especially stroke. Lone atrial fibrillation should perhaps not be regarded as benign, since the risks of peripheral embolisation are just as high as in other causes of atrial fibrillation (Brand et al, 1985).

Atrial fibrillation complicating myocardial infarction is usually transient and self-limiting. It may be preceded by prodromal atrial dysrhythmias such as frequent and multifocal atrial ectopics, atrial flutter or PAT. No P waves are visible on the ECG, and the ventricular response is irregular and variable, and in the untreated patient between 100 and 180 beats per minute (figure 10.14). The QRS complexes are usually normal except when the ventricular response is too rapid and aberration may occur. The ventricular response is irregular but when the rate is very fast may appear to be regular.

Symptoms usually depend upon the ventricular rate. Slow rates may be asymptomatic, but faster rates may give rise to palpitations, angina and syncope. Loss of

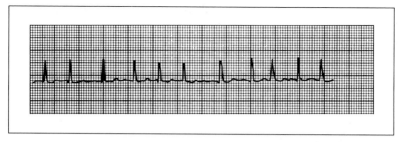

Fig. 10.14   ECG: atrial fibrillation

atrial systole may seriously compromise cardiac output and precipitate heart failure. Thrombosis in the left or right atrial appendage results from stasis, and may give rise to systemic or pulmonary embolisation. This typically occurs when the rhythm changes from fibrillation to sinus rhythm, either spontaneously or as a result of electrical or pharmacological cardioversion. Recent work from the Framingham study (Brand et al, 1985) suggests that all patients with atrial fibrillation (irrespective of cardiac disease) are at risk of stroke, and should receive long-term anticoagulant therapy, provided there are no contraindications.

In acute onset atrial fibrillation, sinus rhythm should always be the aim using d.c. cardioversion and/or drugs.

In patients with atrial fibrillation of more than a few days, the risk of systemic embolisation following cardioversion is 3 to 5 per cent. As such it is probably better to anticoagulate for two to three weeks before elective cardioversion. The energy required is very variable (100 to 400 J) and drug therapy (e.g. quinidine, disopyramide or amiodarone) may be required before, during and after cardioversion.

Controlling the ventricular rate

Control of the ventricular rate is often used in chronic atrial tachydysrhythmias (especially atrial fibrillation), or may be a prelude to elective conversion to sinus rhythm. However, special consideration should be given to patients with abnormal AV conduction (e.g. via anomalous pathways), when suppression of the accessory pathway rather than the AV node is required. Hence, traditional AV blockers such as beta-blockers, verapamil and digoxin are ineffective in the Wolff–Parkinson–White syndrome, and the last agent is usually contraindicated since there is some evidence that digoxin improves conduction through the anomalous pathway, provoking atrial tachycardias.

Idionodal tachycardia (nodal tachycardia)

The normal nodal discharge rate is about 50 to 60 beats per minute. If there is suppression of sinus or atrial pacemaker function, the AV node may take over pacemaker function, with enhanced automaticity. Hence, the rate is usually between 70 and 100 beats per minute. Because the sinus node usually continues to beat, there is a propensity to AV dissociation and capture beats are often seen.

QRS complexes are usually normal unless there is temporary conduction block in one of the bundle branches.

The significance of idionodal tachycardia is the same as that of an idioventricular tachycardia (see p. 216).

Ventricular dysrhythmias

Ventricular dysrhythmias include ventricular ectopics (VEs), ventricular tachycardia (VT), ventricular flutter and ventricular fibrillation (VF). They are associated with myocardial ischaemia, and virtually all cases of myocardial infarction are accompanied by ventricular ectopic beats (Vetter and Julian, 1975). Although infrequent ventricular ectopics do not adversely affect cardiac output, attention has previously been focused on them as 'warning dysrhythmias' (Lown et al, 1967). These were believed to be precursors of ventricular fibrillation, and included:

● Frequent or multifocal ventricular ectopic beats
● Short runs of ventricular tachycardia
● Ventricular bigeminy
● R-on-T ectopics

However, ventricular fibrillation does not always follow these so-called warning dysrhythmias (El Sherif et al, 1976), and occurs without any warning in at least 50 per cent of cases. In addition, successful abolition of these ventricular dysrhythmias with lignocaine does not affect mortality compared with those who are not treated (May et al, 1983).

Therapy now should probably only be considered for ventricular dysrhythmias producing haemodynamic disturbances, repetitive short episodes of ventricular tachycardia and perhaps R-on-T ectopics. Clinical findings such as a persistent third heart sound, early heart failure and prolonged ST elevation may well be better predictors of malignant dysrhythmias.

Ventricular ectopic beats (premature ventricular complexes, PVCs)

Ventricular ectopic beats occur when an ectopic ventricular focus discharges prematurely anywhere within the His–Purkinje system or the ventricles. It can occur at any time in diastole and is followed by a full compensatory pause (since the SA node is not usually penetrated by retrograde activity). The QRS complex is premature, wide (more than 0.12 second), slurred and usually notched (figure 10.15). There is no preceding P wave and the following T wave normally points in the opposite direction. Ventricular ectopics arising from a single focus are usually identical in shape with a fixed coupling interval (variation less than 0.08 second) between ectopics.

Right ventricular ectopics appear like the complexes in left bundle branch block, and left ventricular ectopics appear like the complexes in right bundle branch block. Organic heart disease is nearly always present in patients with ectopic foci in the left ventricle. Those arising in the right ventricle are usually benign and probably do not need treatment. They may be found in healthy individuals, especially in response to

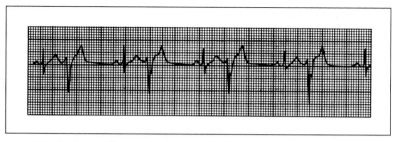

Fig 10.15   ECG: ventricular ectopic beats (ventricular bigeminy)

excitement, tea, coffee, alcohol and cigarettes, and are almost always unifocal in origin.

The *R-on-T phenomenon* refers to the ectopic occurring on the apex of the preceding T wave which sometimes precipitates ventricular tachycardia or fibrillation (Surawicz, 1986).

Therapy

Most ventricular ectopics occur without symptoms and do not require therapy. Reducing the intake of tea or coffee may help. If they produce annoying palpitations, mild sedatives or propranolol may help. Ventricular ectopics complicating congestive heart failure often disappear once the cardiac failure is effectively treated.

Following myocardial infarction, ventricular ectopics exhibiting the R-on-T phenomenon, occurring in salvoes or with multifocal origins probably need treatment. Lignocaine is the usual first line therapy following myocardial infarction, and should be administered to keep the blood levels at 1 to 5 μg/ml. This usually entails a loading bolus of 50 to 100 mg, followed by an infusion of 1 to 4 mg/min. Metabolism of the drug is slow in patients with heart failure and smaller doses will be needed.

Ventricular ectopics complicating digoxin therapy are considered later.

Ventricular tachycardia

Ventricular tachycardia is a life-threatening re-entry dysrhythmia, and may be defined as a succession of three or more beats arising from one or more foci in the ventricles at a rate of over 100 beats per minute. The QRS complexes are widened (longer than 0.12 second) and regular at a rate of 100 to 220 beats per minute (figure 10.16). The atria continue to beat independently, and dissociated P waves may be

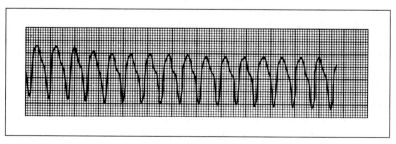

Fig 10.16   ECG: ventricular tachydysrhythmia

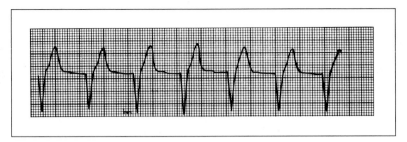

Fig. 10.17   ECG: idioventricular tachydysrhythmia

seen. The atrial rhythm may be faster or slower than the ventricular rate, and usually arises from the sino-atrial node. However, there may be a co-existing atrial tachycardia, atrial fibrillation or junctional rhythm. Occasionally ventricular beats can pass through the node to stimulate the atria retrogradely, and are seen as P waves after the QRS complex. Fusion and capture beats may also appear.

A *capture beat* occurs when an atrial stimulus reaches the AV node when it is not refractory, and is carried through to the ventricles in the normal way.

A *fusion beat* occurs when a normal stimulus meets a ventricular stimulus being conducted retrogradely. The resulting complex looks partly like a normal QRS and partly like a ventricular ectopic.

Both fusion beats and capture beats are preceded by P waves, and considerably help the diagnosis of ventricular tachycardia by proving atrioventricular dissociation.

There are four main types of ventricular tachycardia.

1. *Extrasystolic ventricular tachycardia*   Each paroxysm starts with a ventricular ectopic beat occurring at a fixed interval from the previous QRS complex. At the termination of the tachycardia there is often a long pause before sinus rhythm returns.

2. *Accelerated idioventricular tachycardia*   If the heart rate slows too much, an ectopic pacemaker usually takes over (figure 10.17). When this arises in the ventricles or His–Purkinje system, a slow idioventricular rhythm of less than 60 beats per minute is seen. In certain circumstances (e.g. acute myocardial infarction, hyperkalaemia or digoxin toxicity) this may accelerate for up to 30 beats, when either sinus rhythm takes over or it is replaced by sustained ventricular tachycardia or fibrillation.

3. *Parasystole*   This is a form of dual rhythm where two pacemakers concurrently and independently govern the rhythm of the heart (figure 10.18). Ventricular ectopic beats occur at a fixed rate from another ectopic focus which may be in either the atria or the ventricles. The interval between two premature beats is the same as or a multiple of the interval. Since the parasystolic focus is independent of the regular heart rhythm, there is no fixed relationship and the coupling interval (i.e. the interval between the ectopic beat and the preceding sinus beat) varies.

Normally, the dominant pacemaker in the heart governs and overrides all other pacemakers, and ectopic foci are dominated by faster rhythm. However, in parasystole, the ectopic focus is protected, and cannot be overriden by the faster rhythm. This is because of *entrance block*, a unidirectional block in the vicinity of

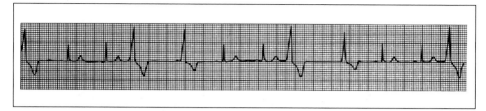

Fig. 10.18 ECG: ventricular parasystole

the ectopic pacemaker. Exit conduction from the focus is however possible from the ectopic stimulus which passes out and acts as a secondary pacemaker. Two pacemakers then exist in the heart, each discharging at its own independent rate, and each activating the heart when the myocardium is in a responsive state. If these two pacemakers discharge at the same time, each activates part of the ventricles, and a fusion beat will arise, giving rise to a QRS complex intermediate between a sinus beat and an ectopic beat. Fusion beats may also be seen in other forms of AV dissociation.

Parasystole is relatively uncommon, and may be seen following myocardial infarction, or in patients taking digoxin. There is no specific therapy, and the dysrhythmia usually resolves spontaneously.

4. *Torsade de pointes (turning of the points)* This is a polymorphous ventricular tachycardia (200 to 250 beats per minute) characterised by paroxysms of ventricular tachycardia or fibrillation following a prolonged QT interval (figure 10.19). The QRS axis undulates every 5 to 30 beats with a marked change of direction. These episodes may be precipitated by drugs which affect the QT interval, such as Class I antidysrhythmics (quinidine, procainamide, disopyramide) and phenothiazines, or by hypokalaemia, hypomagnesaemia and hypocalcaemia. It is likely that severe left ventricular dysfunction predisposes to this dysrhythmia, which is often self-terminating, but may progress to ventricular fibrillation.

Ventricular tachycardia is usually associated with coronary artery disease, although it may sometimes be seen in otherwise normal individuals. Myocarditis, cardiomyopathy, mitral valve prolapse and intracardiac instrumentation (e.g. pacing or Swan–Ganz catheterisation) may also produce ventricular tachycardia, as may drugs such as digoxin, sympathomimetic amines and phenothiazines. Metabolic causes (electolyte imbalance, hypoxia and acidaemia) should also be considered.

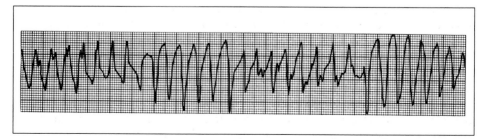

Fig 10.19 ECG: Torsade de Pointes

Table 10.2.   Features that help in the differentiation of ventricular tachycardia from an aberrantly conducted supraventricular tachycardia (SVT).

	Ventricular tachycardia	SVT
Rate	140–180	150–240
Rhythm	Regular or irregular	Regular or irregular
RBBB pattern	Rare	Common
P waves	AV dissociation	Usually 1 : 1
Morphology of preceding ectopics	Same	Different
Capture/fusion beats	Present	Absent
Vagal stimulation	No effect	May help
QRS in V leads	Concordant	Discordant
QRS axis	$< -30°$	Normal

Diagnosis

Differentiating ventricular tachycardia from other broad complex tachycardias is important both in the management of the acute dysrhythmia and for long-term therapy to prevent recurrence. Other dysrhythmias that may give rise to broad complex tachycardias include supraventricular tachycardia with bundle branch block, and SVT with rate-related aberrant conduction.

Ventricular tachycardia is frequently misdiagnosed as a supraventricular tachycardia (Dancy et al, 1985), which is of major concern since the treatment and prognosis are different. Differentiation (table 10.2) often relies heavily upon demonstrating atrioventricular dissociation.

1. *Clinically*
   a. The venous pulse rate is slower than the arterial pulse rate.
   b. There is varying intensity of the first heart sound.

2. *Electrocardiographically*
   a. The QRS axis is $< -30°$ (left axis).
   b. The QRS duration is longer than 0.140 second.
   c. There are multiple QRS morphologies.
   d. There is concordance of the QRS vector in the chest leads (i.e. they are all in the same direction).
   e. In chest lead V1, the R wave is taller than the R1 wave (i.e. the left 'rabbit's ear' is longer).
   f. Dissociated P waves may be visible (best seen in leads II and V1).
   g. Blocked, fusion or capture beats may be present.

A 12-lead ECG should always be recorded provided the patient is well enough during the tachycardia. *Ventricular concordance* (uniformly positive or negative deflections in all chest leads) is virtually diagnostic of ventricular tachycardia. Since the right bundle branch takes longer to recover than the left, aberration leads to the QRS complex appearing as in right bundle branch block (RSR in V1). The RR interval is usually regular and, in contrast to supraventricular tachycardias, does not vary by more than 0.04 second. A QRS duration of longer than 0.14 second indicates a ventricular origin if the sinus rhythm QRS duration is normal (Wellens et al, 1978).

Therapy

Treatment of ventricular tachycardia depends on the haemodynamic status of the patient. Most ventricular dysrhythmias are accompanied by moderate to severe haemodynamic decompensation and require rapid termination. The treatment of choice in such circumstances is cardioversion, with an initial shock of 25 to 50 J. If unsuccessful, the energy level should be doubled. Where a defibrillator is not immediately available, a precordial blow is sometimes effective.

Stable ventricular tachydysrhythmias in the presence of good cardiac output and stable blood pressure can be treated either electrically or pharmacologically. Many antidysrhythmic drugs have been used, but those from Class I are the most effective.

Lignocaine remains the first choice in most coronary care units. A 50 to 100 mg bolus is followed by a continuous infusion of 1 to 4 mg/min. Side effects are rare, but include dizziness, tremor and agitation. Hypotension and conduction disturbances are occasionally seen. Refractory tachycardias may require other agents, and it is best to substitute a drug from another subclass (e.g. procainamide or flecainide). Amiodarone, whilst highly effective (Rosenbaum et al, 1983), may have long-term effects, and its use must be carefully considered, especially in the long term. Other choices include disopyramide and mexiletine.

Special attention should be directed to metabolic imbalance and concurrent drug therapy, particularly if the QT interval is prolonged.

Ventricular flutter

Ventricular flutter is characterised by a rapid ventricular rate (180 to 250 beats per minute, or faster) when it is possible to differentiate the QRS complex from the ST segments (figure 10.20). It often precedes ventricular fibrillation, and therapy is by d.c. cardioversion.

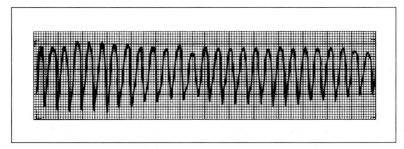

Fig 10.20   ECG: ventricular flutter

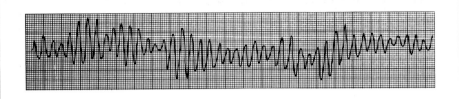

Fig. 10.21   ECG: ventricular fibrillation

Ventricular fibrillation

This is the most serious dysrhythmia since death results if it is not rapidly terminated. The ECG shows fine or coarse waves which are irregular in size, shape and rhythm (figure 10.21). Treatment is by d.c. cardioversion, although a precordial blow is often effective. Several types of ventricular fibrillation have been described.

1. *Sudden death in ambulatory patients:*
   a. without acute myocardial infarction, although evidence of coronary artery disease is usually present,
   b. within a few minutes of typical ischaemic pain.

2. *Primary ventricular fibrillation*   This occurs within the first 24 hours (most within six hours) of acute myocardial infarction in the absence of cardiogenic failure or shock, and accounts for about 80 per cent of in-hospital cases of ventricular fibrillation.

3. *Secondary ventricular fibrillation*   This occurs in the presence of heart failure or cardiogenic shock.

4. *Late onset ventricular fibrillation*   This usually occurs three to seven days after acute myocardial infarction, when the patient has been discharged from the coronary care unit, but is still in hospital. These cases make up 10 to 30 per cent of total hospital deaths.

Identification of high-risk patients and treatment of malignant ventricular dysrhythmias by drugs may help in decreasing the incidence of sudden death. However, caution should be employed when prescribing antidysrhythmic agents because some have the potential for inducing potentially fatal dysrhythmias (e.g. torsade de pointes with Class I antidysrhythmic agents). Invasive electrophysiological testing may be useful in identifying high-risk patients and selecting appropriate therapy.

Clinically, those patients at risk of developing ventricular fibrillation have extensive infarcts, heart failure, persistent tachycardia, intraventricular conduction defects or recent-onset atrial fibrillation. This group of patients could benefit from an intermediate 'step-down' coronary care unit.

Sudden death

Recent evidence now suggests that most out-of-hospital sudden deaths in patients following myocardial infarction are initiated by ventricular tachycardia and not ventricular fibrillation as previously thought (World Scientific Group, 1985). The fatal event may be precipitated by acute ischaemia, or more probably occur by re-entry around relatively discrete circuits that form during the healing of the infarct. The risk of death following myocardial infarction from sudden death is 3 to 8 per cent in the first year, and up to 4 per cent per annum thereafter. Identification of patients at risk and finding satisfactory treatment remains a major goal in treating post-infarct patients (Josephson, 1986).

Digoxin and acute myocardial infarction

The chief role of digoxin is in the treatment of rapid atrial fibrillation. Although it has been used for many years in the treatment of heart failure, it does not have a major place for those in sinus rhythm.

The role of digoxin in the acute phase of myocardial infarction is questionable. Administration increases myocardial work and oxygen consumption, and may increase the size of the infarction. It also provides a relative contraindication to defibrillation should it be later required. Sudden-onset atrial fibrillation complicating acute myocardial infarction is probably better treated with amiodarone and/or d.c. cardioversion. Heart failure will usually respond to diuretics, vasodilators or sympathomimetic agents.

Dysrhythmias are the commonest complication of acute myocardial infarction, and may be worsened by digoxin therapy. Although gastrointestinal symptoms such as anorexia, nausea and vomiting are usually the first signs of toxicity, various rhythm disturbances can be precipitated before these symptoms appear. Toxicity is more common in the elderly, hypokalaemic and hypoxic patient, who is the typical in-patient on the coronary care unit. Plasma levels of digoxin can be assayed, but unfortunately toxicity can occur even when the levels are within the therapeutic range. Assays are only really required to check compliance, to see whether the correct dose is being prescribed and to confirm clinical toxicity. If toxicity is suspected (it may occur in up to 15 per cent of treated patients) the drug can be stopped, but clearance may take many hours or days, and will depend on many factors including the age and renal function of the patient. Signs of toxicity may be present for up to a week.

Digoxin-induced dysrhythmias

Digoxin can produce any rhythm disturbance including ventricular fibrillation. The more common types are ventricular ectopics (especially ventricular bigeminy), sinus bradycardia, heart block and paroxysmal atrial tachycardia. Atrial flutter and rapid atrial fibrillation have been described, but are uncommon.

Ventricular ectopic beats are the most common sign of digoxin toxicity. The ECG usually shows other signs of toxicity (ST/T wave changes, increased PR interval). Ventricular tachycardia is usually precipitated by short runs of ventricular ectopics. Nodal tachycardias usually occur in patients previously in atrial fibrillation, and should be suspected if the pulse rate becomes rapid and regular.

All degrees of heart block at both the atrioventricular and sino-atrial nodes can arise. Extreme sinus bradycardias and slow atrial fibrillation are common.

Treatment

Potassium chloride is very effective in the treatment of digoxin-induced tachydysrhythmias, particularly if there is hypokalaemia. It may be given orally or intravenously, but ECG monitoring is desirable during parenteral administration to observe for signs of hyperkalaemia. Propranolol (2 mg i.v.) or procainamide is especially useful for supraventricular dysrhythmias. Lignocaine will usually abolish ectopic ventricular activity, although phenytoin is particularly effective in digitalis-induced ventricular dysrhythmias. For serious ventricular dysrhythmias d.c. cardioversion may occasionally be required, and pretreatment with lignocaine or phenytoin is recommended.

In the case of digoxin-related bradydysrhythmias, potassium supplements should be stopped because they potentiate heart block. Symptomatic bradycardias may require intravenous atropine, isoprenaline or even temporary cardiac pacing.

Prophylactic antidysrhythmic therapy

Ventricular fibrillation is common in otherwise uncomplicated cases of myocardial infarction. The incidence of ventricular fibrillation not associated with shock or heart failure is about 7 per cent (Noneman and Rodgers, 1978; Ribner et al, 1978). It carries a significant mortality although it is not known whether prevention of this disorder will improve prognosis. Many cardiologists feel that prophylactic measures against ventricular fibrillation are not necessary once the patient has reached coronary care, since d.c. cardioversion is readily available and effective. However, this may be a little optimistic, since even in the best run units some minutes may elapse between the onset of fibrillation and effective defibrillation. Although external cardiac massage may be instituted in the interim period, myocardial perfusion during this time is poor. The ensuing ischaemia and myocardial damage may then have long-term prognostic implications. This is not only a consideration for pre-hospital care but also within hospital, where the relapse rate of primary ventricular fibrillation is in the region of 25 per cent (Lie, 1985). Unfortunately, there is no way of identifying these patients at risk. The so-called 'warning dysrhythmias' occur only in 57 per cent of patients who develop ventricular fibrillation (Noneman and Rodgers, 1978), and many others may develop ventricular fibrillation without any warning.

In an attempt to prevent primary ventricular fibrillation, lignocaine is probably the most frequently and most controversially utilised prophylactic agent. Early studies suggested that it was effective in treating a variety of ventricular dysrhythmias, including ventricular fibrillation, and was particularly advocated for the 'warning' dysrhythmias which have since been shown to be of limited clinical value. From the large numbers of trials reviewed by Kertes and Hunt (1984), it seems that the administration of lignocaine before hospital admission is probably not justified, although it may be of value if instituted in hospital within six hours of onset of the myocardial infarct (Lie, 1985). Nevertheless, dose-related side-effects are common, including hypotension, heart block, heart failure and adverse actions on the central nervous system (nausea, peri-oral paraesthesia, fits). Care is therefore needed in the elderly and those with conduction defects. The dosage for lignocaine prophylaxis is shown in table 10.3 and may be of value following cardiac arrest due to ventricular

Table 10.3.   Recommendations for intravenous lignocaine prophylaxis.

1. Loading dose: 100 mg over 10–20 minutes, given as:
   - 2 × 50 mg boluses at 5–10 minute intervals
   - 1 × 100 mg injection given over 10–20 minutes
   - 100 mg infusion over 20 minutes

2. Maintenance dose: 1–4 mg/min for 48 hours
Notes: ● Reduce doses by 50 per cent in the elderly and those
           with heart failure or liver and kidney disease
       ● Plasma levels are desirable at 12–24 hours (1–5 μg/ml)

fibrillation to prevent recurrence. The trend these days is to give smaller doses for shorter times (12 to 24 hours) than in the past (Harrison, 1978). The incidence of side-effects is then very much reduced without an apparent increase in further episodes of ventricular fibrillation.

Alternative drugs

Many other drugs have been tried as prophylaxis against ventricular dysrhythmias, including quinidine, procainamide, disopyramide, mexiletine and tocainide. Only tocainide has been shown to reduce the incidence of ventricular fibrillation. However, short-term mortality does not seem to differ with or without treatment.

Although the aim of treatment is suppression of the initiating ventricular ectopic beats, agents such as beta-blockers seem to increase the threshold for ventricular tachycardia without suppressing all ventricular ectopics. It may be this non-specific activity that reduces the recurrence of ventricular dysrhythmias and the incidence of sudden death. The use of beta-blockade in the acute phase of myocardial infarction is still being investigated. This seems to reduce the incidence of serious dysrhythmias (attributable to its inherent antidysrhythmic properties) as well as possibly limiting infarct size (due to a sympatholytic effect). Unfortunately, this does not help improve the post-infarction survival, and present evidence suggests that acute administration of beta-blockers is of limited value (Mauro and Zeller, 1985).

If recurrent ventricular tachycardia or fibrillation has complicated myocardial infarction, antidysrhythmic therapy should be continued for about three months. Patients with ventricular aneurysms may benefit from surgery. Patients with chronic recurrent ventricular tachycardia may also need surgery. Scarred or ischaemic areas of the myocardium may act as a focus for dysrhythmias, and coronary artery bypass grafting with or without removal of an irritable focus may be of benefit (Anderson and Mason, 1983). Epicardial and endocardial mapping is often required to locate these areas.

Antidysrhythmic agents

Suppression of serious dysrhythmias following acute myocardial infarction should be associated with a reduced mortality and morbidity, as well as relieving much of the anxiety in the patient with symptomatic dysrhythmias. The ideal antidysrhythmic agent should:

● Be available both parenterally and orally
● Have a rapid onset of action
● Be effective against both ventricular and supraventricular dysrhythmias
● Not depress myocardial contractility
● Be free of short-term and long-term side-effects

Unfortunately, we are still some way away from the ideal agent. Despite large advances in our understanding of the pathogenesis and pharmacological treatment of cardiac dysrhythmias (Rosen and Wit, 1983; Wit and Rosen, 1983; Zipes et al, 1983), treatment is still largely unsatisfactory. Most therapies are based upon empiricism and the avoidance of adverse effects and drug interactions.

Antidysrhythmic drugs basically work by one or more mechanisms.

1. *Blocking the underlying stimulus that provoked the dysrhythmia* Certain exogenous factors are known to precipitate dysrhythmias in the sensitised heart. Increased levels of circulating catecholamines (from metabolic stress or anxiety), hypoxia, increased circulating free fatty acids and hyperglycaemia have all been implicated in provoking dysrhythmias. Therapy aimed at correcting these factors may reduce the incidence of dysrhythmias.

2. *Blocking impulse formation* Many dysrhythmias are initiated or maintained by spontaneous ectopic activity (enhanced automaticity) and suppression of these abnormal impulses plays a major role in the treatment of dysrhythmias.

3. *Inhibiting impulse transmission* Impulse transmission can be blocked by interfering with different electrophysiological mechanisms, and hence preventing impulse transmission.

Classification

There are many ways of classifying antidysrhythmic drugs. They may be classed by the type of rhythm disturbance they may be used to treat, the anatomical site of action (see below) or their electrophysiological action on isolated myocardium. This latter classification (Vaughan Williams, 1984) is extensively used today, and provides many theoretical and practical benefits for a rational approach in the treatment of dysrhythmias (table 10.4). Initial selection of a drug can often be simplified, and should a second agent be required, selection from a different action group is frequently more successful than if an agent from the same group were employed. In addition, side-effects may be reduced.

There are four classes of drug, grouped on the basis of their effects in vitro on the action potentials of normal cardiac cells (chapter 2).

Class I   *Local anaesthetic agents*
       (Examples: quinidine, procainamide, lignocaine, phenytoin, disopyramide)

These agents depress membrane responsiveness and slow myocardial conduction by their membrane stabilising activity. The fast sodium current is inhibited, and thus the phase 0 rise is reduced. These drugs also depress the rate of diastolic depolarisation (phase 4) which reduces spontaneous automaticity.

Table 10.4.   Classification of anti-arrhythmic drugs.

Class	Action	Examples
I Membrane-stabilising agents		
a	Moderately slow conduction Prolong repolarisation Depress phase 0 of the action potential	Disopyramide Quinidine Procainamide
b	Have minimal effect on phase 0 Shorten repolarisation	Lignocaine Mexiletine Phenytoin Tocainide
c	Markedly depress phase 0 Markedly slow conduction Have minimal effect on repolarisation	Flecainide Encainide
II Beta-adrenergic blocking agents		Atenolol Metoprolol Propranolol Sotalol*
III Agents that prolong repolarisation	Have no effect on phase 0	Amiodarone Bretylium Sotalol*
IV Calcium-channel blockers	Depress phases 2 and 3	Diltiazem Verapamil

*Sotalol has both Class II and Class III actions

The group is subdivided into Classes Ia, Ib and Ic on the basis of overall effect on the action potential. Class Ia drugs (quinidine, disopyramide, procainamide) prolong it; Class Ib drugs (lignocaine, tocainide, mexiletine) shorten it; and Class Ic drugs (flecainide, encainide) have no effect. Class Ia drugs are more cardiodepressant.

Class II   *Beta-blockers*
(Examples: propranolol, metoprolol, etc.)
These drugs block catecholamine stimulation of the myocardial cells which may induce cardiac dysrhythmias. They also produce direct effects on the membrane similar to those of Class I drugs (membrane stabilising activity).

Class III   *Drugs sustaining depolarisation*
(Examples: amiodarone, sotalol)
The major action of these drugs is to prolong the duration of the action potential with consequent lengthening of the effective refractory period. The membrane responsiveness, conduction velocity and rate of rise of the action potential in phase 0 are not affected. They impressively suppress ventricular ectopic activity, and may be capable of chemical defibrillation (i.e. restoring sinus rhythm in patients with ventricular fibrillation).

Class IV   *Calcium channel blockers*
(Examples: verapamil, diltiazem)
These agents inhibit the slow inward calcium current and depress phase 2 and phase 3 (plateau phase) of the action potential. These actions are of particular importance

Table 10.5.   A classification of antidysrhythmic drugs by site of action.

1. *Sino-atrial node*	2. *Atrioventricular node*
Class II drugs	Class Ic drugs
Class IV drugs	Class II drugs
Cardiac glycosides	Class IV drugs
3. *Atria*	Cardiac glycosides
Class Ia and Ic drugs	4. *Ventricles*
Class II drugs	Class I drugs
Class III drugs	Class III drugs

5. *Accessory pathways*
   Class Ia drugs
   Class III drugs

in the upper part of the atrioventricular node and will block circus movements during re-entry tachycardias.

This classification is based on presumed alterations in ionic conduction in normal myocardial fibres. However, these drugs probably have differing effects on the diseased myocardium, and many have properties of more than one class. It is perhaps clinically better to have a classification based on the action of the drugs on differing cardiac tissues (table 10.5).

Although this classification may help in selecting a type of drug, the final choice of agent is still often largely based on familiarity, and avoidance of side-effects (Aronson, 1985). The aims of drug therapy of dysrhythmias are:

1. To terminate the acute dysrhythmias by suppressing automaticity or interrupting circus movement

2. To slow the ventricular rate if the dysrhythmia cannot be terminated (e.g. digoxin in rapid atrial fibrillation)

3. To prevent the emergence of a dysrhythmia by suppressing provoking events (e.g. ectopics) or cardiac irritability

4. To prevent sudden paroxysms of the dysrhythmia. If the dysrhythmia (e.g. atrial fibrillation) cannot be suppressed, maintaining it may be associated with fewer symptoms.

Most cardiac dysrhythmias are not primary events, and therapy should always be directed towards the underlying cause.

Dysrhythmogenic effect

Most antidysrhythmic drugs have the potential for causing abnormalities of cardiac rhythm. Most agents are negatively inotropic, and thus reduce coronary perfusion which may predispose to pre-existing or new dysrhythmias. This is more common when more than one drug is being used (e.g. beta-blockers with verapamil). Hence, the first choice of drug needs careful consideration, since a rapid sequence of drugs may be unwise. The best second line approach may be d.c. cardioversion.

CARDIAC FAILURE

About 25 per cent of patients with cardiovascular disease have cardiac failure, and the long-term prognosis is determined by the degree of left ventricular dysfunction. Although a very common complication of myocardial infarction, left ventricular failure or congestive cardiac failure is often the presenting problem of patients admitted directly to the coronary care unit. A thorough understanding of its causes and management is therefore highly desirable (Willerson, 1982).

Definition

Cardiac failure is a clinical syndrome which results from an inability of the heart to provide an adequate cardiac output for the body's metabolic requirements. However, symptoms are not usually due to low cardiac output, but rather to the compensatory mechanisms that the body brings about to maintain an adequate cardiac output. These compensatory responses include fluid retention and increased sympathetic activity which may lead to pulmonary and peripheral oedema. In the later stages, the heart adapts to increased intraventricular tension by dilatation and hypertrophy. These changes predispose to subendocardial ischaemia and may precipitate angina.

Aetiology

Heart failure is caused by any factor or combination of factors that reduces the cardiac output below the body's requirements. This of course does not always mean a low cardiac output. 'High-output failure' may exist (e.g. in thyrotoxicosis) where an increased metabolic demand requires a supranormal cardiac output.

Causes of cardiac failure may be subdivided into:

1. *Loss of myocardial tissue*
   - Myocardial ischaemia and infarction

2. *Decreased myocardial contractility*
   - Cardiomyopathy
   - Hypertrophy
   - Ischaemia
   - Metabolic depression (e.g. acidosis)
   - Amyloidosis

3. *Inappropriate heart rates*
   - Bradycardias
   - Tachycardias

4. *High-output failure*
   - Intracardiac shunts
   - Aortic regurgitation
   - Thyrotoxicosis
   - Beriberi

5. *Increased wall tension*
- Hypertension
- Cardiac dilatation
- Aortic and mitral stenoses

6. *Drugs*
- Cardiodepressants (e.g. antidysrhythmics, beta-blockers)
- Sodium-retaining drugs (e.g. indomethacin)

The response to heart failure

In response to heart failure, several compensatory mechanisms are activated to maintain cardiac output and tissue perfusion. The fall in blood pressure caused by a fall in cardiac output leads to stimulation of the baroreceptors, with increased sympathetic activity (tachycardia and increased myocardial contractility). However, the cardiac catecholamine supplies soon become exhausted, so selective arterial vasoconstriction redistributes the cardiac output. Flow to the gut and liver is reduced so that supply to the heart and skeletal muscle may be increased. Dilatation of the heart causes a reflex increase in cardiac output in accordance with Starling's Law, where increased myofibril stretching increases the force of myocardial contraction. If heart failure is long-standing, the left ventricle hypertrophies to maintain pump action. This latter compensation is counterproductive, since the increased mass requires more oxygen and impairs normal contractility such that stroke volume falls. A further adaptation is seen in the arterioles, particularly those supplying skeletal muscle and the kidneys. The vessel walls become oedematous and less responsive to circulating vasodilators, such as adenosine. As a result systemic vascular resistance is high and the reduced blood flow to the kidneys causes sodium retention by activation of the renin–angiotensin system. Plasma vasopressin and aldosterone levels increase, but the role of other hormones (such as atrial naturetic hormone) is unclear. Angiotensin II causes widespread vasoconstriction and secretion of aldosterone which causes sodium and water retention to expand the plasma volume. This maintains preload, but usually results in oedema.

Symptoms of heart failure

The signs and symptoms of heart failure are caused by reduced cardiac output (*forward heart failure*) and an increased venous pressure in the lungs and peripheries because of inadequate ventricular emptying (*backward failure*).

An increased awareness of respiration is the usual presentation of left ventricular failure; dyspnoea is caused by increased pulmonary vascular engorgement with decreased compliance of the lungs. Paroxysmal nocturnal dyspnoea results when nocturnal absorption of oedema fluid increases the intravascular volume, waking the patient with gasping respiration, cough and wheeze. Fatigue and lethargy are marked, caused by low blood flow to exercising muscles.

Heart failure has been graded according to exercise limitation by the New York Heart Association Criteria Committee (1964). Symptoms such as fatigue, palpitations, dyspnoea and angina are used to record the degree of symptomatic heart failure.

Class 1 Heart disease with no limitation on ordinary physical activity.

Class 2 Slight limitation. Ordinary physical activity (e.g. walking) produces symptoms.

Class 3 Marked limitation. Unable to walk on the level without disability. Less than ordinary activity produces symptoms.

Class 4 Dyspnoea at rest. Inability to carry out any physical activity.

Acute left ventricular failure (pulmonary oedema)

Acute left ventricular failure is often precipitous and may lead to pulmonary oedema as a result of transudation of fluid into the pulmonary alveoli. This occurs when the pulmonary capillary pressure exceeds the pulmonary oncotic pressure (25 to 30 mmHg), secondary to high left atrial pressures. There is decreased airflow to and from the alveoli because oedema of the pulmonary membranes causes airway narrowing. The lung compliance ('stiffness') increases, making breathing more difficult, and alveolar flooding reduces gaseous exchange within the alveoli. This leads to dyspnoea with arterial hypoxaemia. Increased mucus production may precipitate cough and wheeze (*cardiac asthma*) and the sputum may be blood tinged from small haemorrhages in the congested bronchial mucosa.

Right heart failure

Right heart failure usually occurs secondary to left heart failure. Isolated right-sided heart failure may result from tricuspid or pulmonary valve disease, right ventricular infarction, pulmonary embolism, or secondary to pulmonary disease (*cor pulmonale*).

Symptoms are due to pulmonary hypertension which leads to an elevation of the systemic venous pressure. Oedema with elevation of the jugular venous pressure is usual. The liver becomes engorged producing hepatomegaly with right hypochondrial discomfort. Functional tricuspid incompetence may occur and be heard, and the dilated or hypertrophied right ventricle often causes a right parasternal heave. Pleural effusions and ascites are common.

Treatment

The aim of therapy is to:

● Increase salt and water excretion
● Reduce pressure and volume overload in the heart
● Increase myocardial contractility

The underlying cause should always be treated where possible. Following acute myocardial infarction, meticulous attention should be paid to ventilation, since hypoxaemia will further impair left ventricular function by increasing areas of critical myocardial ischaemia. The combined action of reduced pulmonary compliance, pulmonary vascular congestion and respiratory depression (from opiates) will impair arterial oxygenation and respiratory function. Although positive inotropic agents (such as digoxin or dopamine) would seem to be the logical first-line therapy to aid the failing left ventricle, they may increase the size of the infarcted area. Over stimulation with positive inotropic agents may cause an increase in myocardial work in areas of borderline perfusion, and the increased oxygen consumption could lead to an extension of the original myocardial infarction. Treatment should therefore be aimed primarily at reducing intravascular volume which will reduce cardiac preload and, as a consequence, afterload.

Rest

Bed rest promotes a diuresis and reduces myocardial work. Passive leg exercises are needed to prevent deep vein thrombosis.

Diet

In severe cases, sodium and water restriction are required. Drugs that retain sodium (e.g. indomethacin) must be avoided.

Diuretic therapy

Diuretics provide the mainstay of treatment for left ventricular failure, although they are frequently unhelpful in pure right-sided heart failure. Diuretics inhibit sodium resorption by the kidney, and reduce intravascular volume and hence left ventricular load. There is a loss of sodium from arteriolar walls, leading to vasodilatation and hence reduced cardiac afterload.

The reduction in pulmonary capillary pressure eases dyspnoea, and the reduction in left ventricular tension reduces myocardial work and oxygen requirement. The filling pressures, however, must not be lowered too much: a pressure of more than about 18 mmHg is required to optimise left ventricular function. Reducing cardiac output too far will increase the blood urea and lead to fatigue. Filling pressures can be titrated against cardiac output acutely if a Swan–Ganz catheter is being used (Stokes and Jowett, 1985). Potassium intake should be increased since hypokalaemia can initiate dysrhythmias in patients with ischaemic heart disease, especially those taking digoxin.

Diuretic therapy in heart failure includes the following.

Thiazide diuretics

These act on the distal convoluted tubule of the kidney and increase permeability to sodium and chloride. Metabolic abnormalities such as hypokalaemia, diabetes and hyperuricaemia (gout) may complicate long-term use.

'Loop' diuretics

These are potent diuretics with rapid onset of action. They inhibit sodium absorption in the ascending loop of Henlé. Intravenous frusemide reduces pulmonary congestion and pulmonary venous pressure within 15 minutes. This is before the onset of a diuresis, and is probably due to a direct vasodilator effect on systemic arterial beds. Increasing doses may be required in heart failure, especially if there is renal impairment. They may deplete plasma volume, leading to hypokalaemia and provoking an accentuated renin–angiotensin response. In severe heart failure the gut wall becomes oedematous, limiting the absorption of orally administered drugs. A switch from oral to intravenous diuretics is often rewarded by an increased diuresis.

Spironolactone

Spironolactone is a competitive inhibitor of aldosterone, and is particularly of value in congestive heart failure where there is an increased secretion of aldosterone (*secondary aldosteronism*). Its onset of action is slow (two to three days), and its use has fallen since the introduction of the ACE inhibitors (see below).

Vasodilator therapy

The change in cardiac output during vasodilator therapy results from a reduction in filling pressures (preload) and blood pressure (afterload), but the effect in patients with heart failure differs from that in normal individuals. In normal subjects, preload is mainly affected, and there is little effect on cardiac output. In patients with heart failure, afterload is predominantly affected and, despite an additional fall in preload, cardiac output rises. In patients with established left ventricular failure following myocardial infarction, vasodilators will reduce filling pressures and increase cardiac output, but in patients with normal filling pressures cardiac output will fall (Bussmann, 1978). If any clinical doubt exists, haemodynamic assessment with a Swan–Ganz catheter is desirable (Stokes and Jowett, 1985).

Vasodilator therapy is particularly useful when acute myocardial infarction is complicated by hypertension, or rupture of the mitral valve or interventricular septum. In the latter mechanical problems, the vasodilators may act as a holding measure until definitive surgical therapy can be instituted. Vasodilators were originally thought to increase the size of the myocardial infarct as a consequence of hypotension, but their administration may actually limit the size of infarction. The reduction in afterload limits myocardial work and oxygen consumption and additionally improves efficiency of the left ventricular pump (Epstein et al, 1978).

The haemodynamic effect of individual vasodilator agents (table 10.6) depends on their ability to affect arterioles or venules (Franciosa et al, 1984).

Hydralazine raises cardiac output by arteriolar dilatation, but may cause a reflex tachycardia. This may be counterproductive by increasing myocardial work and oxygen consumption.

Prazosin is an alpha-adrenergic blocker which produces both venous and arteriolar dilatation. It works rapidly, and has been used in the acute phase of acute myocardial infarction complicated by heart failure. Unfortunately, in the long term, tachyphylaxis occurs, which limits its use.

Nitrates predominantly affect venous capacitance vessels, but their use is limited by poor bio-availability. The recently introduced isosorbide mononitrate has helped since it is less affected by the first passage through the liver. Intravenous and cutaneous nitrate preparations are useful acutely.

Sodium nitroprusside has been widely used in the treatment of left ventricular failure and acute mitral incompetence following acute myocardial infarction, although there

Table 10.6. Commonly used Vasodilators.

Drug	Mechanism	Dosage	Onset of action	Precautions
Nitroprusside	Direct action	IV only 0.5–1µg/kg/min Titrate for effect	Immediate	Sudden hypotension – requires close monitoring Cyanide and thiocyanate toxicity
Nitrates	Direct action	IV, SL, B, O, TD Wide range of doses	Minutes	Headache, flushing, hypotension
Hydralazine	Direct action	IV, 10–20 mg IM, 10–20 mg O, 25–100 mg tid	Minutes	Tachycardia may produce angina Lupus-like syndrome Blood dyscrasias
Prazosin	Alpha-adrenergic blocker	O, 0.5–5 mg tid	0.5–2 h	First dose hypotension Tachyphylaxis in heart failure
Captopril	ACE inhibitor	O, 6.25–50 mg tid	0.5–1.5 h	First dose hypotension Altered taste Rashes Proteinuria
Enalapril	ACE inhibitor	2.5–40 mg daily	1–2 h	Hypotension if patient is sodium depleted
Nifedipine	Calcium-channel blocker	O, 5–160 mg tid SL, 5 mg	15–30 min 2–5 min	Hypotension and tachycardia Headache Ankle oedema Negative inotropic effect in high doses
Nicardipine	Calcium-channel blocker	O, 20–30 mg tid	30–60 min	As nifedipine, but little inotropic effect

IV = intravenous, IM = intramuscular, B = buccal, O = oral, SL = sublingual, TD = Transdermal.

have been reports of extension of infarcts as a consequence of a 'coronary steel' effect (Chiarello et al, 1976), with blood being drawn away from the area of myocardial ischaemia. However, given with care, sodium nitroprusside will reduce myocardial oxygen demand and ischaemic pain by diminishing arteriolar resistance, wedge pressures and oxygen requirements, while leading to an increased cardiac output. Sodium nitroprusside is useful in hypertensive heart failure and myocardial infarction complicated by hypertension, and in patients with severe heart failure. Its administration requires close supervision.

Calcium channel blockers may be useful in heart failure if hypertension is a complicating feature. Verapamil and nifedipine have negative inotropic effects, but the newer agents nicardipine and felodipine may have little cardiodepressant effect.

Angiotensin converting enzyme (ACE) inhibitors

These agents have rapidly become the most widely prescribed vasodilators for severe heart failure. They work by inhibition of the angiotensin converting enzyme (ACE) so that the formation of the powerful vasoconstricting angiotensin II is blocked, as is the formation of aldosterone. Since the renin–angiotensin system is activated in most patients with marked heart failure, increased levels of angiotensin II are probably responsible for peripheral vasoconstriction and fluid retention. ACE inhibitors lower venous and arterial blood pressure, increase cardiac output and renal blood flow, and lead to a prolonged exercise time.

The effect of ACE inhibition in heart failure seems to be long term in contrast to many of the other vasodilators which appear to have limited long-term effects (Bayliss et al, 1985). This is probably because direct-acting agents (e.g. prazosin) provoke compensatory vasoconstriction. The ACE inhibitors reduce angiotensin II-induced thirst and the production of anti-diuretic hormone (ADH), reducing the incidence of hyponatraemia. Aldosterone levels fall too, reducing fluid retention and allowing a reduction in the dose of diuretics.

Positive inotropic agents

Digoxin

The mainstay of positive inotropic treatment remains digoxin. There is no doubt that it has an acute effect in strengthening the force of myocardial contraction, but its long-term value is the subject of much controversy (Arnold et al, 1980; *Lancet*, 1985). Its principal use today is for controlling the ventricular rate in atrial fibrillation. Digoxin toxicity is a frequent problem, particularly if there is renal impairment or hypokalaemia. The plasma half-life of digoxin is about 36 hours, although the myocardial half-life is longer. This may lead to problems if defibrillation is required. The limitations put upon digoxin have led to a search for other potent oral agents, including non-glycoside sympathomimetics and those with beta-adrenergic activity (Johnston, 1985).

Table 10.7. Comparison of different inotropic agents.

Receptor effects	Adrenaline	Dopamine	Dobutamine	Isoprenaline
Alpha				
Arteriolar vasoconstriction	+ + + +	+ + low dose + + + high dose	+	0
Dopaminergic				
Vasodilation in gut and kidney	0	+ +	0	0
Beta-1				
Increased myocardial contractility	+ + + +	+ + + +	+ + + +	+ + + +
Increased heart rate	+ + +	+ + +	+ +	+ + + +
Increased AV conduction	+ +	+ +	+ +	+ +
Beta-2				
Arteriolar vasodilation	0	+ +	+ +	+ + + +

Amrinone

Amrinone is an orally active agent which acts predominantly as a vasodilator. However, it is probably able to increase the force of myocardial contractility without significantly increasing oxygen requirements. Side-effects are common, but it is very useful in severe or refractory heart failure. A related compound, milrinone, is about 20 times more powerful and may have fewer side-effects.

Beta-adrenergic agonists

Beta-adrenergic agonists produce a short-term haemodynamic improvement in patients with congestive cardiac failure, but long-term use is limited by peripheral vasoconstriction. Dopamine and dobutamine are relatively cardioselective beta-1 stimulants, which are especially useful in patients with heart failure and cardiogenic shock following acute myocardial infarction (table 10.7). The potentially deleterious side-effect of alpha-adrenergic vasoconstriction exerted by dopamine is fortunately only present at higher doses than those required to increase contractility. Its vasodilator effect on splanchnic and renal arterioles, with its positive inotropic effect, generally improves cardiovascular haemodynamics and renal function. Dobutamine is similar and, although it does not have such marked chronotropic effect, it does not specifically increase renal perfusion other than by its positive inotropic effect. Dopamine and dobutamine can only be given intravenously, so that oral therapy for continuing therapy is desirable.

Two oral agents of recent interest are xamoterol and pirbuterol. Xamoterol is a partial beta-1 agonist with a modest inotropic effect which may be useful in patients with heart failure and co-existing angina. Pirbuterol differs from most beta-agonists in possessing vasodilator properties, as well as a positive inotropic action. Long-term value in heart failure is unpredictable.

Prenalterol is available for intravenous use and may be of particular value in patients developing heart failure as a result of beta-blocker therapy.

Ultrafiltration

There is increasing interest in mechanical methods of removing fluid in cardiac failure (Simpson et al, 1986). Ultrafiltration allows controlled removal of body water without the adverse haemodynamic effects of haemodialysis, since only venous access is required. The best results so far have been obtained using a new highly permeable biocompatible filter.

Anticoagulation

Anticoagulation should perhaps be considered routine in patients with dilated or akinetic hearts, marked congestive cardiac failure and unstable rhythm, to prevent thromboembolic complications.

Prognosis

The prognosis of patients with Class I, II or III heart failure is very similar: a five-year survival of about 50 per cent. However, those with Class IV failure have a mortality of 50 per cent in six months, and 80 per cent within three years. Cardiac mortality is usually due to refractory heart failure or sudden death. It is not clear whether drug therapy greatly improves the prognosis. Although short-term therapy in heart failure is excellent, long-term efficacy usually deteriorates. The reason for this is unknown, but may be due to drug tolerance, altered drug metabolism, hormonal reflexes or perhaps deterioration in cardiac performance (Lipkin and Poole-Wilson, 1985).

Inotropic agents such as digoxin, amrinone and milrinone improve symptoms, increase cardiac output and lower filling pressures. However, they may possibly 'overstimulate' the heart, leading to myocardial hypoxia with ventricular dysrhythmias and sudden death. There is no evidence that prognosis is improved.

Vasodilators probably have little influence on prognosis (Furberg and Yusuf, 1985) although there is now preliminary evidence that there may be moderate improvement with the use of ACE inhibitors (Consensus Trial Study Group, 1987).

DISSECTING AORTIC ANEURYSM

An *aneurysm* is a sac produced by dilatation of the walls of an artery or vein, filled with blood and forming a pulsatile tumour. It can present with leakage or rupture (producing shock), or may be found on routine examination.

An acute *dissecting aneurysm* is the most frequent and most lethal acute disorder of the thoracic aorta. There is an incidence of 5 to 10 per million, and it is thus twice as common as rupture of an abdominal aortic aneurysm. It is most common in men and there is usually a previous history of hypertension.

Dissection is initiated by a small tear in the aortic intima, which is a degenerative event. Most dissections (66 per cent) arise in the ascending aorta, and blood passes into the medial layer of the wall. Flow can be proximal to include the pericardium (with rapidly fatal tamponade) or distal to involve the arch and the descending and abdominal aorta.

Clinical features

The presentation is dramatic and virtually always associated with pain. There is sudden excruciating ('tearing') pain felt anywhere from the epigastrium to the neck. It classically radiates through to the back and gives rise to pain in both the upper and lower limbs. The patient is cold, clammy and paradoxically hypertensive, with systolic blood pressures often in excess of 200 mmHg. Subsequent signs depend on which branches of the aorta are involved in the dissection. For example, there may be hemiplegia due to involvement of the carotid arteries, or myocardial infarction when the coronary arteries are involved. A pericardial friction rub is frequently heard, or the murmur of aortic incompetence caused by dilatation of the aortic root. These features may confuse the diagnosis, as does the ECG, which may show ST changes, dysrhythmias, left ventricular hypertrophy or conduction defects.

The chest radiograph is diagnostic in two-thirds of cases, showing widening of the superior mediastinum, and sometimes a left pleural effusion (caused by extravasated blood). Care must be taken when interpreting an emergency anteroposterior (portable) chest film, however, as this may show apparent mediastinal widening in normal patients.

A CAT scan helps localise the dissection, although angiography is the usual definitive investigation.

Management

There are two leading problems: pain and shock. Large doses of intravenous diamorphine are usually required to control the pain, sometimes by continuous infusion. Shock may be produced by pain during dissection (when there may be only slight blood loss) or by profound blood loss from aortic rupture. A central venous pressure line is therefore often helpful. Many cases are complicated by dysrhythmias and acute heart failure, and ECG monitoring is required.

Systemic and pulmonary blood pressures should be reduced immediately using sodium nitroprusside, titrated to keep the systolic blood pressure below 100 mmHg. Beta-blockade helps to reduce the force of contraction and may prevent further intimal tearing. If hypertension is successfully controlled, 40 to 50 per cent of patients will survive with conservative management unless other cardiovascular complications emerge. In this case, or if the blood pressure cannot be easily controlled, surgical exploration with subsequent repair may be possible. All cases that involve the ascending aorta are probably better treated surgically. The most successful surgical techniques are fenestration and circumferential intimal anchorage. Fenestration involves opening the aorta and cutting a window in the intimal dissection flap, enabling blood to re-enter the aortic lumen. In the second procedure, the aorta is opened and the dissection flap is divided and circumferentially sutured to the outer wall of the aorta.

Prognosis

Untreated, the mortality is nearly 30 per cent in the first day, increasing to 70 per cent by seven days and 90 per cent at three months. With medical and surgical therapy, this has now been reduced to less than 15 per cent, many patients surviving for more than three years.

CARDIOGENIC SHOCK

Shock is a complex syndrome associated with inadequate perfusion of vital organs, most significantly the brain, the kidneys and the heart. The cardiac output is usually low, but may be normal or even high. There are four main types of shock.

1. *Neurogenic (vasovagal) shock* occurs immediately after a sudden fright, severe pain or after prolonged standing in a warm environment. There is a pooling of blood in splanchnic and peripheral vascular beds, with a consequent fall in the cardiac output and hypoxia of the vital centres. It is usually associated with profound slowing of the heart (hence 'vasovagal' shock).

2. *Hypovolaemic shock* follows significant loss of circulating body fluid as might complicate severe haemorrhage, trauma, burns or emesis.

3. *Septic shock* complicates septicaemia where bacteria produce endotoxins that damage capillaries and produce stasis and pooling of plasma. Cardiac output is usually high.

4. *Cardiogenic shock* usually results from acute myocardial infarction, but can occur with pulmonary emboli, cardiac tamponade or following cardiac surgery. Massive myocardial infarction can produce such a profound effect on left ventricular function that shock results, but smaller infarcts in patients with previous extensive ischaemic heart disease may equally result in cardiogenic shock. Patients who do not rapidly die develop varying degrees of multiple system dysfunction, with respiratory, hepatic and renal failure, neurological impairment and eventually brain death.

Cardiogenic shock and myocardial infarction

Cardiogenic shock complicates about 10 per cent of cases of acute myocardial infarction admitted to coronary care (Rackley et al, 1977). It is essentially a disease of inadequate pump function, and is nearly always associated with massive damage involving more than 40 per cent of the left ventricular myocardium.

There are four subgroups of patients with cardiogenic shock.

1. *Recent massive myocardial infarction* The affected vessel is usually the left main stem coronary artery which results in 40 to 50 per cent of the left ventricular myocardium being damaged.

2. *Acute-on-chronic infarction* This occurs when there is a smaller myocardial infarction which takes the cumulative damage to more than 40 per cent of the ventricular myocardium. These patients have often been previously hypertensive.

3. *Myocardial infarction with mechanical complications* Here the myocardial infarction is complicated by mechanical defects, such as a ruptured mitral valve, ruptured septum or acute left ventricular aneurysm. These lesions compromise the pumping action of the heart and lead to cardiogenic shock.

4. *Myocardial infarction with recurrent dysrhythmias* Dysrhythmias (especially ventricular tachycardia) reduce cardiac output, increase myocardial work and oxygen

Table 10.8. Assessment of cardiogenic shock.

Determinant	Method
Preload	Swan–Ganz catheter
Afterload	Arterial catheter
Heart rate	ECG monitoring
Contractility	Echocardiography
Infarct size	ECG, cardiac enzymes and ventriculography

consumption, and thus may extend the size of the originally infarcted area. Extension of infarction is commonly seen in the patients dying from cardiogenic shock (Page et al, 1971).

Mortality from cardiogenic shock is in excess of 90 per cent in spite of recent advances in therapy. Some patients are admitted in shock, and 50 per cent develop the syndrome in the first 24 hours. A small proportion (15 per cent) may develop shock much later (more than seven days).

Definition

The syndrome presents with clinical signs of shock, usually in a patient following acute myocardial infarction. The clinical signs are marked by:

● Systemic hypotension (systolic BP less than 90 mmHg)
● Oliguria (less than 20 ml/h of urine)
● Arterial vasoconstriction leading to hypoperfusion of vital organs and the peripheries

The patient is therefore cold and cyanosed, with rapid shallow respiration, hypotension and tachycardia. Mental changes reflecting poor cerebral perfusion are present, including irritability, restlessness and later coma.

The basic mechanical disturbance in cardiogenic shock is the extensive necrosis of left ventricular myocardium. The abrupt loss of contractility results in a significant rise in intracardiac pressures and critical falls in arterial blood pressure and cardiac output. Left ventricular filling pressures and the cardiac index can vary widely, and it is not wise to assume that cardiac output is low, or the filling pressures high. Clinical assessment and invasive monitoring are therefore highly desirable (table 10.8).

Treatment

The greatest difficulty in preventing cardiogenic shock arises because patients are seldom seen early enough following myocardial infarction. Avoiding cardiogenic shock and its associated high mortality relies on early intervention to bring about reperfusion of ischaemic or infarcting myocardium. This approach (*infarct limitation*) may arrest the inevitable progress to myocardial necrosis leading to loss of left ventricular myocardium (see chapter 9).

When first seen in coronary care, reversible causes of shock must be considered, the commonest of which is hypovolaemia. This is often found in patients with right ventricular infarction and patients taking diuretics or antihypertensive agents. Cardiac dysrhythmias may also precipitate shock in patients with borderline left ventricular function, and should be rapidly terminated.

If found to be hypovolaemic, the patient should be placed flat in bed with the feet raised slightly. High oxygen concentrations (100 per cent) are required and toxicity rarely occurs because of arteriovenous shunting in the lungs.

After pain relief with opiates, the first priority is to increase the circulating blood volume using haemodynamic measurements (pulse, blood pressure and intracardiac pressures) as a guide. A Swan–Ganz catheter should be inserted for assessment of intracardiac pressures, and an arterial line is desirable for measurement of blood pressure and frequent blood gas estimation (see chapter 5). A urinary catheter should be inserted to record hourly urine output.

Forrester et al (1976) have demonstrated the importance of haemodynamic subsets in acute myocardial infarction, and this has particular relevance to cardiogenic shock. Cardiovascular haemodynamics should be stabilised using a combination of intravenous fluids, vasodilators and sympathomimetic agents (see table 5.9).

Intra-aortic balloon counterpulsation

Intra-aortic balloon pumping has been used in the management of:

- Haemodynamically unstable patients requiring support during preoperative investigation
- Cases of crescendo angina unresponsive to maximal medical therapy
- Cardiogenic shock

Balloon pumping has a unique role in treating patients with cardiogenic shock. A narrow balloon catheter is inserted via the femoral artery and advanced retrogradely to lie in the descending (thoracic) aorta (figure 10.22). When blood is ejected from

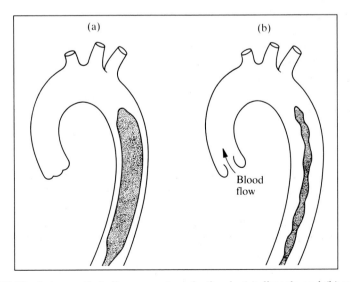

Fig. 10.22   Intra-aortic balloon counterpulsation in (a) diastole and (b) systole

the left ventricle it passes unobstructed around the deflated balloon. At the onset of diastole, a trigger from the ECG causes the balloon to inflate so that it occludes the aorta. Since coronary blood flow occurs predominantly in diastole, the presence of the balloon aids myocardial perfusion, and additionally improves cerebral blood supply. It also reduces cardiac afterload so that, when the balloon deflates again, the intra-aortic pressure is low, and blood is ejected with minimal extra cardiac work. Pulmonary congestion is rapidly relieved, and myocardial perfusion is improved through collateral vessels. Blood flow to peripheral tissues increases as myocardial function improves, and shock rapidly stabilises.

Unfortunately, although pumping may improve the initial mortality for patients in cardiogenic shock, 'balloon dependence' is common, so that when this support is withdrawn shock returns. Since weaning patients off the pump is usually not possible, insertion should only be considered where surgical intervention is possible. Those who survive are those in whom surgery can be undertaken to repair mechanical defects (e.g. repair of the mitral valve, excision of an acute aneurysm). Such surgery is usually combined with simultaneous coronary artery bypass grafting (Johnson et al, 1977).

Summary

Cardiogenic shock is a life-threatening complication of acute myocardial infarction which may become irreversible if not treated early enough. Modern invasive monitoring techniques and strategies aimed at salvaging left ventricular myocardium may help reduce its unacceptably high mortality. The ideal approach is to restore coronary artery perfusion and limit the size of infarction (see chapter 9). Concomitant pharmacological and mechanical assistance will buy time and reduce the risk of multiple system dysfunction and failure.

Initial therapy should be by correction of hypoxaemia, treatment of cardiac failure and restoration of cardiovascular haemodynamics. This may then be followed by coronary thrombolysis, coronary angioplasty or open heart surgery. The ideal management of cardiogenic shock is as follows.

- Rapid admission to a coronary care unit
- Immediate invasive haemodynamic assessment
- Intracoronary or systemic thrombolysis
- Cardiac catheterisation to define coronary anatomy and mechanical defects
- Cardiac surgery or coronary angioplasty

DEEP VEIN THROMBOSIS

The cause of deep vein thrombosis is still not fully understood. Three classical risk factors (slowing of blood flow in the extremities, damage to the vessel walls and increased blood coagulability) are important, and there are thus many reasons why deep venous thrombosis is more likely following myocardial infarction (e.g. immobility, increasing age, obesity and heart failure). Deep vein thrombosis is thought to complicate as many as one-third of cases of myocardial infarction. Many cases are asymptomatic and the first sign may be a fatal pulmonary embolus. Prophylaxis and rapid diagnosis are therefore of major importance.

Diagnosis

Clinical signs are not always reliable, but include swelling, tenderness and redness of the affected limb. Venography is the best method of demonstrating thrombosis in the deep veins, although the iliac veins are not always well shown unless femoral angiography is carried out as well. The investigation is invasive and has the risk of producing thrombophlebitis in some patients.

Impedance phlebography is useful for detecting thrombosis of the great veins, but is not very sensitive for calf vein thrombosis. It is easy to perform, but is associated with a high number of false positive results.

^{125}I–Fibrinogen scanning detects thrombi that are laying down fibrin, but this may be delayed for up to 72 hours.

Management

Prevention

Subcutaneous low-dose heparin (5000 units 8 to 12 hourly) should be routinely used for all admissions to coronary care, and full anticoagulation considered for those with prolonged immobilisation and heart failure. Graded pressure stockings (TD stockings) may additionally be useful. Early mobilisation is highly desirable for all patients (especially the elderly), provided there are no contraindications (Hirsh, 1981).

Therapy

A bolus of heparin 5000 units followed by an infusion of about 40 000 units per day is required, adjusted to keep the coagulation time (PTTK) between two and three times normal. Oral anticoagulants may be given at the same time and take about two to three days for effect.

PULMONARY EMBOLISM

Pulmonary emboli are common and about one-quarter are fatal (West, 1986). They are considered massive if they involve more than 50 per cent of the pulmonary arteries, and minor if less than 50 per cent, the size being determined by angiography, embolectomy or, regrettably, autopsy. By far the commonest sources of emboli are the deep veins of the legs, although clinical evidence will be present in only 50 per cent of cases (Kistner et al, 1972).

The signs and symptoms of pulmonary emboli will depend on their size. Chest pain and dyspnoea will be present in 85 per cent of cases, and the pain is typically pleuritic. However, pulmonary embolism may also masquerade as acute coronary insufficiency. Acute massive emboli have profound and dramatic effects since the outflow from the right ventricle is severely obstructed. This results in an almost total loss of cardiac output with circulatory arrest, collapse and syncope. There is hypotension, tachycardia, a high central venous pressure (measured by the JVP) and a gallop rhythm. Tachypnoea and cyanosis are usual.

Spontaneous lysis is a slow process, so the right ventricle gradually develops higher systolic pressures to increase the cardiac output. Hence, the late presentation of massive pulmonary embolism may be as pulmonary hypertension with a high jugular venous pressure, a loud pulmonary heart sound (P2) and a right ventricular gallop. There will be a persistent sinus tachycardia and dyspnoea.

Smaller emboli usually present with haemoptysis and pleuritic pain caused by the resulting pulmonary infarct. Examination may reveal a tachycardia, a pleural rub and perhaps evidence of pulmonary consolidation.

Diagnosis

It is well recognised that the diagnosis of pulmonary embolism is not easy. Probably half the patients diagnosed clinically as having sustained an embolism have negative investigations. Many diagnostic tests are non-specific and are prone to misinterpretation (Hull et al, 1983).

Electrocardiogram

The ECG is useful for excluding chest pain due to myocardial infarction, but there are no changes diagnostic of pulmonary embolism. Non-specific findings include sinus tachycardia, widespread T wave inversion (especially in leads V1–V4), right axis deviation, right bundle branch block and the classical S1, Q3, T3 pattern (acute cor pulmonale). Atrial fibrillation is precipitated in about 5 per cent of cases.

Chest radiograph

The chest radiograph is frequently normal, but may show pulmonary opacities (not necessarily wedge-shaped) or linear atelectasis with a small pleural effusion. Larger emboli will produce areas of oligaemia and a 'plump' hilum.

Loss of lung volume (e.g. an elevated hemidiaphragm) is the most common sign of pulmonary embolism.

Arterial blood gases

Acute emboli produce both airway and vascular changes, and both mechanical and gas exchange abnormalities may be present. Arterial blood gas abnormalities may provide additional support to the diagnosis of pulmonary embolism, but normal gases do not exclude an embolus. Mild abnormalities are common in patients with other disorders, especially in those with heart failure and chronic obstructive airways disease. Blood gases are therefore non-specific but may be useful in assessing the severity of the disorder. Hypoxaemia and hypocapnia are usually found in massive embolism because of the ventilation–perfusion imbalance, and hyperventilation.

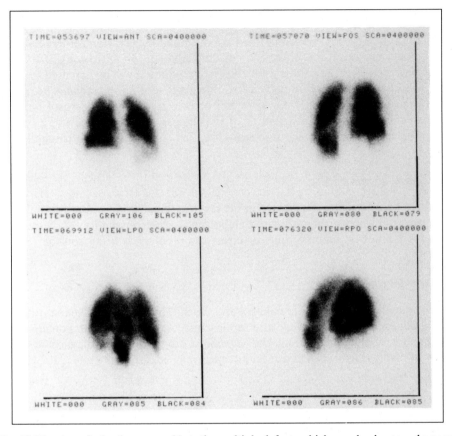

Fig. 10.23 A perfusion lung scan. Note the multiple defects which may be due to pulmonary embolism; a ventilation scan is required for confirmation

Lung scans

Perfusion scan

Although pulmonary angiography (see below) is the definitive way of diagnosing pulmonary embolism, it is highly invasive, and not without risk. The best diagnostic technique generally available at present is therefore the combined perfusion/ventilation lung scan. The patient is injected with technetium-labelled macro-aggregates of albumin, which lodge in the pulmonary capillaries. The distribution of trapped macro-aggregates is determined with a gamma-scanner producing multiple views of pulmonary perfusion. Significant perfusion defects are seen as 'cold' areas on the scan (figure 10.23). A normal perfusion scan excludes the diagnosis of pulmonary embolism but, unfortunately, false positive scans are common. Perfusion defects are produced by numerous conditions that affect pulmonary flow distribution, including chronic obstructive airways disease (including asthma), pneumonia, atelectasis and pleural effusion. If this is the case, a ventilation scan is additionally needed to make the diagnosis of pulmonary embolism.

Ventilation scan

Ventilation should be preserved in the areas of impaired perfusion if there has been a pulmonary embolism (i.e. there is a ventilation/perfusion mismatch). If the area of malperfusion is due to primary lung disease, ventilation will be impaired too, and there will be matching perfusion/ventilation defects seen on the scans. The patient inhales radioactive xenon (^{133}Xe or ^{127}Xe) or uses a technetium aerosol, and the gamma-camera records the distribution of alveolar gas with a multi-view series of pictures. The ventilation and perfusion scans are then compared for matching defects.

Pulmonary angiography

Pulmonary angiography is indicated in the severely ill patient in whom the diagnosis is not clear but where an acute massive embolism is a high possibility. This especially applies if pulmonary embolectomy or direct thrombolysis is being considered.

Differential diagnosis

This includes the other causes of collapse and shock. The high central venous pressure (CVP) will exclude haemorrhage and septicaemia. Acute cardiac tamponade is not associated with a gallop rhythm, and an echocardiogram will be diagnostic. Other causes of pleuritic pain such as a chest infection may be difficult to elucidate without a lung scan.

Treatment

The management is determined by the degree of haemodynamic upset. Most emboli resolve with time, and management is directed towards sustaining life and preventing recurrence. Pain and anxiety should be treated by diamorphine, and 100 per cent oxygen should be given. Vasodilators are contraindicated, and a high central venous pressure must be maintained.

Anticoagulation

Heparin should be given by infusion of 1000 units/h following a loading dose of 10 000 units, and therapy should be monitored by coagulation studies. Heparin should be given continuously until the patient has stabilised (and probably for about a week), after which warfarin can be substituted.

Thrombolysis

Thrombolytic therapy with streptokinase and other similar agents may be effective in massive embolic episodes, and are best delivered via a pulmonary arterial catheter. Bleeding and allergic complications are a frequent problem (see coronary thrombolysis).

Surgery

Embolectomy is very effective in selected cases, but requires cardiopulmonary bypass and carries a high mortality (over 50 per cent). Cases normally considered are those that continue to deteriorate despite thrombolytic therapy and those with persistent shock and respiratory failure.

Prognosis

Most deaths occur within the first hour, and the overall mortality is about 10 per cent. Resolution of clots is rapid, and starts within hours. Smaller emboli will be undetectable at five days and 50 per cent of lung scans are back to normal by two weeks.

PERICARDIAL DISEASE

Pericardial disease presents as pericarditis with or without effusion. There are many causes (table 10.9), the commonest of which are acute viral pericarditis and post-infarction pericarditis. Large effusions may cause tamponade and some types of pericarditis lead to pericardial constriction. Although evidence of pericarditis can be found in about 5 per cent of all autopsies, its true incidence is not known, since mild cases may be asymptomatic or overlooked in the ill patient.

Table 10.9.   Causes of pericardial disease.

Infective
    Viral
    Bacterial (including TB)
    Fungal
    Parasitic

Post-myocardial infarction

Metabolic
    Uraemia
    Hypothyroidism

Autoimmune
    Connective tissue disease
    Dressler's syndrome

Traumatic
    Crush injuries
    Post-cardiac surgery
    Post-radiotherapy

Neoplastic
    Primary and secondary

Idiopathic

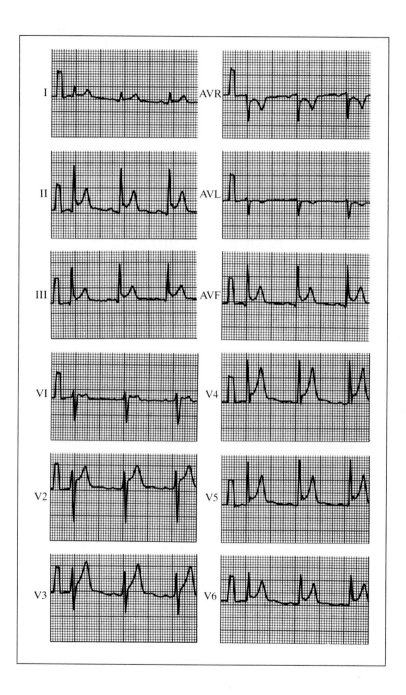

Fig. 10.24 ECG: acute viral pericarditis. Note widespread concave 'saddle-shaped' ST segment elevation

Acute pericarditis

Acute viral pericarditis is common in young adults. The usual viruses are Coxsackie B, echovirius, influenza and infectious mononucleosis. A typical flu-like illness is followed by fever and chest pain, which is characteristically worsened by inspiration and lying flat. The pain is mostly retrosternal and radiates to the left shoulder but not the left arm. Sometimes it is mainly felt in the epigastrium and may be confused with peptic ulcer pain. The pain is sharp, and may be from mild to excruciating. Atrial dysrhythmias are frequent, possibly caused by inflammation of the superficially located sino-atrial node.

The best clinical sign is the *pericardial rub*, which is high pitched, superficial and scratchy and is similar to the sound made by stroking the hair above the ear. It is best heard with the diaphragm of the stethoscope, and has a to-and-fro sound which passes from systole into early diastole as the ventricles fill. It is often missed as it can be localised, soft and transient.

The ECG may show sinus tachycardia and widespread episodes of ST elevation which are concave upwards in the leads facing the affected surface (figure 10.24). The chest radiograph is usually normal, but echocardiography may demonstrate a small pericardial effusion.

Post-infarction pericarditis

This is common (20 per cent) in the first week following acute transmural myocardial infarction and is associated with larger infarcts, left ventricular failure and dysrhythmias. A small effusion may be detectable on echocardiography. Sometimes pericarditis (and pleurisy) recurs two weeks to three months after myocardial infarction (*Dressler's syndrome*). The mechanism is thought to be autoimmune, and the condition responds dramatically to steroid therapy. A similar illness can follow cardiac surgery (*post-cardiotomy syndrome*).

Therapy

Treatment depends on the severity of symptoms. Bed rest and anti-inflammatory agents such as aspirin and indomethacin may reduce the pain and decrease any fever. If pain relief occurs, it is within 48 hours. The illness is self-limiting, but may recur. More severe cases may require steroid therapy. This will rapidly reduce pain, reduce the ESR, and cause resorption of small pericardial effusions. Resistant atrial dysrhythmias caused by the pericarditis may stop or become controllable. If there is an associated myocarditis, management should be as for myocardial infarction.

Pericardial effusion

Small effusions may complicate acute pericarditis or heart failure. They are hard to detect clinically, but larger ones are associated with an impalpable apex beat and increased cardiac dullness on percussion. In developing countries and immigrants therefrom, pericardial effusion is often infective in origin (usually tuberculosis). Pericardiocentesis is seldom necessary unless the aetiology is in doubt or there is evidence of tamponade.

Clinically significant pericardial effusions are uncommon after myocardial infarction. Using echocardiography, effusions may be found in patients with larger infarcts (especially anterior) or in those with heart failure. They often persist for up to six months, but anticoagulants are not contraindicated (*Lancet*, 1987).

Cardiac tamponade

Cardiac tamponade is compression of the heart by fluid accumulating within the pericardial sac. The pericardium is not very compliant and, as fluid collects, the intrapericardial pressure rises, hindering venous return to the heart. The heart is additionally unable to expand in diastole, and thus filling is impaired, with a secondary diminution of stroke volume, cardiac output and blood pressure. The heart rate increases in an attempt to maintain cardiac output but, as intrapericardial pressure rises above 15 cm H_2O, the clinical signs of shock appear.

The most common cause of acute tamponade is intrapericardial haemorrhage caused by cardiac rupture, aortic dissection or perforation during cardiac catheterisation. Tamponade can also arise from pericardial effusions secondary to infection (especially tuberculosis), but these usually accumulate more slowly.

Clinical presentation

The signs and symptoms of pericardial effusion depend on the rapidity with which the fluid accumulates. Although large amounts of fluid are usually associated with tamponade, as little as 200 ml may be lethal if it accumulates suddenly.

Acute tamponade is most commonly due to cardiac rupture which typically occurs in the first three to five days following myocardial infarction and is often rapidly fatal. There is a rise in the central venous pressure (as shown by a raised JVP) with a fall in systemic blood pressure. The patient becomes shocked, hypotensive, cold, clammy and restless. The liver is not acutely enlarged, nor are there signs of peripheral oedema unless the effusion is subacute or chronic. The apex beat cannot be localised, and heart sounds are quiet or muffled. The pericardial rub does not always disappear, even in the presence of large effusions. *Pulsus paradoxus* (table 10.10) and *Kussmaul's sign* (distension of the neck veins on inspiration) may be present (Shabetai, 1983).

Table 10.10.   Measurement of pulsus paradoxus.

---

1. Apply blood pressure cuff and measure the blood pressure
2. Reinflate the cuff to above the systolic point
3. Gradually deflate until the first Korotkoff sound can only be heard during expiration
4. Continue to deflate until the first Korotkoff sound is heard throughout the respiratory cycle
5. The difference between the two pressures is the degree of paradox and should not normally exceed 10 mmHg

---

Investigation

The chest radiograph may be normal if the fluid has accumulated suddenly. Volumes of less than 250 ml cannot easily be seen. Larger effusions distort the cardiac shadow which gives it a globular appearance, and makes a very sharp angle between the right border of the heart and the diaphragm. The lung fields are clear, differentiating the enlarged cardiac shadow from a dilated heart complicating congestive heart failure.

The ECG shows low-voltage QRS complexes, and blood within the pericardial sac often causes tall peaked T waves. *Electrical alternans* is rare but diagnostic. This is the alteration of cardiac electrical axis from beat to beat, said to be caused by the heart's swinging freely in a bag of fluid. An echocardiogram will show small effusions as echo-free spaces around the heart. Mostly, this is posterior with the patient lying supine.

Treatment

A pericardial tap should be carried out immediately if there are signs of tamponade. Fluid is withdrawn under local anaesthesia via a needle inserted under the xiphisternum. Many other routes have been described with their own relative merits. An ECG electrode (V1) is attached to the needle, and other standard limb leads to the patient. If the ECG machine is allowed to run continuously, normal complexes are seen unless the needle makes contact with the epicardium. If this happens, an injury current is obtained (ST elevation) and the needle should be withdrawn a little. Fluid can be aspirated via this needle or a soft cannula. If a bloody aspirate is obtained, it should be sent for a routine blood count and a further sample should be observed for clotting. This enables a bloody effusion to be differentiated from a ruptured heart; effusions do not clot, and have a lower haematocrit than a venous blood sample.

Since the pericardial compliance curve is exponential, relief of tamponade can usually be achieved by removal of approximately 20 per cent of the fluid. A larger quantity is usually removed, however, and is sent for cytology, biochemistry and bacteriology if the origin of the effusion is in doubt. In some centres, 500 ml of air is injected into the pericardial sac to delineate the parietal pericardium in tuberculous pericarditis. Thickening of this membrane by greater than 2 mm is a good sign of the need for pericardectomy to prevent constrictive pericarditis. The underlying cause of the effusion will need specific therapy, and chronic effusions may require pericardotomy to break down loculations and drain viscous fluid.

Constrictive pericarditis

This is usually caused by tuberculosis, but may be secondary to haemopericardium (traumatic), radiation, uraemia or rheumatoid arthritis. Clinically, signs are similar to those of tamponade, but the cardiac shadow is usually not dilated and there may be evidence of calcification of the pericardial sac. Pericardectomy is needed in the symptomatic patient.

References

Alpert J and Braunwald E (1984) Pathological and clinical manifestations of acute myocardial infarction. In: *Heart Disease: A Textbook of Cardiovascular Medicine,* ed. Braunwald E. Philadelphia: W B Saunders.

Anderson K P and Mason J W (1983) Surgical management of ventricular tachydysrhythmias. *Clinical Cardiology,* **6:** 415–425.

Arnold S B, Byrd R C, Meister W, Melmon K, Cheitlin M D, Bristow J D, Parmley W W and Chatterjee K (1980) Long-term digitalis therapy improves left ventricular function in heart failure. *New England Journal of Medicine,* **303:** 1443–1448.

Aronson J K (1985) Cardiac arrhythmias: theory and practice. *British Medical Journal,* **290:** 487–488.

Bayliss J, Norrel M S, Canepa-Anson R, Reid C, Poole-Wilson P and Sutton G (1985) Clinical importance of the renin-angiotensin system in chronic heart failure: double blind comparison of captopril and enalapril. *British Medical Journal,* **290:** 1861–1865.

Bigger J T, Dresdale F J, Heissenbuttel R H, Weld F M and Wit A (1977) Ventricular arrhythmias in ischaemic heart disease: mechanism, prevalence, significance and management. *Progress in Cardiovascular Diseases,* **19:** 255–300.

Brand F N, Abbott R D, Kannel W B and Wolf P A (1985) Characteristics and prognosis of lone atrial fibrillation: 30 year follow up in the Framingham study. *Journal of the American Medical Association,* **254:** 3449–3453.

Bussmann W D (1978) Effect of sub-lingual nitroglycerine in emergency treatment of severe pulmonary oedema. *American Journal of Cardiology,* **41:** 577–583.

Chiarello M, Gold H K, Leinbach R C, Davis M A and Maroko P R (1976) Comparison between the effects of nitroprusside and nitroglycerine on ischaemic injury during acute myocardial infarction. *Circulation,* **54:** 766–773.

Cohn J N, Guiha N H, Broder M I and Limas C J (1974) Right ventricular infarction; clinical and haemodynamic features. *American Journal of Cardiology,* **33:** 209–214.

Consensus Trial Study Group (1987) Effects of enalapril on mortality in severe congestive heart failure. *New England Journal of Medicine,* **316:** 1429–1435.

Dancy M, Camm A J and Ward D (1985) Misdiagnosis of chronic recurrent ventricular tachycardia. *Lancet,* **ii:** 320–323.

El Sherif N, Myerburg R J, Scherlag B J, Befeler B, Afanda J M, Castellanos A and Lazzara R (1976) Electrographic antecedents of primary ventricular fibrillation. Value of the R on T phenomenon in myocardial infarction. *British Heart Journal,* **38:** 415–422.

Epstein S E, Kent K M, Borer J S, Goldstein R E, Smith H J and Capurro W C (1978) Vasodilators in the management of acute myocardial infarction. *Advances in Cardiology,* **22:** 138–146.

Forrester J S, Diamond G, Chatterjee K and Swan H J C (1976) Medical therapy of acute myocardial infarction by application of haemodynamic subsets. *New England Journal of Medicine,* **295:** 1356–1362.

Franciosa J A, Dunkman W B and Leddy C L (1984) Haemodynamic effects of vasodilators and long term response in heart failure. *Journal of the American College of Cardiology,* **3:** 1521–1530.

Furberg C D and Yusuf S (1985) Effect of vasodilators on survival in chronic congestive heart failure. *American Journal of Cardiology,* **55:** 1110–1113.

Harrison D C (1978) Should lidocaine be administered routinely to all patients after acute myocardial infarction? *Circulation,* **58:** 581–584.

Herlitz J et al (1984) The Gotenburg metoprolol trial. *American Journal of Cardiology,* **53:** 3D–50D.

Hirsh J (1981) Prevention of deep vein thrombosis. *British Journal of Hospital Medicine,* **26:** 143–147.

Hull R, Hirsh J and Carter C (1983) Pulmonary angiography, ventilation lung scanning and venography for clinically suspected pulmonary embolism with abnormal lung perfusion scan. *Annals of Internal Medicine,* **98:** 891–899.

Johnson S A, Scanlon P J, Loeb H S, Moran J M, Pifarre R and Gunnar R M (1977) Treatment of cardiogenic shock by intra-aortic balloon counterpulsation and surgery. *American Journal of Medicine,* **62:** 687-692.

Johnston G D (1985) Alternatives to the digitalis glycosides for heart failure. *British Medical Journal,* **290:** 803-804.

Josephson M E (1986) Treatment of ventricular arrhythmias after myocardial infarction. *Circulation,* **74:** 653-658.

Kannel W B and Abbott R D (1984) Incidence and prognosis of unrecognised myocardial infarction: an update on the Framingham Study. *New England Journal of Medicine,* **311:** 1144-1147.

Keenan D J M, Monro J L, Ross J K, Manners M, Conway N and Johnson A M (1985) Left ventricular aneurysm. *British Heart Journal,* **54:** 269-272.

Kertes P and Hunt D (1984) Prophylaxis of primary ventricular fibrillation in acute myocardial infarction. The case against lignocaine. *British Heart Journal,* **52:** 241-247.

Kistner R L, Ball J J, Nordyke R A and Freedman D G (1972) Incidence of pulmonary embolism in the course of thrombophlebitis of the lower extremities. *American Journal of Surgery,* **124:** 169-176.

Lancet (1985) Needless digoxin. *Lancet,* **ii:** 1048.

Lancet (1987) Pericardial effusion after acute myocardial infarction. *Lancet,* **i:** 1015-1016.

Lie K J (1985) Lidocaine and prevention of ventricular fibrillation complicating acute myocardial infarction. *International Journal of Cardiology,* **7:** 321-325.

Lipkin D P and Poole-Wilson P A (1985) Treatment of chronic heart failure: a review of recent drug trials. *British Medical Journal,* **291:** 993-996.

Lown B, Fakhro A M, Hood W B and Thom G W (1967) The coronary care unit: new perspectives and developments. *Journal of the American Medical Association,* **199:** 188-198.

Matsuda Y, Toma Y, Ogawa H, Matsuzaki M, Katayama K, Fuji T, Yoshino F, Moritani K, Kumada T and Kusukawa R (1983) Importance of left atrial function in patients with myocardial infarction. *Circulation,* **67:** 566-571.

Mauro V F and Zeller F P (1985) Early use of beta-adrenergic blocking agents in acute myocardial infarction. *Drug Intelligence and Clinical Pharmacology,* **20:** 14-19.

May G S, Furburg C D, Eberlein K A and Geraci B J (1983) Secondary prevention after acute myocardial infarction: a review of short-term acute phase trials. *Progress in Cardiovascular Diseases,* **25:** 335-359.

Mundth E D (1972) Rupture of the heart complicating myocardial infarction. *Circulation,* **46:** 427-429.

New York Heart Association Criteria Committee (1964) *Diseases of the Heart and Blood Vessels; Nomenclature and Criteria for Diagnosis.* 6th edn. Boston: Little, Brown.

Noneman J W and Rodgers J F (1978) Lidocaine prophylaxis in acute myocardial infarction. *Medicine (Baltimore),* **57:** 501-515.

Page D L, Caulfield J B, Kastor J A et al (1971) Myocardial changes associated with cardiogenic shock. *New England Journal of Medicine,* **285:** 133-137.

Rackley C E, Russell R O, Mantle J A and Moraski R E (1977) Cardiogenic shock: recognition and management. *Cardiology Clinics,* **7:** 251-259.

Ribner H S, Isaac E S and Frishman W H (1978) Lidocaine prophylaxis against ventricular fibrillation in acute myocardial infarction. *Progress in Cardiovascular Diseases,* **21:** 287-313.

Rodrigues E A, Dewhurst N G, Smart L M, Hannan W J and Muir A L (1986) Diagnosis and prognosis of right ventricular infarction. *British Heart Journal,* **56:** 19-26.

Rosen M R and Wit A L (1983) Electropharmacology of antiarrhythmic drugs. *American Heart Journal,* **106:** 829-839.

Rosenbaum M B, Chiale P A, Haedo A, Lazzari J O and Elizari M V (1983) Ten years experience with amiodarone. *American Heart Journal,* **106:** 957-964.

Shabetai R (1983) Changing concepts in the treatment of cardiac tamponade. *Modern Concepts in Cardiovascular Disease,* **52:** 19-23.

Simpson I A, Rae A P, Simpson K, Gribben J, Boulton Jones J M, Allison M E and Hutton I (1986) Ultrafiltration in the management of refractory congestive heart failure. *British Heart Journal,* **55:** 344-347.

Stokes P H and Jowett N I (1985) Haemodynamic monitoring using the Swan–Ganz catheter. *Intensive Care Nursing,* **1:** 9–17.

Surawicz B (1986) R-on-T phenomenon: dangerous and harmless. *Journal of Applied Cardiology,* **1:** 39–61.

Vaughan Williams E M (1984) A classification of antiarrhythmic actions reassessed after a decade of new drugs. *Journal of Clinical Pharmacology,* **24:** 129–147.

Vetter N J and Julian D G (1975) Comparison of arrhythmia computer and conventional monitoring in coronary care units. *Lancet,* **i:** 791–797.

Vlodaver Z, Coe J I and Edwards J E (1975) True and false left ventricular aneurysms: propensity for the latter to rupture. *Circulation,* **51:** 567–572.

Wartman W B and Hellerstein H K (1948) The incidence of heart disease in 2000 consecutive autopsies. *Annals of Internal Medicine,* **28:** 41–65.

Webb S W, Adgey A A J and Pantridge J F (1972) Autonomic disturbance at the onset of acute myocardial infarction. *British Medical Journal,* **3:** 89–92.

Wellens H J, Bar F W and Lie K I (1978) The value of the electrocardiogram in the differential diagnosis of tachycardia with a widened QRS complex. *American Journal of Medicine,* **64:** 27–33.

West J W (1986) Pulmonary embolism. *Medical Clinics of North America,* **70:** 877–893.

Willerson J T (1982) What is wrong with the failing heart? *New England Journal of Medicine,* **307:** 243–245.

Wit A L and Rosen M R (1983). Pathophysiologic mechanisms of cardiac arrhythmias. *American Heart Journal,* **106:** 798–811.

World Scientific Group (1985) *Sudden Cardiac Death.* WHO Technical Report Series No. 726. World Health Organisation: Geneva.

Zipes D P, Heger J J and Prystowyski E N (1983) Pathophysiology of arrhythmias: clinical electrophysiology. *American Heart Journal,* **103:** 812–828.

11

Cardiopulmonary Resuscitation

Cardiorespiratory arrest occurs when there is sudden cessation of spontaneous respiration and circulation. The commonest reason is a cardiac dysrhythmia secondary to coronary heart disease. Other causes include pulmonary emboli, massive haemorrhage and trauma. Coronary care units were developed primarily to treat ventricular fibrillation and other serious dysrhythmias in the first few hours following myocardial infarction. Unfortunately, many episodes occur before admission to hospital, and 40 per cent of deaths relating to coronary heart disease occur within the first hour following onset of symptoms (63 per cent in young and middle-aged patients), of which 90 per cent are due to ventricular fibrillation. In addition, a large proportion of cardiac arrests occur on the hospital wards, or after discharge from specialist units where it is the nursing staff who have the responsibility for carrying out basic life support before the arrival of the 'arrest team'. Undoubtedly, open-plan wards permit the rapid recognition of circulatory arrest and, from the point of view of resuscitation, it is a shame that so many four-bed or single-bed wards now exist. Simulated cardiac arrests may help in identifying any deficiencies or difficulties in resuscitation within such areas (Sullivan and Guyatt, 1986).

Since resuscitation by nurses is usual on high-dependency units, and early steps are commonplace on general medical wards (especially at night), it is essential that the nursing staff can cope with this task competently. Although chances of resuscitation should be optimal within hospital, there are often deficiencies in the knowledge of basic resuscitation skills (Hershey and Fisher, 1982). Studies both in the UK and the USA have highlighted this inadequacy, not only in nursing staff but also in the junior medical staff (Gass and Curry, 1983; Casey, 1984; Skinner, 1985; Kaye and Mancini, 1986, Wynne et al, 1987). One of the principal functions of the coronary care unit and its specialist staff must be to train personnel in the basic resuscitation procedures (Jowett and Thompson, 1988a). All hospital staff, whatever their work, need to learn the rudiments of cardiopulmonary resuscitation; it is one of the main life-saving procedures that can be carried out by everybody (Resuscitation Council, 1984). In addition, those in specialist areas (e.g. CCU, ITU, casualty) and junior medical staff need to be checked in their proficiency of these basic skills, the use of simple equipment (oxygen, suction and airways) and defibrillation procedures (Royal College of Physicians, 1987). As staff become more senior and more experienced at attending arrests, increased confidence is not necessarily matched by an increase in skills (Gass and Curry, 1983), so that periods of retraining and retesting are required.

THE ETHICS OF RESUSCITATION

Most of the moral difficulties of resuscitation surround whether or not it should be undertaken in cases where there is serious underlying disease or debility. Resuscitation is best not attempted if a patient is found dead, or if he is known to have a distressing or inevitably fatal illness. The age of the patient is immaterial. Failed attempts do little to enhance the dignity of death, and may subject the patient and his relatives to added pain and misery (Baskett, 1986).

CARDIOPULMONARY RESUSCITATION

The basic principles of modern cardiopulmonary resuscitation (CPR) have arisen only from research work over the last 25 to 30 years, and the sequence of airway management, artificial respiration and external cardiac massage is now well established. Early manual methods of ventilation (e.g. Holger–Neilson) have been surpassed by expired air resuscitation methods (mouth-to-mouth) which have been shown to improve arterial oxygenation (Safar et al, 1958; Elam and Greene, 1961; Nolte, 1968), but support of the arrested circulation has changed little since early descriptions (Kouwenhoven et al, 1960; Jude et al, 1961). Much more is now known about resuscitation physiology, and modifications to traditional resuscitation methods have been suggested in recent years, with more efficient methods of providing circulatory and ventilatory assistance (Jowett and Thompson, 1988b).

When conventional CPR was first introduced, it was believed that the heart was emptied by being squeezed between the sternum and the thoracic spine. However, this 'cardiac pump' hypothesis assumes that the heart valves remain competent during external compression which is not the case (Chandra et al, 1980). Two-dimensional echocardiography has shown that the heart valves remain open, and there are no changes in left ventricular size as might be expected if the heart were acting as a pump (Rich et al, 1981). The heart therefore seems to act as a passive conduit rather than a pump (Werner et al, 1981). Although there is no difference in pressure within intrathoracic organs during compression (Chandra et al, 1981a), there is between intrathoracic and extrathoracic vessels (Niemann et al, 1981). The current idea is that the whole of the chest acts as a pump during external compression, and blood is probably ejected by the production of an intermittent pressure gradient between the inside of the chest and the rest of the body (the *thoracic pump mechanism*), with the heart and the great vessels constituting the pump (Rudikoff et al, 1980). The mitral and aortic valves remain open, and partial closure of the pulmonary valve with collapse of the great veins helps prevent retrograde blood flow (Rudikoff et al, 1980; Werner et al, 1981).

External chest compression only produces a cardiac output of about 25 per cent of normal (MacKenzie et al, 1964), which provides poor perfusion of the carotid and coronary arteries (Niemann, 1984), and hence methods to augment this have been sought. The term 'new CPR' has arisen following recent research into new techniques for improving blood flow during resuscitation. These include:

● Simultaneous chest compression and ventilation
● Abdominal compression with synchronised ventilation

● Interposed abdominal compression
● Continuous abdominal binding

Inflation of the lungs at the same time as chest compression may increase cerebral and coronary perfusion, and has been shown in animal experiments using simultaneous ventilation and compression at a rate of 40 per minute using high airway pressures (Chandra et al, 1980). However, once endotracheal intubation is accomplished, ventilation and compression are better performed asynchronously (Melker and Cavallaro, 1983).

Abdominal binding may help by raising intra-abdominal aortic diastolic pressure and promoting coronary and cerebral perfusion (Chandra et al, 1981b). However, the central venous pressure is also elevated, and this may compromise coronary perfusion (Niemann et al, 1984). Abdominal binding is preferred to abdominal compression which may cause intra-abdominal trauma, including laceration of the liver. Binding of the abdomen also takes time, and abdominal compression (either synchronised or interposed) requires a third resuscitator (Rosborough et al, 1981; Babbs and Tacker, 1986) and might delay more formal resuscitative measures. No study has demonstrated that interposed abdominal compression improves survival in man, and as such the technique remains experimental.

DEFINITIONS AND AETIOLOGY

Cardiac arrest is the cessation of effective cardiac contraction, with a consequent lethal fall in cardiac output. In clinical practice this implies either ventricular standstill (asystole) or ventricular fibrillation, although there may be virtual circulatory arrest with profound bradycardias or ventricular tachycardia.

Electromechanical dissociation (EMD) describes a state where normal electrical complexes continue to show on the electrocardiograph, but there is no effective pulse or blood pressure. This may be seen in:

● Massive myocardial infarction
● Severe haemorrhage (when there will be a tachycardia on the ECG, and a low CVP)
● Pulmonary embolism (tachycardia and high CVP)
● Cardiac rupture or tamponade

The majority of cardiac arrests occur outside hospital, and 'sudden deaths' are usually due to ventricular dysrhythmias. Cardiac arrest may be due to problems arising within the heart (e.g. myocardial infarction) or to problems elsewhere in the body (e.g. hypovolaemia, hypoxia or hyperkalaemia). Common precipitating causes are acute myocardial ischaemia, valvular heart disease (especially aortic stenosis), cardiomyopathy, chronic obstructive airways disease and drugs. In hospital, conditions commonly associated with cardiac arrest include myocardial infarction, pulmonary embolism, valvular heart disease, postoperative patients and investigative procedures.

There are often warning signs preceding cardiac arrest which experienced nurses on coronary care can recognise, and certain rhythm disturbances have long been associated with onset of ventricular fibrillation, especially:

● R-on-T ectopic beats
● Frequent left ventricular ectopics
● Multifocal ectopic beats

Unfortunately, many cases of ventricular fibrillation occur with no warning. There are two main phases of CPR:

● Basic life support (BLS)
● Advanced cardiac life support (ACLS)

BASIC LIFE SUPPORT

The main objective of CPR is to provide oxygen to the vital organs (brain, heart, kidneys) until spontaneous oxygenation returns, or until definitive medical treatment (advanced cardiac life support) can be initiated. The lungs can withstand long periods of anoxia, although the heart and kidneys can only survive for 30 minutes before irreversible ischaemic changes result. However, the cerebral cortex can only withstand anoxia for about five minutes (Heymans, 1950).

The critical factor in basic life support is therefore speed. The most impressive reports showing success of CPR are in those cases where resuscitation was initiated within four minutes of collapse, with advanced resuscitation techniques being commenced within eight minutes (Cobb et al, 1980). This applies not only within hospital, but also in the community where bystander resuscitation may be utilised to good effect (Myerburg et al, 1982; Hanson, 1984).

Basic life support (BLS) is designed to:

1. Prevent circulatory or respiratory arrest through prompt recognition and intervention.

2. Support circulation and ventilation, if required, by CPR.

The ABCs of basic life support

Basic life support traditionally follows several ABC sequences (Evans, 1986). The first of these is as follows.

A: Ascertain arrest

An assessment phase is critical, and must start with the recognition and confirmation of cardiopulmonary arrest.

Recognition

During cardiac arrest there is ineffective mechanical activity of the heart, a reduced cardiac output and cerebral hypoperfusion. Loss of consciousness, apnoea (or gasping respiration) and loss of pulses occur within seconds. Other signs such as cyanosis and dilatation of the pupils take much longer, and should not be awaited. Speed in initiating CPR is essential and any delay may be fatal; a false alarm is better than a dead patient. In the context of acute myocardial infarction, cardiac arrest does not necessarily reflect serious myocardial damage. However, the neurones of the cerebral cortex undergo irreversible changes after three to five minutes, and if prompt and efficient CPR is not started within this time permanent cerebral damage will occur. Hence, cardiac arrest must be assumed to have occurred with:

- Any sudden loss of consciousness
- Sudden onset of a seizure in a non-epileptic patient
- Sudden onset of cyanosis or respiratory distress

Other underlying causes may of course be responsible (syncope, cerebrovascular accidents, haemorrhage or epilepsy), but where there is any doubt CPR should be immediately instituted.

Confirmation

Immediate clinical assessment will reveal the following in a patient who has suffered a cardiac arrest.

- Rapidly deteriorating level of consciousness
- Change in skin colour: pallor or cyanosis
- Absence of a pulse (put an ear to the chest: time should not be wasted in trying to feel peripheral pulses)
- Absence of respiration (note that a spontaneous 'gasping' ineffective respiration may occur for a few minutes following circulatory arrest)

B: Bang on chest

A mechanical method for restoring sinus rhythm was reported in 1920 by Schott, who terminated a Stokes–Adams attack with a precordial blow. This method of restoring sinus rhythm was widely practised until it was suggested that such a manoeuvre might convert ventricular tachycardia to ventricular fibrillation (Adgey and Webb, 1979). However, the potential benefit of the precordial thump to mechanically cardiovert ventricular fibrillation to sinus rhythm greatly outweighs its risks and it should always be used (Caldwell et al, 1985). A similar mechanical stimulus may be given by raising the legs to promote venous return.

Conscious patients with ventricular tachycardia may restore sinus rhythm by forceful coughing, and some patients can maintain cerebral circulation by repeated coughing (*cough-CPR*). Arterial pressures of 100 mmHg are achieved using the pressure changes in the chest, and give support to the thoracic-pump mechanism (Criley et al, 1976; Niemann et al, 1980).

C: Call for help

Once cardiac arrest is confirmed, help will be required for basic and advanced cardiac resuscitation. Shout for immediate help, and make sure that an 'arrest call' is put out.

The second ABC

The second ABC refers to the basic resuscitation skills of Airway clearance, initiating artificial Breathing and Circulation.

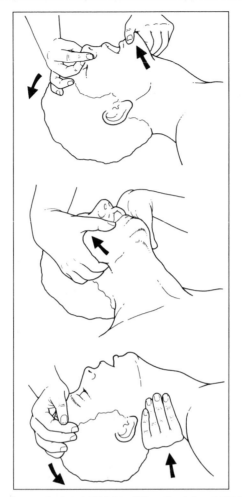

Fig. 11.1   Opening the airway: the head-tilt/chin-lift method, head-tilt/jaw-thrust method and head-tilt/neck-lift method

A: Airway

Effective CPR requires the patient to be supine and on a flat, firm surface. The head must never be raised above the level of the thorax or the brain will not be perfused. The patient should be placed on his back on a hard surface. If there is no board under the mattress, the patient is best pulled onto the floor. The rescuer should kneel at the patient's shoulders to allow access to both mouth and chest.

The most important initial action is to open the airway. In 90 per cent of unconscious patients, the upper airway will be obstructed, usually by the tongue which falls back into the pharynx when muscle tone is lost, allowing its supporting structures to relax. Since the tongue is attached to the lower jaw, moving the jaw forward will lift the tongue away from the back of the throat and open the airway. There are three ways of opening the airway (figure 11.1):

- The head-tilt/chin-lift method

● The head-tilt/jaw-thrust method
● The head-tilt/neck-lift method

Since it may be a lay-person who is first on the scene, it is necessary for the manoeuvre to be simple, safe, easily learned and effective. The widely taught head-tilt/neck-lift method does not fulfil these criteria (Guildner, 1976), and is no longer recommended (National Conference on Cardiopulmonary Resuscitation and Emergency Cardiac Care, 1986). The simplest method is the head-tilt/chin-lift method, although medical staff may find the jaw thrust more useful. It is technically more difficult and tiring (Guildner, 1976), but is highly effective, and especially useful if neck injury is suspected, since it may be used without hyperextending the neck.

Head-tilt/chin-lift manoeuvre

The head is tilted back by firm backward pressure on the patient's forehead with the palm of the hand. The fingers of the other hand are used to lift the chin forward so that the teeth almost close together. This supports the jaw and helps hold the head back.

Head-tilt/jaw-thrust

The mandible is pulled forward by grasping the angle of the jaw on both sides and tilting the head back. This may be made easier if the rescuer's elbows are allowed to rest on the floor close to the patient's head.

B: Breathing

The absence of respiration is deduced by the lack of chest movement, and by feeling and listening for expired air from the mouth and nose. The presence of vomit or foreign bodies (e.g. dentures) should be suspected if the airway is not cleared after proper positioning of the head and neck. A finger should be swept around the mouth to locate and remove any obstruction. If none is found, the possibility of inhalation exists. The application of chest or abdominal thrusts are more efficient than traditional blows to the back for dislodging foreign bodies in the airway (National Conference on Cardiopulmonary Resuscitation and Emergency Cardiac Care, 1986). Basic life support often needs to be instituted when equipment is not always to hand, and the use of mouth-to-mouth and mouth-to-nose respiration is of great emergency benefit. However, not only does the sight of vomit and blood usually deter the most hardened resuscitator, the theoretical risks of serum hepatitis and AIDS (the acquired immune deficiency syndrome) have now to be contended with. Nevertheless, delay should not be allowed to occur, since the risk of infection is small. Outside hospital, most cardiac arrests occur at home, and the previous health of the victim is often known. Within hospital, the number of occasions upon which any individual is called to administer mouth-to-mouth ventilation are few, and again the health of the patient is usually known.

Mouth-to-mouth ventilation should therefore be started immediately, and may be made easier with an oropharyngeal airway, if available.

Whilst maintaining the airway using the head-tilt/chin-lift technique, the nose is pinched, and one or two slow breaths are delivered in succession (1 to 1.5 seconds each) with the lips sealed over the patient's mouth. Pre-oxygenation with up to four quick full breaths without allowing the chest to deflate, previously recommended, should not be used. It is almost impossible to inflate the lungs in under a second (Safar, 1963), and attempts at faster inflation simply force air down the oesophagus, leading to gastric dilatation, which promotes vomiting and limits full expansion of the lungs. The chest should be observed for equal and satisfactory movements, and expiration of air should be heard when the chest falls. If these do not occur, the airway is obstructed and should be cleared. Subsequent inflation of the patient's lungs should be slow to produce less pressure on the pharynx, and hence reduce the risk of gastric dilatation (Melker, 1985). The expired volume should not be greater than 1200 ml. The normal adult tidal volume is 400 ml, and the forced vital capacity is 4500 ml (3200 ml in women), so that it can be seen that a full, forced expiration is not required, but rather a slow exhalation, following a quick intake of breath.

Mouth-to-nose respiration may be more effective than mouth-to-mouth ventilation, and is associated with a lower incidence of regurgitation of gastric contents (Ruben, 1964). It is additionally of great value in cases of oral trauma or trismus. The mouth is covered with the bottom hand which maintains the chin-lift. The rescuer's mouth is sealed around the patient's nose, and ventilation is carried out as previously described.

Cricoid pressure

The 'Sellick manoeuvre' (Sellick, 1961) may be useful in preventing gastric regurgitation during artificial respiration. Pressure is applied over the cricoid cartilage, to displace it backwards and occlude the oesophagus. It is probably best only learned and applied by advanced rescuers.

C: Circulation

Circulatory arrest should be assessed by palpation of the carotid artery which lies in the groove between the trachea and the sternomastoid (strap) muscles in the neck. Peripheral pulses should not be used, as low-output states may masquerade as cardiac arrest. If there is no pulse, and the precordial thump is unsuccessful, external cardiac massage should be started.

External cardiac massage

The application of compressions over the lower half of the sternum has been used to effect artificial circulation for over 25 years (Kouwenhoven et al, 1960). The heel of the hand nearest the patient's head is placed over the lower half of the sternum,

Table 11.1. *Compression/ventilation intervals.*

One rescuer
Cycle of 15 compressions at 80–100 per minute (one-and-two-and-three, etc.) with 2 breaths (15 : 2), with reassessment of the carotid pulse after every 4 cycles

Two rescuers
The compression/ventilation ratio should be 5 : 1, with a pause for ventilation of 1–1.5 seconds

---

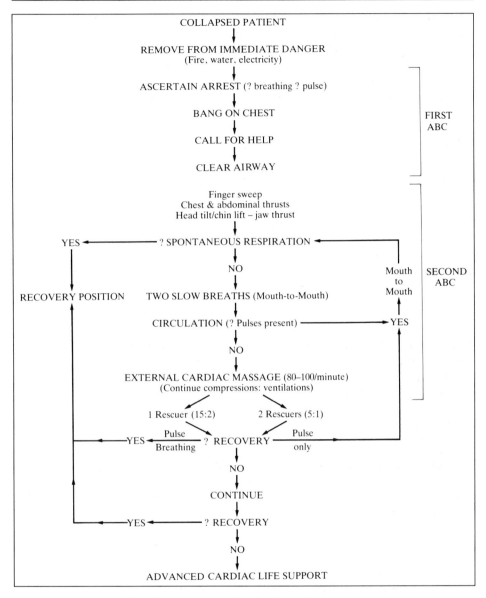

Fig. 11.2   An algorithm for basic life support

and the other hand is placed over the top with the fingers either extended or interlocked (but not in contact with the chest). Pressure of the fingers on the ribs or lateral pressure increases the possibility of rib fractures or costochondral separation. The arms should be kept straight, with the elbows locked, so that pumping action is delivered in a straight line from the shoulders by pivoting at the hips to depress the sternum 4 to 5 cm in adults.

Compressions should be smooth, regular and uninterrupted (except during artificial respiration) at a rate between 80 and 100 per minute. Recent studies (Maier et al, 1986) have suggested that the compression rate should be even faster (*high-impulse CPR*), and approaching 120 per minute.

At the end of each compression, relaxation must be complete to allow adequate refilling of the thoracic pump, although the hands should not lose contact with the patient, in case correct position is lost. Applying cardiac massage at the wrong site may lead to laceration of the liver, fractured ribs, pneumothorax or lung contusion. The optimal compression to relaxation ratio is between 50 : 50 and 60 : 40, so that at least half the cycle is spent in systole (Taylor et al, 1977), although high-impulse CPR makes timing difficult. Coronary blood flow takes place during the relaxation phase, and cerebral blood flow in the compression phase, and thus such a ratio gives priority of blood flow where it is needed.

The ratio of ventilation to number of compressions depends upon whether there is one rescuer or two. The recommended ratios are shown in table 11.1. A single breath of two seconds may be preferable to the two breaths (Melker, 1985), especially if the compression rate is greater than 100 per minute.

Changing the initial sequence of ventilation and compression (CAB rather than ABC) is taught by the Dutch Heart Association (Crul et al, 1985), since most patients with cardiac arrest are well oxygenated up until the time of cardiac standstill. The application of an early stimulus to the heart may lead to a return in spontaneous cardiac activity, rather as in the case of the precordial thump (Caldwell et al, 1985). This line of argument makes sense within hospital in the case of a witnessed arrest, but in other cases the period of anoxia is not always known and the lay bystander would be best to use the ABC approach to avoid applying cardiac massage inappropriately.

An algorithm for basic life support is shown in figure 11.2.

The arrival of help should ideally lead to advanced resuscitative measures. These include:

- Securing an airway (oropharyngeal airway, oesophageal obturator airway or endotracheal tube)
- Augmentation of oxygenation with portable oxygen, a self-inflating bag and face mask
- Recognition of cardiac rhythms with an ECG
- Treatment of dysrhythmias with drugs and electrical defibrillation
- Cardiovascular stabilisation to allow transport of the patient to a high-dependency unit

ADVANCED CARDIAC LIFE SUPPORT

Advanced cardiac life support (ACLS) combines basic life support with the use of specialist techniques and equipment for maintaining circulation and respiration. The key components are:

- Ensuring an adequate airway
- Early defibrillation
- Establishing intravenous access
- Electrocardiographic monitoring
- Pharmacological therapy

The design of basic life support does not require the use of equipment, although the highest priority must be given to early defibrillation. The use of other adjuncts is useful, though not so critical, and basic resuscitation should never be neglected because of the absence of medical aids.

Once instituted, therapy should be continued until admission to a specialist unit, or until a decision is made for life support to be terminated.

Airway management

The airway can be cleared in most patients by correct positioning of the head and neck, the finger-sweep manoeuvre and suction. There are many adjuncts which may be utilised to secure an airway and improve oxygenation. Expired air has a fractional inspired oxygen (FIo_2) of about 17 per cent, so that enrichment with portable oxygen is highly desirable. All airways should utilise 100 per cent oxygen wherever possible. Oropharyngeal airways should be used only in unconscious patients, as they may otherwise induce vomiting. Care and practice is required for correct insertion, or the tongue may be displaced backwards into the pharynx and obstruct the airway.

Laerdal pocket masks are extremely effective, and should be carried by all would-be resuscitators. They allow bag-and-mask and mouth-to-mask ventilation (Stewart et al, 1985), and can deliver an FIo_2 of 100 per cent oxygen if a flow rate of 30 l/min is used.

Self-inflating bag-valve-mask units can deliver an FIo_2 of 100 per cent at flow rates of 15 l/min, but ideally need two people to be effective. One rescuer maintains the jaw-thrust position and ensures a tight seal between the mask and the patient's face, whilst the other inflates the lungs by squeezing the bag. There is no doubt that the pocket mask is superior to the bag-valve-mask unit in all but the most experienced hands (Maull, 1984).

The main disadvantage of mask ventilation is gastric distension, leading to diaphragmatic splinting and oesophageal regurgitation (Melker, 1985). Hence these methods should be converted to endotracheal intubation as soon as possible.

The oesophageal obturator airway

The oesophageal obturator airway (OOA) consists of a soft plastic cuffed tube mounted through a traditional face mask which is passed into the oesophagus. Jaw-lift is maintained with the other hand, and the OOA is gently inserted into the oesophagus. It should never be forced, or oesophageal lacerations or rupture may occur. The distal orifice of the tube is blocked, but several upper openings at the upper end allow air to flow out at the pharyngeal level (figure 11.3). When the cuff is inflated, the oesophagus is occluded, thus preventing gastric distension and regurgitation. Mouth-to-mask or bag-and-mask ventilation can then be administered, provided a good seal is obtained between the mask and the face (Donen et al, 1983). If the trachea is intubated by mistake, it will be impossible to ventilate the patient, so auscultation of the chest is required before the cuff is inflated. This will additionally prevent damage to the walls of the trachea.

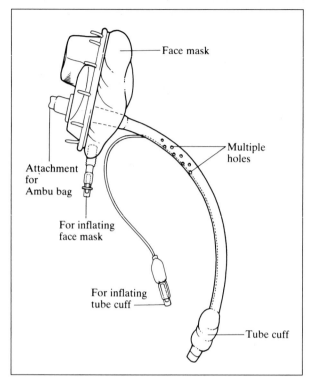

Fig. 11.3 The oesophageal obturator airway (From Jowett and Thompson, 1988. Reproduced by kind permission of Churchill Livingstone)

A modification of the OOA is the oesophageal gastric tube airway (OGTA) which has a distal opening in the oesophageal tube to allow decompression of the stomach by passage of a gastric tube (Gordon, 1977). A spring-loaded valve prevents gastric contents being accidentally forced up the tube (figure 11.4).

Endotracheal intubation

The best means of securing and maintaining an airway is endotracheal intubation (Stoelting, 1981). This additionally ensures delivery of high concentrations of oxygen, and provides an alternative route for drug administration. The procedure requires skill which can only be gained by practice; repeated attempts to intubate should not be made, and the maximum interruption in ventilation should be 30 seconds. Endotracheal tubes are labelled with the internal diameter in millimeters, and should be cut to appropriate lengths. Female patients will require the 7.5–8.0 mm size, and male patients 8.0–8.5 mm. Passage of the tube may sometimes be aided by external pressure on the cricoid cartilage (the Sellick manoeuvre) which occludes the upper part of the oesophagus and prevents aspiration of gastric contents (Sellick, 1961). After intubation the position of the tube should be verified by watching for equal

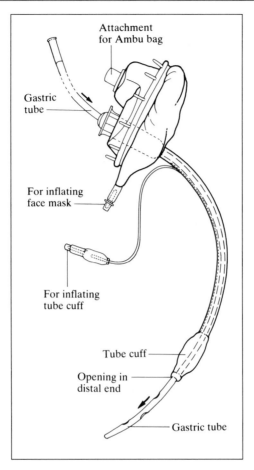

Fig. 11.4 The oesophageal gastric tube airway (From Jowett and Thompson, 1988. Reproduced by kind permission of Churchill Livingstone)

expansion of both sides of the chest, and listening over the lungs with a stethoscope. Ventilation should be at about 12 to 15 inflations per minute, and there is no need for synchronised compression of the heart (Melker and Cavallaro, 1983).

Intravenous access

Intravenous access is essential for administration of fluids and drugs. Peripheral lines are the simplest, since the veins are easily seen despite their tendency to collapse following cardiac arrest. The site of choice is the antecubital fossa, since cannulation of the subclavian and neck veins needs practice, and may require a temporary halt of CPR. However, peripheral administration of drugs may cause significant delay (one to two minutes) in arrival at the heart, even with optimal external cardiac massage (Doan, 1984). A large volume of flushing solution is therefore required, or the passage of a long line through a peripheral cannula. Although peripheral administration of adrenaline has been found to be as effective as central administration

(Gueugniaud et al, 1987), this is probably because peripheral lines can be set up more quickly. An additional central line is therefore highly desirable, since the larger veins allow faster infusion of fluids and drugs into the central circulation. They may additionally be utilised for transvenous pacing if required (Hazard et al, 1981).

Regardless of the aetiology of the arrest, increased vascular permeability allows plasma proteins and water to pass into the extravascular spaces, leading to intravascular hypovolaemia (Safar, 1984). However, caution is advised in administering large volumes routinely, since cerebral and myocardial blood flow may be diminished (Ditchey and Karliner, 1981). Expansion of circulating blood volume is of course critical in patients with severe acute blood loss, and cardiac arrest in these patients is often marked by electromechanical dissociation (see below).

Cardiac monitoring

Most sudden deaths are due to malignant ventricular dysrhythmias, especially in the early period following myocardial infarction, when rhythm disturbances are usually abrupt and without warning (Adgey and Webb, 1979). Electrocardiographic monitoring should be established as soon as possible in all patients following myocardial infarction or sudden collapse (Jowett et al, 1985). 'Quick-look' paddles on defibrillators may be used initially to avoid delay.

Three lethal dysrhythmias are commonly associated with cardiac arrest (asystole, ventricular fibrillation and electromechanical dissociation) although there are other serious dysrhythmias which may be precursors of cardiac arrest, or associated with a critical fall in cardiac output (e.g. ventricular tachycardia).

Arrest rhythms

Ventricular fibrillation

This is the commonest arrest dysrhythmia. There is a total breakdown of ordered electrical activity within the heart, and contraction of individual myocardial fibres is random and independent. The generated work is counterproductive and cardiac output falls dramatically. The ECG shows random waves which will usually diminish into asystole if left untreated. Consciousness is lost within 20 seconds, and rapid resuscitation is required as cerebral damage results after three to five minutes of circulatory standstill.

Ventricular tachycardia is another allied dysrhythmia, which in the context of acute myocardial infarction does not differ practically from ventricular fibrillation.

Asystole

Asystole is characterised by ventricular standstill due to suppression of the cardiac pacemakers by myocardial disease, anoxia, electrolyte imbalance or drugs. Strong cholinergic activity may depress the sino-atrial and atrioventricular nodes following myocardial infarction or episodes of myocardial ischaemia.

Asystole may occur without warning, or may be preceded by various types of heart block, and is found in about 25 per cent of hospital cardiac arrests (10 per cent outside hospital). It often represents massive cardiac damage or sometimes appears as the last dying rhythm of the heart following prolonged ventricular fibrillation. Survival is less than 4 per cent (Thompson et al, 1984). The ECG shows a flat trace which must be differentiated from fine ventricular fibrillation or sometimes from faulty connection of the leads and monitor.

Electromechanical dissociation

This is characterised by sinus rhythm on the ECG in the presence of circulatory failure; the ECG trace is an indication of the heart's electrical activity and not its contractile state. Electromechanical dissociation (EMD) may complicate anoxia, hypovolaemia, tension pneumothorax, severe acidosis or pulmonary embolism. The occurrence of EMD following myocardial infarction usually signifies a terminal event, such as rupture of the heart or cardiac tamponade.

EMD is rare outside hospital practice, but occurs in about 5 per cent of hospital cardiac arrests. The prognosis is very poor.

Treatment

Effective myocardial function depends on coordinated contraction of myocardial fibres. Ventricular fibrillation is the extreme example of disorganisation, which will result in death due to total abolition of cardiac output. Prompt therapy is mandatory. There are essentially two methods of restoring normal cardiac rhythm: electrical and pharmacological. Defibrillation is probably the cornerstone of advanced resuscitation (Zoll et al, 1956), and the earlier this is performed the more likely sinus rhythm is to result (Friesen et al, 1982). Any delay allows further myocardial ischaemia, anoxia and acidaemia, which will inhibit the restoration of normal rhythm. Defibrillation should therefore be carried out with or without ECG confirmation of ventricular fibrillation (Creed et al, 1983).

Defibrillation

The defibrillator basically consists of a large capacitor for storing electrical energy, and two conductive paddles, positive ($+$ve) and negative ($-$ve), for delivering this energy to the heart. The energy delivered is usually measured in joules (volts $\times$ amps $\times$ time), which is displayed on a meter. Older models are usually calibrated from 0 to 400 J as energy 'stored', but recent machines are calibrated for energy 'delivered'. Stored values of 100, 200 and 400 J will deliver 80, 160 and 320 J respectively. The pulse width is usually fixed at 3 ms, and is not variable. The shock is delivered by two hand-held paddles which are well insulated. A button is usually built into the handle of one of the paddles for delivery of the defibrillating shock. In many machines these paddles can act simultaneously as electrodes for ECG monitoring, and when not transmitting electricity to the patient can convey the heart's electrical activity back to a conventional oscilloscope to show the cardiac rhythm ('quick-look paddles').

A paddle diameter of 10 cm is recommended for adults (Kerber et al, 1981). Conductive electrocardiographic paste should be applied to the conducting surfaces, or preferably a solid conducting gel should be placed directly onto the skin. This is quicker, less messy, aids electrode contact and prevents 'jelly-bridging'. The paddle position is important to maximise the energy delivered to the heart. Standard placement requires one paddle to be placed to the right of the upper sternum inferior to the clavicle (2nd–3rd intercostal space), with the other in the anterior axillary line, just lateral to the left nipple (figure 11.5a). The paddles should be placed firmly against the skin with at least 25 lb pressure to prevent loss of current, flying sparks and skin burns. Obese patients have increased transthoracic resistance, and the chest-to-back method is advised (figure 11.5b). Here, the patient is rolled into the right lateral position and one electrode is placed over the left precordium at the base of the sternum, with the other posteriorly, slightly to the left of the spine (which would otherwise prevent good skin contact). Transthoracic resistance can also be overcome by using higher energies or multiple discharges, or by shortening the intervals between shocks (Kerber et al, 1981). The amount of energy required to restore sinus rhythm without producing myocardial damage is very difficult to calculate, and depends upon such variables as paddle size and position, blood pH and drugs (Kerber et al, 1981). It is not dependent upon body weight, and there is no need for defibrillators delivering more than 320 J (Patton and Pantridge, 1979). An initial shock of 160 J will defibrillate most patients, and there is no advantage for the initial use of higher energies. If the first shock is not effective, it should be repeated before proceeding to higher energies (Kerber, 1986). A defibrillation algorithm is shown in figure 11.6.

The operator should stand well clear of the patient and bed, and ensure that colleagues do too. This especially applies to the anaesthetist who may be hand-ventilating the patient, and will not thank the operator for delivering the current to him. Automatic and semi-automatic defibrillators have been designed for paramedical staff (Cummins et al, 1986). Once adhesive chest leads are applied, a defibrillator computer decides whether a shock should be delivered or not, based upon the recorded cardiac rhythm. This is delivered either automatically or semi-automatically (i.e. by an operator). Energy levels are preset, and warning buzzers sound to make sure that no-one is in contact with the patient at the time of defibrillation. Occasionally, antidysrhythmic drugs are needed between shocks to help restore sinus rhythm, and these are always worth trying if the first three attempts fail.

Drug therapy

Pharmacological intervention is utilised during cardiac arrests to:

- Correct hypoxia and acidosis
- Accelerate or reduce the heart rate
- Suppress ectopic activity
- Stimulate the strength of myocardial contraction

Definitive intravenous drug therapy should be started whilst CPR is in progress, and central venous cannulation will allow faster transit of drugs to the heart (Doan, 1984).

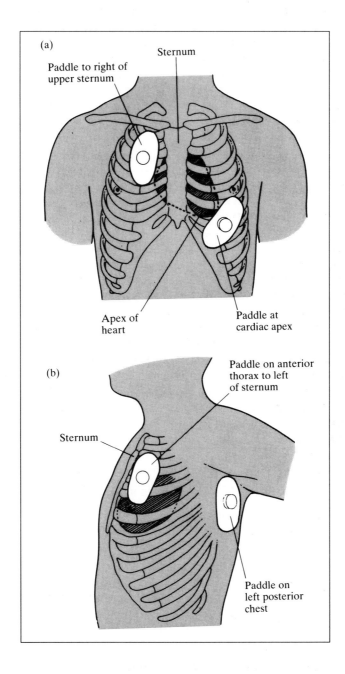

Fig. 11.5   Positioning of defibrillation paddles for (a) a normal weight patient and (b) an obese patient (From Jowett and Thompson, 1988. Reproduced by kind permission of Churchill Livingstone)

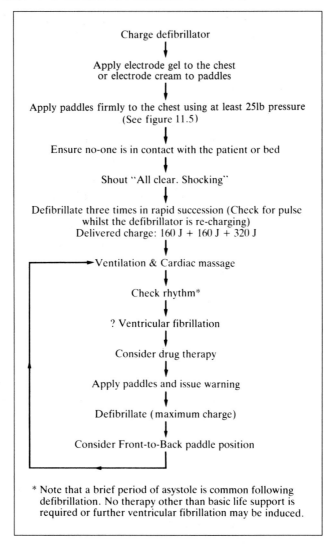

Fig. 11.6   Procedure for defibrillation

The first pharmacological consideration must be correcting the metabolic acidosis that inevitably accompanies poor tissue perfusion, with a build-up of lactic acid and increased levels of carbon dioxide. This acidosis depresses myocardial contractility, produces vasodilatation and capillary leakage, inhibits catecholamine activity, and increases the likelihood of dysrhythmias (Cingolani et al, 1975).

Sodium bicarbonate

Intravenous sodium bicarbonate has been widely utilised in the past for correcting the metabolic acidosis that follows cardiac arrest, but there is little evidence that this therapy improves outcome. Indeed the recent guidelines from the National

Conference on Cardiopulmonary Resuscitation and Emergency Cardiac Care (1986) no longer recommend its use because of the frequent occurrence of deleterious side-effects, including:

- Hyperosmolarity and hypernatraemia
- Creation of an extracellular alkalosis
- Shift of the oxygen dissociation curve to the left
- Inactivation of concurrently administered catecholamines
- Increasing carbon dioxide levels
- Tissue necrosis if accidentally given extravascularly

Critically ill patients in hospital may warrant early therapy with sodium bicarbonate if there is developing hyperkalaemia or acidosis which might precede a cardiac arrest, but these occasions are now the exception rather than the rule. The principal method of correcting the acidosis is thus by establishing adequate alveolar ventilation. Hyperventilation corrects respiratory acidosis by removing carbon dioxide which freely diffuses across cellular membranes. Optimal oxygenation, ventilation and airway control are therefore vital.

Calcium chloride and calcium channel blockers

The critical role of calcium ions in myocardial contraction and impulse formation is well established. However, the routine administration of calcium salts during cardiopulmonary resuscitation is questionable (Carlon et al, 1980; Dembo, 1984). Calcium may cause coronary and cerebral vasospasm, as well as increasing ventricular irritability in patients taking digoxin. Doses of 2 to 4 mg/kg (2 ml 10 per cent calcium chloride solution) may be useful for cardiac arrest complicated by:

- Hypocalcaemia
- Hyperkalaemia
- Electromechanical dissociation
- Patients on high doses of calcium channel blocking agents (e.g. nifedipine, verapamil or nicardipine)

The therapeutic role of calcium channel blockers for the relief of vasospasm is of current interest. Although no value has been shown during cardiac arrest, they may be useful in post-resuscitation care for relieving cerebral vasospasm in the post-anoxic state.

Adrenaline

Adrenaline has strong alpha- and beta-adrenergic agonist activity with a powerful vasoconstrictor action. Administration will result in peripheral vasoconstriction which augments the effect of chest compression, leading to increased cerebral and coronary perfusion. It may also increase the likelihood of defibrillation by converting fine ventricular fibrillation into more vigorous and rapid coarse fibrillation. The beta-agonist properties (positive chronotropic and inotropic effects) certainly help myocardial stimulation following attainment of sinus rhythm. The recommended dose in adults is 0.5 to 1 mg (5 to 10 ml of a 1 : 10 000 solution), which may be repeated every five minutes.

Lignocaine

Lignocaine has been used for over 20 years for the control of ventricular dysrhythmias complicating cardiac arrest and myocardial infarction. Its major action during cardiac arrest is to inhibit the initiation of re-entry dysrhythmias in the ischaemic myocardium (Kupersmith et al, 1975). Bolus therapy may be used during CPR every 8 to 10 minutes (0.5 mg/kg). Reduced hepatic circulation may make lignocaine toxicity more likely, and no more than 3 mg/kg should be administered.

Atropine

Atropine lowers vagal tone, although its value after the first few minutes following cardiac arrest is unclear, since significant vagotonia is unlikely to be present. However, 0.6 to 1.2 mg is still recommended in asystolic and bradycardic arrest, and may be repeated if there has not been a favourable response in a few minutes. Large doses should be avoided since they may reduce the electrical stability of the heart, making ventricular fibrillation more likely (Cooper and Abinader, 1979).

Treatment of ventricular fibrillation (figure 11.7)

Since spontaneous reversion from ventricular fibrillation is rare, immediate defibrillation gives the best chance of restoring normal rhythm. The precordial thump is advised in witnessed arrests, or in monitored ventricular fibrillation. Basic life support should be immediately instituted, until the defibrillator arrives (Jowett and Thompson, 1988a).

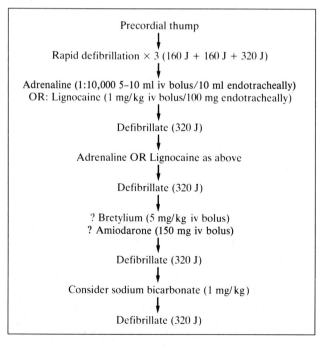

Fig. 11.7   Treatment of ventricular fibrillation

The initial shock delivered should be 160 J (200 J stored), which should be repeated before higher energies are employed (Patton and Pantridge, 1979). Three initial shocks should be given in fairly rapid succession (160 + 160 + 320 J), since this will lower transthoracic resistance and hence maximise energy delivery to the heart. The pulse and/or ECG rhythm should be checked between shocks, and if there is no pulse 15 further cardiac compressions should be given whilst the defibrillator is recharging. The Resuscitation Council for the United Kingdom recommends that the third shock should be 320 J (Chamberlain, 1986), although 240 J may be sufficient (Kerber, 1986).

The following agents may then be tried between shocks.

● Lignocaine (1 mg/kg) after the third shock
● Adrenaline (10 ml of 1 : 10 000) after the fourth shock
● Sodium bicarbonate (50 ml 8.4 per cent) after the fifth shock

Bretylium (5 to 10 mg/kg) and amiodarone (300 mg) are alternative agents, and phenytoin (150 to 300 mg) may be of value if the patient has been taking digoxin.

Treatment of ventricular tachycardia

Ventricular tachycardia may respond to the precordial thump or other mechanical methods such as coughing or raising the legs (Caldwell et al, 1985). Otherwise, treatment is the same as for ventricular fibrillation, especially if there is haemodynamic decompensation.

Treatment of torsade de pointes

Torsade de pointes is a polymorphic ventricular tachycardia associated with a prolonged QT interval, and is characterised by gradual alteration in the amplitude and direction of the electrical activity. Whilst treatment is as for ventricular fibrillation, intravenous magnesium sulphate may be useful.

Treatment of asystole (figure 11.8)

Fine ventricular fibrillation may often appear as asystole, so that a defibrillatory shock is always worthwhile (Thompson et al, 1984). If an additional monitor lead is connected, the rhythm can be checked, and if quick-look paddles are being used they should be rotated through 90° to confirm the rhythm. Adrenaline (0.5 to 1 mg i.v. every five minutes) is now recommended for first-line drug therapy because of its alpha- and beta-agonist activity. The alpha-activity helps maintain cerebral and coronary perfusion by intense vasoconstriction of non-essential vascular beds, and the beta-adrenergic action increases nodal activity. Early administration of atropine (0.6 to 1.2 mg) may be useful to relieve cholinergic overactivity on the conducting tissues (Brown et al, 1979), and can be repeated after five minutes.

The place of calcium salts is disputed (see above) and, if given, the injection should be slow and at lower doses than previously recommended (2 ml of 10 per cent calcium chloride). Sodium bicarbonate may be considered (1 mg/kg), but certainly not in the first 10 minutes following cardiac arrest (Jaffe, 1986).

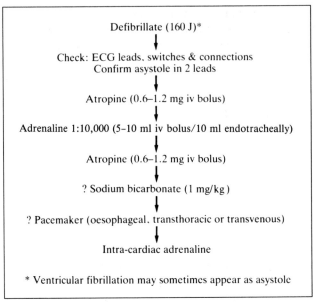

Defibrillate (160 J)*

↓

Check: ECG leads, switches & connections
Confirm asystole in 2 leads

↓

Atropine (0.6–1.2 mg iv bolus)

↓

Adrenaline 1:10,000 (5–10 ml iv bolus/10 ml endotracheally)

↓

Atropine (0.6–1.2 mg iv bolus)

↓

? Sodium bicarbonate (1 mg/kg)

↓

? Pacemaker (oesophageal, transthoracic or transvenous)

↓

Intra-cardiac adrenaline

* Ventricular fibrillation may sometimes appear as asystole

Fig. 11.8   Treatment of asystole

Pacing is perhaps a more logical approach to treating asystole and may be carried out transoesophageally, transvenously or transthoracically (Roberts and Greenberg, 1981; Hazard et al, 1981). Pacing is usually ineffective if the arrest is due to extensive myocardial damage, but may be of value in patients with impaired impulse formation or conduction.

Treatment of electromechanical dissociation (figure 11.9)

The prognosis of EMD is grave, and an aggressive search for possible underlying causes should be taken. These include severe acidosis, hypoxia, hypovolaemia, tension pneumothorax, cardiac tamponade and pulmonary embolus.

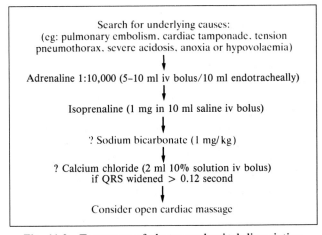

Search for underlying causes:
(eg: pulmonary embolism, cardiac tamponade, tension
pneumothorax, severe acidosis, anoxia or hypovolaemia)

↓

Adrenaline 1:10,000 (5–10 ml iv bolus/10 ml endotracheally)

↓

Isoprenaline (1 mg in 10 ml saline iv bolus)

↓

? Sodium bicarbonate (1 mg/kg)

↓

? Calcium chloride (2 ml 10% solution iv bolus)
if QRS widened > 0.12 second

↓

Consider open cardiac massage

Fig. 11.9   Treatment of electromechanical dissociation

Treatment is with adrenaline in the first instance (0.5 to 1 mg). Calcium may help, especially if the QRS complex is widened to greater than 0.12 second (Camm, 1986). Sodium bicarbonate may be needed to correct severe acidosis, which itself may precipitate EMD.

INTRACARDIAC AND TRANSBRONCHIAL ADMINIS-TRATION OF DRUGS

Adrenaline can be given intravenously or directly into the heart. It can also be given transbronchially via the endotracheal tube in twice the intravenous dose, diluted with 5 to 10 ml of water (Greenberg et al, 1981). Lignocaine can also be given in this way. Its onset of action is as rapid as an intravenous bolus, and its effect is twice as long. Other agents which can be given transbronchially are atropine and naloxone. Bicarbonate, calcium carbonate and noradrenaline should not be given via the endotracheal tube as they are very irritant to the tissues.

The use of intracardiac adrenaline is controversial. Direct ventricular puncture is performed via the 4th intercostal space on the left or via the subxiphisternal route. Aspiration of blood confirms cardiac puncture. However, since major complications may occur, including coronary laceration, pericardial effusion and tamponade, this approach should only be used as a last resort (Boike and Rybak, 1983).

CHANCES OF SUCCESS WITH CPR

The likelihood of survival following cardiac arrest is dependent on many variables, the most important of which are:

- The patient's overall physical fitness
- The underlying illness
- Where the arrest takes place
- The patient's condition after arrest

The development of out-of-hospital resuscitation has been shown to be of benefit in reports from the USA, the UK and Sweden (Geddes, 1986), with immediate by-stander CPR doubling the percentage of survivors. The improved prognosis noted in these speedily resuscitated patients may be because early CPR limits the extent of myocardial damage by establishing early reperfusion.

Most patients who arrest in hospital have recently sustained a myocardial infarction and warrant special observation, especially those with hypotension and heart failure (Hollingsworth, 1969). Ventricular fibrillation will not always be preceded by warning dysrhythmias. 'Step-down' coronary units have been advocated for these patients for their care between the coronary care unit and the ward (Karliner and Gregoratos, 1981). The prognosis of patients resuscitated within hospital is often governed by where the arrest takes place. The time between collapse and initiation of resuscitation is critical (Friesen et al, 1982). A recent report suggests that the long-term survival in ward patients is only 2 to 3 per cent (Hershey and Fisher, 1982), probably reflecting the increased time spent in confirmation of diagnosis and initiation of definitive therapy. Initial success rates in all cases of adult resuscitation may be as low as 30 per cent, falling to 10 per cent long-term (Peatfield et al, 1977). Nevertheless, these poor results should not discourage attempts at resuscitation since there are many full cardiac arrests that can be averted in the early stages when warning dysrhythmias or pure respiratory arrest has occurred. The best results may be obtained if resuscitation equipment is readily available and the nursing staff are able to defibrillate on their own initiative. The resuscitation rate then approaches 75 per cent, with 50 per cent of all arrest cases being discharged from hospital (Mackintosh et al, 1979).

POST-ARREST MANAGEMENT

The treatment of a patient following resuscitation depends on the initial outcome of CPR. Full recovery from cardiac arrest is rarely immediate, and can only be said to have occurred when the patient is fully conscious, with full cardiac, cerebral and renal function. These will be more likely if prompt CPR and defibrillation (within two to five minutes) is carried out, and if the underlying dysrhythmia is ventricular fibrillation. After stabilisation, all standard care should be given, although the amount of care patients require following a cardiac arrest varies enormously (table 11.2).

Patients may be broadly divided into four groups.

1. Immediate recovery with no sequellae.

2. Unconscious for a few hours. These patients may well be amnesic, but some suffer anxiety, confusion, delusions and difficulty in concentrating for several months.

3. Unconscious for more than 24 hours. These patients often exhibit signs of spasticity, stroke or incoordination. The prognosis is variable.

4. Decerebrate. Death is usual within a few days.

Table 11.2.   First steps after resuscitation.

  1. Check ventilation is adequate:
     ● Endotracheal tube is correctly placed
     ● 100 per cent oxygen
     ● Air entry is going to all areas of the chest
  2. Obtain blood gases and potassium
  3. Insert urinary catheter
     ● Measure hourly output
  4. Insert nasogastric tube
     ● Aspirate gas and fluid
  5. Obtain ECG and chest radiograph
  6. Consider need for:
     ● Low-dose dopamine infusion
     ● Lignocaine infusion

The patient should be thoroughly examined to assess haemodynamic status and to look for complications of the resuscitation procedure such as aspiration of gastric contents, or pneumothorax (secondary to rib fracture, or central venous catheterisation). An underlying cause for the arrest should be considered, such as anoxia or drug toxicity. Elective ventilation and prophylactic drug therapy may be required. Special attention should be given to the following.

Cardiovascular system

A full ECG and chest radiograph should be obtained. Blood should be sent for analysis of blood gases and electrolytes. An adequate blood pressure and cardiac output must be obtained to allow renal, coronary and cerebral perfusion. Formal haemodynamic monitoring with a Swan–Ganz catheter and arterial lines may be needed (Stokes and Jowett, 1985). Low-dose dopamine is often of value in promoting renal perfusion to avert acute renal failure.

Respiratory system

Ventilation–perfusion defects are common in both lungs following resuscitation and oxygen therapy should always be given. Arterial blood gases should be measured and artificial ventilation may be required. Hyperventilation to lower the $P\text{CO}_2$ may be useful in reducing cerebral oedema acutely.

Renal system

Adequate renal perfusion must be obtained as a priority, and an adequate blood pressure should produce 40 to 50 ml of urine per hour. Catheterisation of the bladder will usually be required, with urine output measured at hourly intervals to detect early signs of renal failure. Some authorities advocate the use of frusemide or mannitol to prevent renal shut-down or cerebral oedema. Low-dose dopamine may also be considered. Renal failure should be treated along conventional lines. Careful consideration must be given to the use of drugs excreted by the kidneys, or those with potential nephrotoxic side-effects.

Central nervous system

Primary cerebral damage may be caused by hypoxia during the arrest. Secondary damage may also occur after circulation is restored if the injured brain becomes oedematous. A flat trace on the electroencephalogram (EEG) is seen within 10 seconds of loss of cerebral circulation, and cerebral glucose is used up within one minute. Microthrombi may form in the small cerebral vessels when blood flow ceases, which compromises cerebral perfusion when circulation is restored. Microemboli may also be ejected from the heart and great vessels during cardiac massage. The widespread use of calcium during cardiac arrest is questionable (other than for electromechanical dissociation), since it promotes vasospasm in the cerebral vessels. Calcium antagonists given after the arrest may theoretically be of value to relieve this. Adequate arterial oxygenation is of great importance, if necessary utilising mechanical ventilation. Cerebral oedema may be reduced by the use of intravenous mannitol (200 ml of 20 per cent solution) and dexamethasone (10 mg intravenously, followed by 4 mg orally every six hours). Limitation of intravenous fluids and elevation of the head to 30° to increase venous drainage may also help. An EEG may be of prognostic importance.

Acid-base status

The acid–base balance must be urgently assessed, and plasma potassium must be measured immediately and frequently after the arrest. Both should be corrected as required. Care is required in administration of sodium bicarbonate, since it can lead to rapid falls in plasma potassium levels, and a rise in $P\text{CO}_2$ (thereby worsening cerebral oedema).

Gastrointestinal system

If bowel sounds are absent, a nasogastric tube should be inserted. There is a high incidence of stress ulceration and gastrointestinal haemorrhage. Antacids and cimetidine may help control gastric acidity.

WHEN TO STOP

The decision to terminate CPR is a medical one, and should be made by the most senior physician present. This decision should follow an assessment of the patient's cerebral and cardiovascular status as well as prognosis (Baskett, 1986). Prolonged resuscitation is seldom justified: the mortality following an arrest of over 15 minutes is 90 per cent (Bedell et al, 1983). Deep coma, dilated pupils and absence of spontaneous respirations usually indicate cerebral death.

All patients who die suddenly should be considered as potential organ donors, and visceral perfusion and oxygenation should be maintained until a decision is made.

DEFIBRILLATION AND CARDIOVERSION

The use of an electric current to terminate ventricular fibrillation in man was first reported in 1947 by Beck et al, who applied 120 V directly to the ventricles. Later an alternating current (a.c.) defibrillator was developed for terminating ventricular fibrillation by passing a current across the chest at 720 V (Zoll et al, 1956). The modern direct current (d.c.) defibrillator was developed by Lown et al in 1962, with the advantages of being smaller, chargeable with batteries and (because smaller currents were being employed) less likely to cause myocardial damage or precipitate dysrhythmias. Electrical defibrillation depolarises myocardial tissue ahead of the intrinsic depolarisation wave, making it refractory to conduction. The whole myocardium is thus suddenly depolarised, and awaits intrinsic pacemaker function to return, hopefully from the sino-atrial node. It follows that, if an insufficient current is applied, not all the myocardium will be depolarised, and defibrillation will not be successful. Following its application to ventricular fibrillation, the defibrillator was applied to other dysrhythmias with marked success. Electrical treatment of cardiac dysrhythmias has marked advantages over drugs in that it is free from pharmacological side-effects (especially depression of myocardial contractility), and it is useful against a wide variety of tachydysrhythmias, especially those originating from the ventricles (VT and VF). An early complication of this procedure was ventricular fibrillation, which was believed to occur following delivery of the shock to the heart at a time coincident with the vulnerable 30 ms preceding the apex of the T wave of the cardiac cycle (R-on-T). Synchronised defibrillators have thus been developed which trigger the shock just after the R wave.

Indications for cardioversion

Many cardiologists prefer to treat all tachydysrhythmias with drugs provided there is no contraindication such as profound hypotension or heart failure. There is obviously no choice if the dysrhythmia is causing circulatory collapse.

Elective synchronised cardioversion is useful for treatment of both supraventricular and ventricular dysrhythmias. Typical indications include atrial flutter (which is very sensitive to low energies), ventricular tachycardia and supraventricular tachycardia unresponsive to drug therapy. Atrial fibrillation is usually treated initially with drugs, but cardioversion may be employed:

● For atrial fibrillation unresponsive to drug therapy
● With recent onset atrial fibrillation (especially peri-infarction)
● After thyrotoxicosis has been corrected
● After mitral valvotomy
● After therapy for heart failure has reduced the size of the left atrium

Elective cardioversion for atrial fibrillation is seldom successful in patients with dilated left atria, and it is often of value to assess atrial size by echocardiography beforehand. Anticoagulants should not be necessary for recent onset atrial fibrillation, but other cases should be given warfarin for two to six weeks before cardioversion, and possibly up to a month after. Digoxin should preferably be stopped beforehand, and lower energies will be needed for cardioversion.

Metabolic and drug considerations

Hypoxic and acidotic ventricles are difficult to defibrillate. Attention needs to be directed to these metabolic upsets for successful defibrillation. Careful attention should also be paid to electrolyte levels, particularly those of potassium. Drugs may also influence the heart's response to cardioversion. Digoxin reduces the energy threshold required for defibrillation, and smaller currents should be delivered. In contrast, quinidine, lignocaine and phenytoin all increase the threshold, and higher energies will be needed to restore sinus rhythm.

Technique

The procedure should be explained to the patient, and consent obtained. The patient should be fasted for six to eight hours. A standard 12-lead ECG should be recorded before and after cardioversion, and a rhythm strip should be recorded during the procedure. An anaesthetist should be in attendance to administer a short-acting anaesthetic, and resuscitation equipment must be immediately available (table 11.3). It is usual to pre-oxygenate the patient, and oxygen should also be administered throughout the procedure and during recovery.

There are two main methods of electrode placement, although there appears to be no superiority in either method.

1. *Precordial*   One paddle is applied over the right 2nd–3rd intercostal space, close to the sternum, and the other just below the apex of the heart.

2. *Chest-to-back*   One paddle is placed to the left of the base of the sternum and the other between the scapulae slightly to the left of the spine (which would otherwise prevent good skin contact).

The technique is the same as used for defibrillation, and as in the first part of figure 11.6.

It is best to ensure that the ECG is set so that the QRS complex displays the most upright R wave to aid synchronised discharge of the defibrillator. The discharge will not necessarily occur as soon as the button is pressed, and the operator must not be tempted to release pressure on the paddles until after the shock has been delivered.

Because myocardial damage increases with the amount of energy applied, the shock should be 'titrated' against the type of dysrhythmia. For example, energy levels of greater than 200 J (stored) are required to terminate ventricular fibrillation, whereas most supraventricular tachycardias (with the exception of atrial fibrillation) will revert at between 25 and 50 J. If unsuccessful, a second shock at a higher energy level should be given. It must be remembered that high currents may actually produce dysrhythmias.

Occasionally, antidysrhythmic drugs are needed between shocks to help restore sinus rhythm, and these are always worth trying if the first two or three attempts fail. Administration of a suitable antidysrhythmic agent is particularly recommended if multiple ventricular ectopic beats develop after an unsuccessful shock.

After restoration of sinus rhythm, a further 12-lead ECG should be obtained, vital signs recorded, and arrangements for monitoring for at least eight hours made.

Complications

Dysrhythmias may occur after cardioversion, either because the underlying problem that precipitated the original dysrhythmia is still present, or as a direct consequence of cardioversion.

Bradydysrhythmias frequently occur immediately following cardioversion and are usually self-limiting. Sinus bradycardias, wandering pacemakers and junctional rhythms are not serious, but can be treated with atropine if they persist. A few ventricular ectopic beats may also be seen, and again are usually self-limiting. However, runs of ectopics, ventricular tachycardia and fibrillation need treating along usual lines. Because these complications may develop up to eight hours following cardioversion,

Table 11.3. Typical contents of the cardiac arrest trolley.

A Portable defibrillator and paddles
Electrocardiogram (battery), straps and electrode jelly
Chest electrodes
Defibrillator pads

B *Venous cannulation equipment*
Cannulae for peripheral/central lines
Gauze swabs
Syringes: 4 × 5 ml
4 × 2 ml
2 × 10 ml
Needles
Spinal needles: 2 × size 18
2 × size 20
2 × size 22
Tourniquet
Butterfly needles (19, 21 and 23 gauge)
Giving sets × 5
Cut-down set

C *Ventilation equipment*
Ambu bag and assorted masks
Airways: 1 × size 2
1 × size 3
1 × size 4
Brooks airway
Noseworthy connection
Endotracheal tubes (7.5 mm, 8 mm, 8.5 mm, 9 mm)
Introducer
Artery forceps and syringe
Angled connectors and black rubber tubing
Scissors
Laryngoscopes (1 curved, 1 straight)
Spare bulbs for above
Magill and artery forceps
Ribbon gauze
KY jelly
Oxygen tubing
Suction tubing and catheters

D *Intravenous fluids*
Dextrose 5 per cent
Lignocaine 0.2 per cent
Haemaccel
Normal saline (0.9 per cent)
Sodium bicarbonate 8.4 per cent

E *Drugs*
Adrenaline 1 : 1000 and 1 : 10 000
Atropine 0.6 mg
10 per cent calcium chloride (5 mmol in 10 ml)
Hydrocortisone 100 mg
Isoprenaline 2 mg
Lignocaine 100 mg
Practolol 10 mg
Dextrose 50 per cent (50 ml)
Dopamine

prolonged monitoring is indicated. This is particularly the case if antidysrhythmic drugs have also been used or if hypokalaemia is present. The risk of ventricular fibrillation and ventricular tachycardia is increased if the patient has been taking digoxin, and although it is preferable to discontinue the drug cardioversion should not be witheld provided there are no signs of toxicity (Ditchey and Karliner, 1981). Injury to the myocardium is well documented (Dahl et al, 1974) and makes subsequent dysrhythmias more likely (Jones and Jones, 1980). It is therefore always advisable to start defibrillation at lower energies and allow two to three minutes to elapse before the next shock is given. Rapid repeated countershocks lower transthoracic resistance and are more likely to damage the myocardium. Clinical signs of myocardial injury are not usually evident, even after multiple shocks, but ECG and enzyme changes are frequent. However, the enzymes probably originate from skeletal rather than cardiac muscle.

Thromboembolic complications occur in about 2 per cent of cases restored to sinus rhythm. The risk may be minimised by prior anticoagulation of any patient thought to be at increased risk for a period of two to six weeks. This includes patients with long-standing dysrhythmias, dyskinetic ventricular walls or dilated hearts.

Paddle burns are uncommon if careful attention is paid to application of the electrodes. Any inflammation will quickly respond to topical steroid cream such as 1 per cent hydrocortisone.

References

Adgey A A J and Webb S W (1979) The treatment of ventricular arrhythmias in acute myocardial infarction. *British Journal of Hospital Medicine,* **21:** 356–379.
Babbs C F and Tacker W A (1986) Cardiopulmonary resuscitation with interposed abdominal compression. *Circulation,* **74** (Suppl. IV): 37–41.
Baskett P J F (1986) The ethics of resuscitation. *British Medical Journal,* **293:** 189–190.
Beck C S, Prilchard W H and Feil H S (1947) Ventricular fibrillation of long duration abolished by electric shock. *Journal of the American Medical Association,* **135:** 985–986.
Bedell S E, Delbanco T L, Cook E F and Epstein F H (1983) Survival after cardiopulmonary resuscitation in hospital. *New England Journal of Medicine,* **10:** 569–576.
Boike S C and Rybak M J (1983) Pharmacological intervention in resuscitation. *Emergency Medical Clinics of North America,* **1:** 553–569.
Brown D C, Lewis A J and Criley J M (1979) Asystole and its treatment: the possible role of the parasympathetic nervous system in cardiac arrest. *Journal of the American College of Emergency Physicians,* **8:** 448–452.
Caldwell G, Millar G, Quinn E, Vincent R and Chamberlain D A (1985) Simple mechanical methods for cardioversion: defence of the precordial thump and cough version. *British Medical Journal,* **291:** 627–630.
Camm A J (1986) ABC of resuscitation: asystole and electromechanical dissociation. *British Medical Journal,* **292:** 1123–1124.
Carlon G C, Howland W S, Kahn R C and Schweizer O (1980) Calcium chloride administration in normocalcaemic critically ill patients. *Critical Care Medicine,* **8:** 209–212.
Casey W F (1984) Cardiopulmonary resuscitation: a survey of standards among junior hospital doctors. *Journal of the Royal Society of Medicine,* **77:** 921–924.
Chamberlain D (1986) ABC of resuscitation. Ventricular fibrillation. *British Medical Journal,* **292:** 1068–1070.
Chandra N, Rudikoff M and Weisfeldt M L (1980) Simultaneous chest compression and ventilation at high airway pressure during cardiopulmonary resuscitation. *Lancet,* **i:** 175–178.
Chandra N, Guerci A, Weisfeldt M L, Tsitlik J and Lepor N (1981a) Contrasts between intrathoracic pressure during external and internal cardiac massage. *Critical Care Medicine,* **9:** 789–792.

Chandra N, Snyder L and Weisfeldt M L (1981b) Abdominal binding during CPR in man. *Journal of the American Medical Association*, **246**: 351–353.

Cingolani H E, Faulkner S L and Mattiazzi A R (1975) Depression of human myocardial contractility with respiratory and metabolic acidosis. *Surgery*, **77**: 427–432.

Cobb L A, Werner J A and Trobaugh G B (1980) Sudden cardiac death: parts 1 and 2. *Modern Concepts in Cardiovascular Disease*, **49**: 31–42.

Cooper M J and Abinader E G (1979) Atropine-induced ventricular fibrillation: case report and review of the literature. *American Heart Journal*, **99**: 225–228.

Creed J D, Packard J M and Lambrew C T (1983) Defibrillation and synchronised cardioversion. In: *Textbook of Advanced Cardiac Life Support*. eds. McIntyre K M and Lewis A J, pp. 89–96. Dallas: American Heart Association.

Criley J M, Blaufuss A H and Kissel G L (1976) Cough-induced cardiac compression. *Journal of the American Medical Association*, **236**: 1246–1250.

Crul J F, Neursing B T and Zimmerman A H (1985) The ABC sequence of cardiopulmonary resuscitation (CPR). *Journal of the World Association of Emergency and Disaster Medicine*, **1** (Suppl. 4): 236–245.

Cummins R O, Eisenberg M S and Shultz K R (1986) Automatic external defibrillators: clinical issues in cardiology. *Circulation*, **73**: 381–385.

Dahl C F, Ewy G A and Warner E D (1974) Myocardial necrosis from direct current countershock: effect of paddle electrode size and time interval between discharge. *Circulation*, **50**: 956–961.

Dembo D H (1984) The role of calcium chloride in cardiac arrest. *Journal of the American Medical Association*, **250**: 3327–3329.

Ditchey R V and Karliner J S (1981) Safety of electrical cardioversion in patients without digoxin toxicity. *Annals of Internal Medicine*, **95**: 676–679.

Doan L A (1984) Peripheral versus central venous delivery of medications during CPR. *Annals of Emergency Medicine*, **13**: 784–786.

Donen N, Tweed W A, Dashfsky S and Guttormson B (1983) The esophageal obturator airway: an appraisal. *Canadian Anaesthetists Society Journal*, **30**: 194–200.

Elam J O and Greene D G (1961) Mission accomplished. Successful mouth to mouth resuscitation. *Anesthesia and Analgesia (Current Research)*, **40**: 440–442, 578–580, 672–676.

Evans T R (1986) *ABC of Resuscitation*, ed. Evans T R. London: *British Medical Journal*.

Friesen R M, Duncan P, Tweed W A and Bristow G (1982) Appraisal of pediatric cardiopulmonary resuscitation. *Canadian Medical Association Journal*, **126**: 1055–1058.

Gass E A and Curry L (1983) Physicians' and nurses' retention of knowledge and skills after training in CPR. *Canadian Medical Association Journal*, **128**: 550–551.

Geddes J S (1986) Twenty years of prehospital coronary care. *British Heart Journal*, **56**: 491–495.

Gordon A S (1977) An improved esophageal obturator airway. In: *Advances in Cardiopulmonary Resuscitation*, ed. Safar P and Elam J O. New York: Springer-Verlag.

Greenberg M I, Roberts J R and Baskin S I (1981) Use of endotracheally administered epinephrine in a pediatric patient. *American Journal of Diseases of Children*, **135**: 767–768.

Gueugniaud P Y, Theurey O, Vaudelin T, Rochette M and Petit P (1987) Peripheral versus intravenous lines in emergency cardiac care. *Lancet*, **ii**: 573.

Guildner C W (1976) Resuscitation – opening the airway: a comparative study of techniques for opening an airway obstructed by the tongue. *Journal of the American College of Emergency Physicians*, **5**: 588–590.

Hanson G C (1984) Cardiopulmonary resuscitation: chances of success. *British Medical Journal*, **288**: 1324–1325.

Hazard P B, Benton C and Milnor J P (1981) Transvenous cardiac pacing in cardiopulmonary resuscitation. *Critical Care Medicine*, **9**: 666–668.

Hershey C O and Fisher L (1982) Why outcome of CPR in general wards is poor. *Lancet*, **i**: 31–34.

Heymans C (1950) Survival and revival of nervous tissue after arrest of circulation. *Physiological Reviews*, **30**: 375–379.

Hollingsworth J H (1969) The results of cardiopulmonary resuscitation: a 3-year university hospital experience. *Annals of Internal Medicine,* **71:** 459–466.

Jaffe A S (1986) Cardiovascular pharmacology I. *Circulation,* **74** (Suppl. IV): 70–89.

Jones J L and Jones R E (1980) Post-shock arrhythmias: a possible cause of unsuccessful defibrillation. *Critical Care Medicine,* **8:** 167–171.

Jowett N I and Thompson D R (1988a) Basic life support. The forgotten skills? *Intensive Care Nursing,* **4:** 9–17.

Jowett N I and Thompson D R (1988b) Advanced cardiac life support: current perspectives. *Intensive Care Nursing,* **4:** 71–81.

Jowett N I, Thompson D R and Bailey S W (1985) Electrocardiographic monitoring I: static monitoring. *Intensive Care Nursing,* **2:** 71–76.

Jude J R, Kouwenhoven W B and Knickerbocker G G (1961) Cardiac arrest. Report of application of external cardiac massage in 118 patients. *Journal of the American Medical Association,* **178:** 1063–1070.

Karliner J S and Gregoratos G (1981) *Acute Coronary Care.* Edinburgh: Churchill Livingstone.

Kaye W and Mancini M E (1986) Retention of cardiopulmonary resuscitation skills by physicians, registered nurses and the general public. *Critical Care Medicine,* **14:** 621–623.

Kerber R E (1986) Energy requirements for defibrillation. *Circulation,* **74** (Suppl. IV): 117–119.

Kerber R E, Grayzel J and Hoyt R (1981) Transthoracic resistance of human defibrillation: influence of body weight, chest size, serial shocks, paddle size and paddle contact pressure. *Circulation,* **63:** 676–682.

Kouwenhoven W B, Jude J R and Knickerbocker G G (1960) Closed chest cardiac massage. *Journal of the American Medical Association,* **173:** 1064–1067.

Kupersmith J, Antman E M and Hoffman B F (1975) In vivo electrophysiological effects of lidocaine in canine acute myocardial infarction. *Circulation Research,* **36:** 84–91.

Lown B, Amarasingham R and Newman J (1962) A new method for terminating cardiac arrhythmias. *Journal of the American Medical Association,* **182:** 548–555.

MacKenzie G J, Taylor S H, MacDonald A H and Donald K W (1964) Haemodynamic effects of external cardiac compression. *Lancet,* **ii:** 1342–1345.

Mackintosh A F, Crabb M E, Brennan H, Williams J H and Chamberlain D A (1979) Hospital resuscitation from ventricular fibrillation in Brighton. *British Medical Journal,* **i:** 511–513.

Maier G W, Newton J R, Wolfe J A, Tyson G S, Olsen G O, Glower D D, Spratt J A, Davis J W, Feneley M P and Rankin J S (1986) The influence of manual chest compression rate on hemodynamic support during cadiac arrest: high impulse cardiopulmonary resuscitation. *Circulation,* **74** (Suppl. IV): 51–59.

Maull K I (1984) Pocket-mask ventilation: a critical appraisal. *Archives of Emergency Medicine,* **1:** 161–163.

Melker R J (1985) Recommendations for ventilation during cardiopulmonary resuscitation: time for a change? *Critical Care Medicine,* **13:** 882–883.

Melker R and Cavallaro D (1983) Synchronous and asynchronous ventilation during CPR. *Annals of Emergency Medicine,* **12:** 142–147.

Myerburg R J, Kessler K M, Zarman L, Conde C A and Castellanos A (1982) Survivors of prehospital cardiac arrest. *Journal of the American Medical Association,* **247:** 1485–1490.

National Conference on Cardiopulmonary Resuscitation and Emergency Cardiac Care (1986) Standards and guidelines for cardiopulmonary resuscitation and emergency cardiac care. *Journal of the American Medical Association,* **255:** 2905–2984.

Niemann J T (1984) Differences in cerebral and myocardial perfusion in closed chest resuscitation. *Annals of Emergency Medicine,* **13:** 849–853.

Niemann J T, Rosborough J P, Brown D and Criley J M (1980) Cough-CPR: documentation of systemic perfusion in man and in an experimental model – a 'window' to the mechanism of blood flow in external CPR. *Critical Care Medicine,* **8:** 141–146.

Niemann J T, Rosborough J P, Hausknecht M, Garner D and Criley J M (1981) Pressure synchronised cine-angiography during experimental CPR. *Circulation,* **64:** 985–991.

Niemann J T, Rosborough J P, Ung S and Criley J M (1984) Hemodynamic effects of continuous abdominal binding during cardiac arrest and resuscitation. *American Journal of Cardiology,* **53:** 269–274.

Nolte H (1968) A new evaluation of emergency methods of artificial ventilation. *Acta Anaesthesiologica Scandinavica,* **29**: 111–125.

Patton J N and Pantridge J F (1979) Current required for ventricular fibrillation. *British Medical Journal,* **i**: 513–514.

Peatfield R C, Sillett R W, Taylor D and McNicol M W (1977) Survival after cardiac arrest in hospital. *Lancet,* **i**: 1223–1225.

Resuscitation Council (1984) *Resuscitation for Citizens.* London: Resuscitation Council.

Rich S, Wix H L and Shapiro E P (1981) Clinical assessment of heart chamber size and valve motion during cardiopulmonary resuscitation by two-dimensional echocardiography. *American Heart Journal,* **102**: 367–373.

Roberts J R and Greenberg M I (1981) Emergency transthoracic pacing. *Annals of Emergency Medicine,* **10**: 600–612.

Rosborough J P, Niemann J T, Criley J M, O'Bannon W and Rouse D (1981) Lower abdominal compression with synchronised ventilation. A CPR modality. *Circulation,* **64** (Suppl. IV): 303.

Royal College of Physicians (1987) Resuscitation from cardiopulmonary arrest. Training and organisation. *Journal of the Royal College of Physicians,* **21**: 175–182.

Ruben H (1964) The immediate treatment of respiratory failure. *British Journal of Anaesthesia,* **36**: 542–549.

Rudikoff M T, Maughan W L, Effron M, Freund P and Weisfeldt M L (1980) Mechanisms of blood flow during cardiopulmonary resuscitation. *Circulation,* **61**: 345–352.

Safar P (1963) Clinical aspects. In: *An International Symposium on Resuscitation,* ed. Safar P, p. 27. Heidelberg: Springer-Verlag.

Safar P (1984) Cardiopulmonary-cerebral resuscitation. In: *Textbook of Critical Care,* eds. Shoemaker W C, Thompson W C and Holbrook P R, p. 15. Philadelphia: W B Saunders.

Safar P, Escarra L and Elam J (1958) A comparison of the mouth to mouth and mouth to airway methods of artificial respiration with the chest pressure arm-lift method. *New England Journal of Medicine,* **258**: 671–677.

Schott E (1920) Uber Ventrikelstillstand (Adams–Stokes'sche Anfalle) nebst Bemerkemgen uber andersartige Arhythmien passagerer. *Deutsches Archiv für Klinische Medizin,* **131**: 211–229.

Sellick B A (1961) Cricoid pressure to control regurgitation of stomach contents during induction of anaesthesia. *Lancet,* **ii**: 404–406.

Skinner D V (1985) Cardiopulmonary skills of pre-registration house officers. *British Medical Journal,* **290**: 1549–1550.

Stewart R D, Kaplan R, Pennock B and Thompson F (1985) Influence of mask design on bag-mask ventilation. *Annals of Emergency Medicine,* **14**: 403–406.

Stoelting R K (1981) Endotracheal intubation. In: *Anesthesia,* ed. Miller R D, pp. 233–255. New York: Churchill Livingstone.

Stokes P H and Jowett N I (1985) Haemodynamic monitoring using the Swan–Ganz catheter. *Intensive Care Nursing,* **1**: 9–17.

Sullivan M J J and Guyatt G H (1986) Simulated cardiac arrests for monitoring quality of in-hospital resuscitation. *Lancet,* **ii**: 618–620.

Taylor G J, Tucker W M, Green M T and Weisfeldt M L (1977) Importance of prolonged compression during cardiopulmonary resuscitation in man. *New England Journal of Medicine,* **296**: 1515–1517.

Thompson B M, Brooks R C, Pionkowski R S, Aprahamian C and Mateer J R (1984) Immediate countershock treatment of asystole. *Annals of Emergency Medicine,* **13**: 827–829.

Werner J A, Green H H L, Janko C L and Cobb L A (1981) Two-dimensional echocardiography during CPR in man: implications regarding the mechanism of blood flow. *Critical Care Medicine,* **9**: 375–376.

Wynne G, Marteau T M, Johnston M, Whiteley C A and Evans T R (1987) Inability of trained nurses to perform basic life support. *British Medical Journal,* **294**: 1198–1199.

Zoll P M, Linenthal A J, Gibson W, Paul M and Norman L (1956) Termination of ventricular fibrillation in man by externally applied counter shock. *New England Journal of Medicine,* **254**: 727–732.

12

Cardiac Pacing

Control over the electrical activity of the heart is frequently made by means of an artificial pacemaker. If pacing is for a short time only, an external power source is used to deliver electricity to the heart either endocardially, via the skin (transcutaneous pacing) or via the oesophagus (oesophageal pacing). Temporary cardiac pacing is often utilised in coronary care and intensive care units to treat transient conduction problems. However, when long-term control is required, a permanent pacemaker is implanted. The first implant was reported in 1959, and now nearly 200 000 permanent pacemakers are implanted worldwide every year.

INDICATIONS FOR PACING

Indications for pacing vary widely both nationally and internationally. Generally considered indications include the following.

Stokes–Adams attacks

Stokes–Adams attacks are frequently associated with second- and third-degree heart block and require pacing without need for further investigation. Less frequently the aetiology is the sick sinus syndrome or paroxysmal tachycardias which should usually be further evaluated by electrophysiological testing.

Low-output states associated with bradycardia

Raising the heart rate to between 70 and 80 beats per minute by inserting a temporary pacemaker can dramatically improve cardiac failure or other symptoms, if these have been associated with bradycardia. Raising the rate of the heart above 80 to 90 beats per minute, however, may be detrimental and result in a fall of the cardiac output. In these circumstances it is preferable to insert an atrial pacing wire and synchronise atrial and ventricular emptying in physiological sequence. Such procedures are not without risk and the extra benefits obtained may be minimal.

Conduction defects following acute myocardial infarction

Temporary and permanent pacing following acute myocardial infarction are considered in detail later.

Inferior myocardial infarction

Pacing is usually indicated if the heart rate falls below 60 beats per minute (unresponsive to atropine) where there are symptoms or signs attributable to low-output cardiac failure. Observation only is needed in the remaining cases.

Anterior myocardial infarction

The prognosis for conduction defects following anterior myocardial infarction is poor, and the indications for pacing are controversial (Norris et al, 1972; Klein et al, 1984). Certainly complete heart block needs pacing, but whether bifascicular, first-degree or second-degree heart block needs insertion of a prophylactic pacing wire is not clear.

Refractory tachycardias

Where tachydysrhythmias are not controlled by medical therapy, permanent pacing may have a beneficial role. Ectopic foci can be suppressed by ventricular pacing at a higher rate than sinus rhythm (*overpacing*). Alternatively, fixed-rate pacing in short bursts either slower (*underdrive*) or faster (*overdrive*) than sinus rate may be effective in preventing dysrhythmias. In the 'brady–tachy' syndrome, where the patient has both fast and slow dysrhythmias, drugs such as beta-adrenergic blocking agents and digoxin can be given to control the faster rates, using a pacemaker to prevent very slow heart rates.

Perioperative heart block

Patients with sino-atrial disease or incomplete heart block may be at risk of developing complete heart block during drug therapy or surgery. General anaesthesia with fluorinated hydrocarbons (e.g. halothane) may adversely affect atrioventricular conduction (Atlee and Alexander, 1977), as can succinylcholine. A pacing wire may therefore need to be inserted for prophylactic reasons perioperatively.

Miscellaneous

Temporary pacing may be required in cases of permanent pacemaker failure, or for extreme bradycardias caused by drugs (e.g. digoxin or beta-adrenergic blocking agents) or electrolyte disturbances. Pacemakers are also sometimes used to aid diagnosis in complex conduction disorders or during electrophysiological testing procedures (Cobbe, 1986).

TEMPORARY CARDIAC PACING

Temporary endocardial pacing has been used since the early 1960s to maintain cardiac output during episodes of extreme bradycardia, heart block and asystole, particularly in association with acute myocardial infarction. Before the advent of cardiac pacemakers, the combination of acute myocardial infarction and complete heart block was usually fatal (Cohen et al, 1958). Although of some value, the use of isoprenaline has now virtually disappeared other than in places where pacing facilities do not exist (Christiansen et al, 1973). Pacing electrodes can now be rapidly passed percutaneously into the right ventricle under local anaesthesia, and in experienced hands this is a safe and simple procedure.

There is little doubt that it may be life saving acutely, but long-term value is a little more difficult to assess. Prognosis is influenced not only by complications of the procedure (dysrhythmias, cardiac perforation, septicaemia), but also by the degree of underlying myocardial damage which originally led to the conduction defect. Many patients effectively treated acutely by temporary pacing die later, whilst still in hospital, from heart failure due to extensive myocardial infarction (Norris et al, 1972). The principal determinant of prognosis is the site of the infarct (Norris, 1969). Anterior infarction may have necrosed the bundle branches as well as a greater part of the left ventricular myocardium which leads to pump failure. Inferior infarcts on the other hand do not usually involve so much critical myocardium, and normally result only in reversible ischaemia and oedema in the region of the atrioventricular node. In patients who have not suffered an acute myocardial infarction, temporary pacing is most often required by patients with chronic atrioventricular block and sick-sinus syndrome. The underlying disease in most of these cases is *Lenegre's disease* (AV fibrosis), and only a small number are due to ischaemic damage. As such, left ventricular function is usually better, and the outcome following pacing is much better (Hayward, 1981). Patients found to have the sick-sinus syndrome, however, may have a coexisting cardiomyopathy which could adversely influence the prognosis.

Pacing and acute myocardial infarction

Pathophysiology (table 12.1)

Inferior myocardial infarction is usually caused by acute occlusion of the right coronary artery which supplies the inferior wall of the heart. The AV node is supplied by the right coronary artery in 90 per cent of cases, and by the circumflex artery in the remainder. As a result, conduction disturbances commonly occur following acute inferior myocardial infarction, and are usually caused by ischaemia or oedema of the conducting system. These effects will be worsened if there is pre-existing damage to the conducting tissues, such as ischaemia or fibrosis of the AV node and bundle branches. Fortunately, for unknown reasons, ischaemic injury to the AV node following inferior myocardial infarction is rarely permanent. Complete heart block usually develops slowly and the escape rhythm is usually high junctional at 40 to 60 beats per minute. This is generally haemodynamically stable and pacing is usually not necessary provided blood pressure and renal perfusion are maintained (Gupta et al, 1976). Conduction disturbances can occur at any time in the first two weeks, but are usually transient, with normal conduction returning in hours or days.

Anterior myocardial infarction is caused by occlusion of the left anterior descending coronary artery, which additionally provides the major blood supply to the His bundle and bundle branches. Proximal occlusion of the left coronary artery leads to

Table 12.1. Characteristics of complete heart block complicating inferior and anterior myocardial infarction.

	Anterior infarction	Inferior infarction
Incidence	25–40%	60–75%
Pathology	Septal necrosis and infarction of the AV node and bundle branches	Ischaemia of the bundle branches
Timing	Usually sudden following sinus rhythm or second-degree heart block	Normally slow following first- and second-degree heart block
Ventricular response	30–40 unstable	40–60 stable
QRS morphology	Widened	Narrow
Risk of asystole	High	Low
Mortality	60–75%	25–40%
Prognosis	Often permanent	Most reverse within 14 days

extensive myocardial damage, often resulting in heart failure and cardiogenic shock. Heart block is a sinister and sudden complication, and is due to ischaemic destruction of the conducting tissues below the AV node. Emergent ventricular escape rhythms are unreliable, slow and irregular; there is a marked tendency to develop asystole. The insertion of a temporary pacing wire under these circumstances probably has little influence on the outcome, although it is usual practice. Mortality is high and late deaths are common (Mullins and Atkins, 1976).

Sudden onset of bundle branch block may warn of impending complete atrioventricular block, and prophylactic pacing wires are sometimes inserted in those who develop second-degree or bifascicular block in the presence of anterior myocardial infarction. Resolution of atrioventricular blockage takes longer than with inferior infarctions, and bundle branch block may persist. The presence of bundle branch block is associated with increased mortality due to heart failure or refractory dysrhythmias (Norris et al, 1972).

Possible indications for pacing in acute myocardial infarction complicated by heart block are shown in table 12.2.

Acute myocardial infarction and complete heart block

Complete heart block (CHB) complicates 9 to 33 per cent of acute myocardial infarctions, and is associated with a high mortality (Norris, 1969; Kostuk and Beanlands, 1970). The lower incidence may reflect the difficulty in recognising CHB electrocardiographically. Atrioventricular dissociation is often confused with complete heart block, and is usually not associated with severe myocardial damage (see figure 10.5). Other episodes of CHB which appear to have a good prognosis could be first-degree heart block with accelerated junctional rhythm.

Table 12.2. Possible indications for temporary pacing in acute myocardial infarction complicated by AV block.

Inferior infarction
Ventricular rate < 40 per minute
Premature ventricular contractions (PVCs)
Ventricular tachycardia (VT)
Ventricular fibrillation (VF)
Cardiac failure
Cardiogenic shock

Anterior infarction
Acute bifascicular block
Second-degree heart block (Mobitz type II)
Complete heart block

Hypertension, pre-existing diabetes mellitus and high blood glucose concentrations on admission to hospital are common risk factors for those requiring temporary pacing following acute myocardial infarction. Disorders of atrioventricular and intraventricular conduction are significantly more common in diabetic patients with acute myocardial infarction than those who are not diabetic (Czyzyk et al, 1980), and this may be due to pre-existing micro-angiopathic damage of the conducting system (Blandford and Burden, 1984). The higher incidence of previous myocardial infarctions and hypertension in those patients requiring pacing is probably an indication of a greater degree of underlying myocardial damage.

The prognosis in patients with complete heart block appears to be related to factors other than conduction abnormality, especially following anterior myocardial infarction where mortality is higher than in those with inferior infarction (Lassers and Julian, 1968; Norris, 1969). Although restoration of stable haemodynamics will affect immediate morbidity and mortality due to bradycardia and asystole, it will not help those with extensive myocardial damage who often have mechanical heart failure and cardiogenic shock.

The benefits of routine pacing for inferior myocardial infarction are also in doubt. Mortality has been reported as 37 per cent without pacing (Cohen et al, 1958), and is almost as high in those who are paced. Insertion of wires for heart block complicating inferior infarction is often routine on many coronary care units, even in the absence of haemodynamic decompensation. However, the majority of cases do not deteriorate, and insertion of a temporary wire is usually not necessary (Gupta et al, 1976).

Temporary pacemakers

It is usual for a special room to be set aside for pacing, so that there are facilities for sterility, fluoroscopy and resuscitation. The procedure should be explained to the patient and a consent form signed if possible. However, many patients will have a compromised cardiac output, and may not be fully conscious. Many different methods have been employed for cardiac pacing.

Transvenous pacing

Transvenous pacing is the most common method employed, and involves the passage of a bipolar electrode into the apex of the right ventricle which is activated by an external impulse generator. The temporary wire is best positioned with the aid of fluoroscopy, but occasionally has to be attempted as a 'blind' procedure in emergency. Any route can be used, but the commonest puncture sites are the veins of the antecubital fossa, the subclavian veins and the femoral veins. The latter site has an increased risk of major venous thromboses and is potentially unsterile. It is not recommended, and will not be discussed further.

Percutaneous subclavian puncture

To achieve success, previous experience of central venous catheterisation is highly desirable. Insertion here requires a higher level of expertise than from the arm, since the veins cannot be visualised and there is a risk of pneumothorax, subclavian artery puncture and damage to the thoracic duct or surrounding brachial nerve roots. However, access to the heart and manipulation after insertion is much simpler, and the final electrode position is much more stable since there is less restriction of the patient's movement (McNeil and Taylor, 1979). The patient must be horizontal, or head-down (particularly if thought to have hypovolaemia) to prevent air embolism.

Median basilic vein

This site offers easy, visible venous access with a low insertion complication rate. The patient does not have to be lying flat since there is no risk of air embolism, which is a distinct advantage if orthopnoea (due to pulmonary oedema) is a problem. However, patient mobility is severely hampered, thrombophlebitis and cellulitis are common, and manipulation of the wire into a good position is difficult. It is therefore not a good route in an emergency.

Method of catheterisation

- Percutaneous needle and sheath techniques
- Percutaneous Seldinger technique using a guide wire
- Cut-down, suitable for the arm veins

The method of choice is probably the Seldinger technique, although once again experience of the technique is desirable. The advantage is that a long cannula is passed into the superior vena cava, which helps the passage of the pacing wire into the heart. In addition, unlike shorter cannulae, it will not become displaced if external cardiac massage is required during the insertion procedure. If there is a cardiac arrest, it can be occluded and pacing resumed following resuscitation. The cannula can also be conveniently used for infusing drugs and other fluids as required.

The pacing wire becomes more pliable as it warms to body temperature, and so should be inserted as quickly as possible. Sometimes, there is difficulty in passing the electrode into the superior vena cava, which may be made easier by moving the

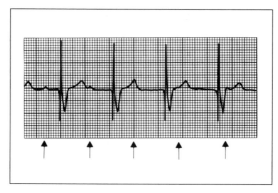

Fig. 12.1 ECG: trace obtained when the cardiac pacing wire is correctly positioned. The pacing spike can be seen preceding each QRS complex. Independent atrial P waves are indicated

patient's shoulders or rotating the arm across the body. Passage through the heart requires experience and the ability to judge position from the fluoroscopic image. Traversing the tricuspid valve is a frequent problem, particularly if the heart rate is fast or if the myocardium is irritable. Gentle manipulation or looping in the right atrium may help. Passage into the right ventricle can be confirmed by observing the characteristic 'bucking' of the catheter by the tricuspid valve about 5 cm from the tip. Wedging the electrode is sometimes made easier by passing it directly into the pulmonary artery (especially if a balloon flotation-type catheter has been used), and then letting it fall back into the apex. This can be seen just medial to the apex on the cardiac silhouette, and the tip of the electrode should point slightly inferiorly. Once wedged, verification of pacing and threshold measurements are necessary. The former is judged from the appearance of a pacing 'spike' preceding the QRS complex on the ECG. Each spike should capture a QRS complex (figure 12.1). The pacing threshold is obtained by determining the lowest pacing voltage that produces a paced beat. This threshold should be less than 1 V, and preferably below 0.5 V. The wire can then be fixed to the skin with a suture. The pacing mode is then selected (usually 'demand') and the voltage set at about twice the threshold.

Problems during transvenous pacing

Dysrhythmias

The major complication of temporary pacing is ventricular tachycardia and fibrillation. It is probably produced by mechanical irritation of the endocardium. The appearance of ventricular ectopics is usually a good sign that the catheter has entered the right ventricle, but the wire should be moved if these are frequent or occur in runs. This complication may also be caused electrically if 'fixed' rather than 'demand' mode is selected on the pacing box, or if an inappropriately high pacing threshold is used. Standard resuscitation is required during ventricular fibrillation, although overpacing can sometimes be used to restore a more stable rhythm in ventricular tachycardia.

Perforation of the heart or septum

This may be an early or late complication, and may be indicated by:

● Failure to pace despite good radiological position
● Signs of pericarditis or tamponade
● Diaphragmatic twitching

A change from the usual left bundle branch block ECG pacing pattern to right bundle branch block indicates that the wire has perforated the septum. This is usually insignificant, but the wire should be moved.

Failure to pace

Pacing failure may be evident from absence of a pacing spike (implying failure in pulse generation), or the spikes failing to capture (implying a displaced electrode or change in threshold). The box or the wire will then need replacing or repositioning.

Pacemaker dependence

Pacing wires not infrequently need repositioning, because they have moved, because of a rapidly increasing pacing threshold or because of dysrhythmias. Unfortunately, pre-existing rhythms are often abolished after pacing for a while, leaving complete asystole as the underlying rhythm (seen if the pacing box is turned off momentarily). Movement of the wire or transient rises in the threshold may then be associated with Stokes–Adams attacks, because the heart has become 'pacemaker dependent'. This problem may need the passage of a second pacing wire which can take over whilst the other is relocated or removed.

Care of patients with temporary pacing wires

Patients often feel much better following temporary pacing, and are in a much better physical and psychological state for discussion about the pacemaker and its implications. Mobility will necessarily be restricted, but if the subclavian approach has been utilised this will be minimal. However, the wire should be secured to the body to prevent accidental pulling. Many pacing boxes are now small and portable, thus enabling early mobilisation of the patient. There is usually not much pain at the site of wire insertion, but this should be routinely observed for signs of bleeding and infection. Routine checks are also required on the equipment, with attention to connections and performance. The threshold and underlying rhythm need charting on a twice daily basis, and settings discussed for the following 12-hour period. This should be documented in the patient's notes and the nursing notes, as well as on the charts beside the bed. Although many pacing units are protected, it is advisable to turn off the pacemaker to prevent electrical damage if the patient needs defibrillation.

Removal of the pacing wire is a simple and straightforward procedure carried out at the patient's bedside. The unit should be turned off, and the dressing and retaining sutures removed. Whilst observing the ECG monitor for ectopic activity, the wire should be slowly withdrawn, and a sterile pad held firmly over the puncture site for a few minutes to prevent bleeding. It may be advisable to remove the tip of disposable pacing wire aseptically, for sending to the bacteriology laboratory, particularly if the patient is pyrexial. Special care is required to ensure that the end is not being detached from a re-usable pacing wire!

Transcutaneous pacing

External temporary cardiac pacing was first introduced in 1952, and was widely used as a temporary measure for the treatment of asystole and bradycardia (Zoll, 1952), until superseded by transvenous pacing with an internal wire in 1959. In recent years, renewed interest has been shown in external cardiac pacing as a rapid, simple and safe method of maintaining cardiac output. Because it is applied externally it can be instituted quickly, and used repeatedly if necessary. It also has applications outside hospital, perhaps as part of standard ambulance equipment. Units are well tolerated, with little more than slight cutaneous discomfort (Zoll and Zoll, 1985).

Transoesophageal pacing

The technique of transoesophageal pacing was originally described in the late 1960s in New York (Burack and Furman, 1969). Although transvenous cardiac pacing is the treatment of choice, the transoesophageal route can often act as a holding measure until a percutaneous wire can be inserted. The electrode is passed transnasally into the oesophagus (rather like a nasogastric tube) and the current switched on, initially at about 30 V. When the diaphragm is reached (producing diaphragmatic twitching) the electrode is slowly withdrawn until ventricular capture is seen on the ECG monitor, and the threshold is then determined. Unfortunately, the method is not very reliable.

PERMANENT PACEMAKERS

The recent development of implantable cardiac pacemakers and other cardio-stimulatory devices has made the selection of the correct unit required for permanent pacing very difficult, and recommendations are rapidly changing. The ever-increasing demand for specialist patient assessment and pacemaker implantation may soon lead to cardiac pacing being established as a subspecialty (Parsonnet, 1982). About 114 new pacemakers are inserted annually for every million people in Britain, and this number is expected to increase to 300 to 400 per million over the next five years.

The indications for pacing are based upon careful evaluation of symptoms, electrocardiograms, Holter tapes and intracardiac electrophysiological tests. Additionally, long-term prognosis and general medical and psychological health need to be taken into account before any decision is made to implant a permanent pacemaker.

Indications for permanent pacing

Patients with abnormal cardiac function may or may not be symptomatic. This applies not only to those with poor left ventricular function, but also in those with disturbances of conduction (see Frye et al, 1984).

Patients with complete heart block and syncope have improved survival following permanent pacing (Edhag and Swahn, 1976), although it makes no difference to those with first-degree AV block. Patients with second-degree block have a more variable prognosis. Mobitz type I AV block is usually benign, but Mobitz type II block usually progresses to complete heart block (Dhingra et al, 1974). The current recommendations are for permanent pacing to be offered to patients with symptomatic complete heart block, second-degree heart block (with or without symptoms) and symptomatic bradycardias (Horgan, 1984). For patients with conduction problems following myocardial infarction, the long-term prognosis is related to the severity of the myocardial injury, and not to the presence or absence of heart block (Ginks et al, 1977). However, consideration is sometimes given to a small group, mostly for conduction abnormalities following anterior myocardial infarction (see p.298).

The permanent pacemaker

The modern pacemaker is a small metal box weighing 30 to 130 g, and powered by a lithium battery which lasts up to 15 years. Two types of pulse generator are currently available for permanent implantation: single chamber pacemakers (electrode placed in either the atrium or the ventricle) and dual chamber pacemakers (electrodes situated in both chambers). Although non-programmable pacemakers are still in use, programmable models are being increasingly used (table 12.3). This enables greater flexibility in pacemaker function (e.g. rate, output, sensitivity and inhibitory functions), which can be altered to meet the specific requirements of the individual patient.

Table 12.3. Programmable functions of cardiac pacemakers.

Rate
    Beats per minute
    Upper rate limit
    Lower rate limit

Energy output
    Milliamperes
    Volts
    Pulse duration

Refractory period

Sensitivity of the sensing electrode(s)

Atrioventricular delay between atrial sensing and ventricular pacing

Mode of function
    DDD
    DVI etc.

These specific requirements change in about 20 per cent of patients following implantation of a permanent pacemaker, and can be altered without need for a second operation or implantation of a different pacemaker.

Many new pacemakers are able to report electronically on their own clinical function and performance (Parsonnet et al, 1981), which allows any physician to determine which unit has been implanted, its programming, battery life and even information about the medication the patient is currently taking.

Single and dual chamber pacing

The original permanent pacemakers were single chamber pacemakers (VVI units), with the electrode being located in the right ventricular apex. However, ventricular pacing results in the reduction of about 20 per cent of the cardiac output because of the loss of the haemodynamic contribution of atrial systole. This may be critical in patients with poor left ventricular function who would benefit from synchronised sequential atrioventricular activity. Atrial pacemakers will obviously overcome this problem provided there is no AV nodal conduction block. These simple pacemakers are useful for those patients with symptomatic sino-atrial disease, and require a single electrode in the right atrial appendage. A second, and often distressing, problem with ventricular pacemakers is the *pacemaker syndrome*, again caused by impairment of cardiac output (Kenny and Sutton, 1986). Although the pacemaker may be functioning correctly, the patient continues to complain of dizzy spells, syncope, exercise limitation and postural hypotension. This is a consequence of episodic mechanical atrioventricular dissociation when the atria contract during ventricular systole. Retrograde conduction from the ventricles to the atria causes them to contract against closed atrioventricular valves, resulting in raised left and right atrial pressures. A fall in cardiac output and systemic blood pressure then follows which is often symptomatic. Drugs such as flecainide and disopyramide can be used to prevent this abnormal conduction, often with complete resolution of these distressing symptoms. However, what is required (and preferred) is sequential atrioventricular contraction as occurs physiologically. This has led to the introduction of dual chamber pacemakers.

Dual chamber pacemakers have separate electrodes. One is situated in the right atrium and the other in the right ventricle, and both can pace and sense. Most patients with complete heart block will have variable atrial rates (depending on, for example, physical activity), and thus the usual arrangement is for ventricular pacing to occur whenever atrial activity is sensed by the atrial electrode. For this reason, they are not a good idea for patients with recurrent supraventricular tachycardias. If there is co-existent sino-atrial disease with a slow atrial rate, the electrodes can be fired sequentially, mimicking normal atrioventricular myocardial contraction.

A generic code has been adopted by the Intersociety Commission for Heart Disease (Parsonnet et al, 1981) to help with identification and description of these multiple units. There is a five letter code which provides a standardised means for identifying the functional operation of a cardiac pacemaker, regardless of its trade make or model. The minimum code length is three letters, with O used if a function is not present. Code letters IV and V are often omitted if they are O. The current system

Table 12.4. Intersociety Commission for Heart Disease Code of Pacing Modes and Functions (Parsonnet et al, 1981).

Position of letter				
I	II	III	IV	V
				Special
Chamber paced	Chamber sensed	Mode of response	Programmable functions	tachyarrhythmia function
V Ventricle	V Ventricle	T Triggered	P Programmable (rate and/or output only)	B Bursts
A Atrium	A Atrium	I Inhibited	M Multiprogrammable	N Normal rate competition
D Double	D Double	D Double O None	C Communicating	S Scanning
	O None	R Reverse	O None	E External

of nomenclature is shown in table 12.4. The first two positions indicate the chambers in which the pacemaker operates, with position I representing the chamber paced, and position II indicating the chamber sensed. If the pacemaker can sense and pace in the same chamber, it is designated D (double).

Code position III describes the mode of response of the pacemaker, such as I for 'inhibited' (when the presence of sensed electrical activity from the heart inhibits the pacemaker) or T for pacemakers that are 'triggered' by spontaneous cardiac electrical activity. D in position III indicates a double response: an atrial-triggered and ventricular-inhibited pacemaker. Reverse pulse generators (R) come into action only during abnormally fast rates, to terminate the dysrhythmia.

Position IV describes the programmable features such as rate and/or output, which may be altered non-invasively. In its simplest form, programming is achieved using a magnet which is applied over the unit. By certain movements, the programming may be altered. More commonly, the programming is transmitted using strings of electronic impulses from a programming head. An increasing number of units can also transmit their present programme values, allowing information to be extracted from the pacemaker (interrogation) for record keeping, determining pacemaker type and function, and to provide physiological data. Several pacemakers have been described as diagnostic units. Some can produce histograms giving the incidence of beats within a preset range, or can report on extreme bradycardia and ventricular ectopic activity.

Position V is used to indicate antidysrhythmic function, the pacemaker being employed to prevent or terminate tachydysrhythmias by inducing changes in heart rate and rhythm using single or multiple stimuli. These pacemakers must be able to differentiate simple physiological sinus tachycardias from abnormal rhythms. The unit is designed to break the re-entrant circuit by making any myocardial cells in the path of the circuit refractory.

Examples of permanent pacemaker coding are shown in table 12.5. The most sophisticated pacemaker system is the DDD ('universal'), where both atria and

Table 12.5. Examples of different permanent pacemakers.

Position of letter			Description of mode
I	II	III	
A	O	O	Asynchronous (fixed-rate) atrial pacing
A	A	I	Demand atrial pacing, output inhibited by sensed atrial signals
A	A	T	Triggered atrial pacing, output pulse delivered into P waves (or any electrical signals sensed by the atrial electrode), paces atrium at preset escape interval
V	O	O	Asynchronous (fixed-rate) ventricular pacing
V	V	I	Non-competitive (demand) ventricular pacing, output inhibited by sensed ventricular signals
V	V	T	Triggered ventricular pacing, output pulse delivered into R waves (or any electrical signals sensed by the ventricular electrode), paces ventricle at preset escape interval
D	V	I	Paces in both atrium and ventricle, does not sense P waves, senses R waves
V	D	D	Paces in ventricle, senses in both atrium and ventricle, synchronizes with atrial activity and paces ventricle after a preset atrioventricular interval
D	D	D	Paces and senses in both atrium and ventricle

ventricles can sense and pace. Hence, they can pace atria on demand in patients with sinus bradycardia and intact AV nodes, ventricles in response to sensed atrial activity, and atria and ventricles sequentially in patients with sinus bradycardia and atrioventricular block.

The implanted defibrillator

This implanted device is able to recognise ventricular tachycardia and fibrillation, and then deliver a corrective defibrillatory charge of about 50 J. It is at present still being evaluated and refined, but has already increased survival of several patients at high risk of sudden death (Mirowski et al, 1980). The main problems at present are prevention of myocardial damage and designing a power source which can deliver more than the present limited 100 shocks per implant.

Permanent pacing following acute myocardial infarction

Permanent pacing is seldom required following inferior myocardial infarction; those who do not regain normal conduction usually do not survive the acute infarct, often dying in cardiogenic shock. The prognosis in terms of conduction is excellent for those who survive. However, following acute anterior myocardial infarction, the mortality in patients who develop heart block is very high, and conduction defects are often permanent in those who do survive. It is likely that all these patients are at risk of

Table 12.6. Possible indications for permanent pacing in patients recovering from acute myocardial infarction with AV block.

Infarct/block	Pace?
Inferior with transient AV block	No
Inferior with permanent second/third-degree block	Yes
Anterior with fascicular block	?No
Anterior with transient second/third-degree block	?Yes
Anterior with permanent second/third-degree block	Yes

further symptomatic rhythm disturbances, although indications for permanent pacing are controversial (Klein et al, 1984; Frye et al, 1984). Possible indications for permanent pacing in this group are shown in table 12.6.

For those who recover normal AV conduction, exercise testing and 24-hour Holter monitoring are useful for post-infarction assessment. Electrophysiological testing, if available, may give early indication of impaired infranodal conduction, allowing consideration for permanent pacing before problems arise (Cobbe, 1986).

Progress continues to be made in the design of permanent pacemakers. The use of microprocessors will allow diagnosis and storage of more data concerning cardiac function and conduction patterns.

Truly physiological pacemakers have not yet been developed, but the capability of units that respond to metabolic needs such as blood pH, temperature, oxygen saturation and respiratory rate exists. A balance will soon have to be struck between what technology can do, and what patients actually require.

References

Atlee J L and Alexander S C (1977) Halothane effects on conductivity of the atrioventricular node and His–Purkinje system in the dog. *Anesthesia and Analgesia,* **56:** 378–86.

Blandford R L and Burden A C (1984) Abnormalities of cardiac conduction in diabetics. *British Medical Journal,* **289:** 1659.

Burack B and Furman S (1969) Trans-oesophageal cardiac pacing. *American Journal of Cardiology,* **23:** 469–472.

Christiansen I, Haghfelt T and Amtorp O (1973) Complete heart block in acute myocardial infarction: drug therapy. *American Heart Journal,* **85:** 162–166.

Cobbe S M (1986) Electrophysiological testing after acute myocardial infarction. *British Medical Journal,* **292:** 1290–1291.

Cohen D B, Doctor L and Pick A (1958) The significance of atrioventricular block complicating myocardial infarction. *American Heart Journal,* **55:** 215–219.

Czyzyk A, Krolewski A S, Szablowska S, Alot A and Kopczynski J (1980) Clinical course of myocardial infarction amongst diabetic patients. *Diabetes Care,* **4:** 526–529.

Dhingra R C, Denes P, Wu D, Chuquimia R and Rosen K M (1974) The significance of second degree atrioventricular block and bundle branch block. *Circulation,* **49:** 638–644.

Edhag O and Swahn A (1976) Prognosis of patients with complete heart block or arrhythmic syncope who were not treated with artificial pacemakers. *Acta Medica Scandinavica,* **200:** 457–463.

Frye R L, Colins J J, DeSanctis R W, Dodge H T, Dreifus L S, Gillette P C and Fisch C (1984) Guidelines for permanent cardiac pacemaker implantation. *Circulation,* **70:** 331A–339A.

Ginks W R, Sutton R, Oh W and Leatham A (1977) Long term prognosis after acute anterior infarction with atrioventricular block. *British Heart Journal,* **39:** 186–189.

Gupta P K, Lichstein E and Chadda K D (1976) Heart block complicating acute inferior wall myocardial infarction. *Chest,* **69:** 599–604.

Hayward R (1981) Who do we pace? *British Journal of Hospital Medicine,* **25:** 466–474.

Horgan J H (1984) Cardiac pacing. *British Medical Journal,* **288:** 1942–1944.

Kenny R A and Sutton R (1986) Pacemaker syndrome. *British Medical Journal,* **293:** 902–903.

Klein R C, Vera Z and Mason T (1984) Intraventricular conduction defects in acute myocardial infarction: incidence, prognosis and therapy. *American Heart Journal,* **108:** 1107–1013.

Kostuk W J and Beanlands D S (1970) Complete heart block associated with myocardial infarction. *American Journal of Cardiology,* **26:** 380–384.

Lassers B W and Julian D G (1968) Artificial pacing in the management of complete heart block complicating acute myocardial infarction. *British Medical Journal,* **ii:** 142–146.

McNeil G P and Taylor N C (1979) Use of the subclavian vein for permanent cardiac pacing. *British Heart Journal,* **40:** 114–116.

Mirowski M, Reid P R, Morton M M, Watkins L, Gott V L, Schauble M S, Kolenik S A, Fischell R E and Weisfeldt M L (1980) Termination of malignant ventricular arrhythmias with an implanted automatic defibrillator in human beings. *New England Journal of Medicine,* **303:** 322–324.

Mullins C B and Atkins J M (1976) Prognoses and management of ventricular conduction blocks in acute myocardial infarction. *Modern Concepts in Cardiovascular Disease,* **45:** 129–133.

Norris R M (1969) Heart block in posterior and anterior myocardial infarction. *British Heart Journal,* **31:** 352–356.

Norris R M, Mercer C J and Croxson M S (1972) Conduction disturbances due to anteroseptal myocardial infarction and their treatment by endocardial pacing. *American Heart Journal,* **84:** 560–566.

Parsonnet V (1982) The proliferation of cardiac pacing: medical, technical and socio-economic dilemmas. *Circulation,* **5:** 841–845.

Parsonnet V, Furman S D and Smyth N P (1981) A revised code for pacemaker identification. Report of a pacemaker study group. *Circulation,* **64:** 60A–62A.

Zoll P M (1952) Resuscitation of the heart in ventricular standstill by external cardiac stimulation. *New England Journal of Medicine,* **247:** 768–771.

Zoll P M and Zoll R H (1985) Non-invasive temporary cardiac stimulation. *Critical Care Medicine,* **13:** 925–926.

13

Rehabilitation after Myocardial Infarction

In the past, strict and prolonged bed rest played a central role in the early management of acute myocardial infarction. However, it soon became clear that prolonged immobilisation had undesirable and sometimes dangerous side-effects, including deep vein thrombosis and pulmonary embolism. Other effects include impaired respiratory function, with a tendency to chest infections, negative nitrogen balance, and a decrease in skeletal muscle mass and muscular contractile strength. Prolonged immobilisation also resulted in marked physical weakness and a reduced ability to exercise. This, in part, was due to a reduction in left ventricular stroke volume, and resumption of activity often resulted in tachycardia and orthostatic hypotension.

Cardiac rehabilitation can be traced back to New York in the early 1940s, when assessing and improving exercise capacity played a prominent role in 'work classification units'. Rehabilitation, however, should not be equated with exercise training alone; no observation or trial has shown that exercise alone reduces morbidity and mortality following myocardial infarction.

In the early 1970s, the World Health Organisation set up a study into rehabilitation and secondary prevention following myocardial infarction, and the results have shown that patients who are involved in formal rehabilitation programmes have a decreased mortality and an earlier return to work (Dorossiev, 1983). However, too much emphasis should not be placed on these end-points alone, and it is preferable to look upon improvements in the quality of life, particularly in the early months following the illness. The following are major areas for rehabilitation.

- Medical therapy
- Psychological adjustment and motivation
- Self-care
- Financial matters and income
- Housing
- Transport
- Occupation
- Recreation
- Sexual activity

The goal of rehabilitation is to restore the patient to an optimum level of recovery (physical, emotional, social, economic and vocational) and, where possible, to prevent progression of ischaemic heart disease. The major components of rehabilitation are early ambulation, health education, and counselling of the patient and family. In theory, the rehabilitation process should begin the moment the patient enters the hospital, and continue after discharge; in practice it rarely does. Many patients leave hospital unaware that they have even had a heart attack, let alone what this means and what to do about it once they get home.

In the UK, there has been progress in early mobilisation and discharge from hospital, but interest in other aspects of cardiac rehabilitation are only just emerging. This is not the case in other countries such as West Germany, where over 80 per cent of patients are admitted to 'heart groups' following myocardial infarction (Scheuermann et al, 1985).

Cardiac rehabilitation involves the use of a wide range of skills from different health professionals including the nurse, doctor, physiotherapist, occupational therapist, clinical psychologist, dietitian and social worker. The nurse assumes a central role by being responsible, directly or indirectly, for controlling the many factors that influence the patient's recovery (Runions, 1985). She is in most frequent contact with the patient and family, and is responsible for planning and coordinating the amount of activity the patient is expected to undertake. The nurse can assist the patient and family to understand, accept and adapt to the illness, and may be able to stimulate them to take an active part in recovery and rehabilitation. In addition, she can assist them in making realistic plans for the future. In order to achieve this, attainable goals need to be defined, with plans being jointly agreed upon by the patient, his family and other members of the health care team. An attitude of optimism should be adopted by staff, remembering that most patients who are going to die from acute myocardial infarction do so before reaching hospital.

From early convalescence in hospital, the patient and his spouse should realise that a return to normality within a matter of a few weeks is not only expected, but is also safe and beneficial, given that the patient's condition warrants it. It is the success of coping and support that often ultimately determines the outcome of the patient's illness; the heart may recover more rapidly than the patient's often depressed mental state.

REHABILITATION PROGRAMMES

Successful rehabilitation should not be viewed narrowly in terms of economic or vocational outcomes, but rather as the achievement of a life-style which enables the patient and his family to enjoy a full and active life (with some allowance for physical limitations) in which he can usefully contribute to his family and society.

Cardiac rehabilitation programmes consist of patient education (often coupled with counselling) and exercise.

The *education* component involves teaching patients and their families to better understand the illness and its management (including the factors that may have caused it), and to enable them to assume a large degree of responsibility for their care.

The *exercise* component involves a graduated programme beginning with passive and low-level activities and aiming for a full return to normal activities.

Patient education

Information provided to patients and their spouses about their stay in hospital is frequently lacking (Wilson-Barnett, 1979). Although patient teaching is increasingly being recognised as an important nursing function, there is little evidence to show that it is being accomplished effectively and consistently. It is the responsibility of the health care team to ensure that the patient and his family understand the illness, the purpose of treatment and how to cope both within and outside the hospital. The nurse is in an ideal position to teach because she frequently becomes the most familiar person to the patient, and is thus often in the best position to communicate with the patient and family.

Teaching programmes during the patient's stay in hospital are designed to decrease the patient's feeling of helplessness, to help restore self-esteem and to bolster the patient's confidence in terms of a successful outcome. Patients who understand the cause and significance of their illness and its management are likely to have improved motivation to comply with therapy and cope with the consequences of their illness (Linde and Janz, 1979; Hogan and Neill, 1982). Patients particularly need information about potential events that may occur after their return home when professional help is not immediately available (Wilson-Barnett and Oborne, 1983).

Teaching and learning is a two-way process, and the individual patient's requirements will vary with his general educational background and intellectual capabilities.

Assessment should include:

- Demographic variables, such as family composition, ethnic and religious background, and educational level
- Pre-existing knowledge and misconceptions of coronary heart disease
- Life-style and habits
- Readiness to learn

Simple language should always be used, and it should be remembered that earlier statements are remembered better than later ones. Repetition increases recall as does specific rather than general advice.

Contemporary approaches to patient teaching are numerous and varied, but information should be tailored to individual needs, and given in a consistent and structured fashion. The comprehension of new information will be at its best when the patient is motivated and when the information is presented clearly, concisely, and in small doses (Redman, 1984). There is no substitute for personal advice, and its value depends heavily upon the attending medical and nursing staff adopting an informed, committed and uniform approach. Similar education of the patient's family is equally important, and giving this at the bedside (when the patient is surrounded by high technology and obvious intensive care) may reinforce the importance of such advice.

Instructional aids (physical, printed and audiovisual) are very useful as part of the educational process. Vocabulary, sentence length, illustrations, type size and style, as well as readability and accuracy of the information presented, should be carefully considered. Visual information is usually assimilated better than the spoken word, so that the use of illustrations, pamphlets and models is a helpful and useful adjunct. A plastic model of the heart is useful for demonstrating cardiac anatomy and the coronary arteries and explaining about the blood supply to the heart. This helps correct the common myth that the heart receives its nourishment by blood flowing through the chambers. The atherosclerotic process may then be described, including plaque formation, progressive narrowing and obstruction of the coronary arteries, and myocardial infarction. The discussion should include an explanation of other symptoms that the patient may have experienced, such as sweating and palpitations. The role of coronary artery spasm can be discussed if the patient has a history of variant angina. The healing process of the heart and the meanings of ECG and laboratory findings should also be briefly explained. It is important to stress that there is no cure for ischaemic heart disease, but that some medical intervention and modification of life-style may be necessary to alleviate symptoms and reduce the risk of further problems.

Structured teaching seems to improve patients' knowledge about their myocardial infarction (Deberry et al, 1975; Rahe et al, 1975; Owens et al, 1978), particularly if booklets and discharge information sheets are given (Gregor, 1981). However, some researchers have found only limited effects with inpatient or outpatient teaching and counselling (Sivarajan et al, 1983). There may be various reasons for this: there may be lack of individual attention, or the patient may have indirectly (and incorrectly) obtained information from other patients while in hospital.

Nurses, doctors and patients generally agree upon certain topics that should be included for discussion, including the recognition of signs and symptoms of myocardial infarction, the names, dosages and side-effects of medications, and knowledge of personal risk factors and how to modify them (Casey et al, 1984). Other aspects that need to be covered are the nature of the disease, emergency treatment, resumption of activities, and physical, psychosocial and financial problems encountered on return to home and work. Aspects frequently neglected include how to take the pulse, sexual activity, and instruction on the normal convalescence (Moynihan, 1984). It is important to try to avoid presenting information in a standardised fashion and the nurse needs to find out what the patient's needs are (Runions, 1985).

Providing information may be made more effective by employing the 'IIFAC scheme' outlined by Nichols (1985).

I   *Initial information check* What do the patient and spouse know, and are they suitable candidates for receiving further information?

I   *Information exchange* An exchange of essential knowledge and information in acceptable terms.

FAC *Final accuracy check* Do the patient and spouse accurately and fully understand the information, or do they require further teaching?

Questionnaires may be useful for evaluating the patient's needs and level of comprehension (Rahe et al, 1975). However, when assessing the efficacy of the education programme, it is important to differentiate between what the patient learns and what he is actually going to do about it; the acquisition of new information does not necessarily result in a change of behaviour (Wenger, 1975).

Involvement of the patient's family

The family can have a direct influence on the rehabilitation process by understanding the illness and helping the patient adapt to it. They can also help in modification of the patient's life-style. They should therefore be included in most, if not all, teaching so that they are equipped with the necessary information. Spouse involvement has been minimal in rehabilitation, despite the widespread opinion that success generally depends upon their support. A programme that involves both patients and spouses provides an ideal opportunity for giving information, instilling hope and redefining health (Dracup et al, 1984). The rest of the family also needs information to feel useful to the patient, and to understand that he is receiving appropriate care (Gaglione, 1984).

Information on the coronary care unit and the ward

Education initiated on the coronary care unit helps the patient understand what has happened, what is immediately being done, and what is likely to happen over the ensuing days. Teaching needs to be relevant to the individuals concerned; vagueness and ambiguity will only result in increased fear and anxiety (Geissler et al, 1985). A programme centred around these principles is likely to improve the patient's attitudes, behaviour and understanding of the illness, and improve his recovery (Halhuber, 1978).

At an early stage, brief explanations regarding the staff, equipment, procedures and routines of the coronary care unit will reduce anxiety and misunderstanding. The nurse should avoid bombarding patients with too much information during the early phase as they invariably retain very few facts during this acute stage. Capacity for learning is impaired by fear, anxiety, pain and fatigue. Patients will, however, benefit from answers to specific questions, and answers should be clear, simple and repeated frequently.

If the patient has to undergo a painful or invasive procedure, information on the patient's likely experiences and sensations will be more effective in alleviating anxiety than details about the procedure alone (Johnson, 1980). When the patient's mental and physical condition permits the assimilation of more detailed and complex information, the nurse can provide information about his condition, its limitations, possible problems and outcome.

Physical activity

Early studies on the role of exercise in prevention of coronary heart disease in the 1940s and 1950s showed that roughly half the number of coronary deaths occurred in those with physically active jobs as opposed to those with sedentary occupations (for example, bus conductors and postmen had lower mortality rates than bus drivers and telephone operators). Since then, favourable associations have been reported between the taking of vigorous physical activity and a reduced risk of coronary heart disease (Morris et al, 1980). Physical fitness also leads to improvements in coronary risk factors; exercise increases HDL-cholesterol concentrations, and reduces weight and often blood pressure too (Paffenbarger and Hyde, 1980).

Emphasising physical exercise following acute myocardial infarction usually represents a major change to the typical patient's sedentary life-style involving the car, labour-saving devices and long hours in front of the television. However, exercise improves mood and morale, and physical fitness allows an earlier return to normal life-style and work. Regular exercise also helps cardiovascular performance, keeps the body supple and helps control body weight. Coronary rehabilitation programmes are to be encouraged to this end.

Regular moderate exercise (30 to 45 minutes three or four times per week) at a level of 75 to 85 per cent of maximal capacity is an ideal way of achieving physical fitness. Vigorous physical activity may be employed later, and is recognised as an important factor in protection against the development of coronary heart disease (Morris et al, 1980); the greater the energy expenditure, the lower the incidence of coronary heart disease seems to be. Paffenbarger and Hyde (1980) estimate that the risk of myocardial infarction is reduced by 5 per cent for each hour spent per week in vigorous activity. However, care is required in those with pre-existing heart disease; exercise is not without hazard and low-level activities are preferable in older and less fit patients.

Formal exercise programmes are very useful following acute myocardial infarction. Early graduated physical activity starting with gentle passive exertion has been designed to avert or minimise the risk of venous stasis and its complications (deep vein thrombosis and pulmonary emboli). When the patient is first allowed out of bed, he is often shocked at the tremendous feeling of physical weakness, which is usually not expected or easily explicable in terms of the short period of bed rest and inactivity. The patient will need reassuring and encouragement to gradually increase the level of activity. Any restrictions thought necessary should be carefully explained in a positive fashion so that the patient does not become frustrated.

Information regarding physical activity will depend on the stage of recovery the patient has reached. Initially, the reasons for temporary restriction of activity will need to be explained, and that the resumption of activity will be gradual to allow the myocardium to heal.

Activity planning

The functional classification of the New York Heart Association provides a crude guide for determining appropriate activities as well as expected symptoms in patients following acute myocardial infarction (table 13.1). Advice about specific activities should be individualised and take into account the extent and severity of the myocardial infarction, the patient's previous level of activity, the extent of recovery and stability of the current condition.

Progress in early rehabilitation has been greatly assisted by the use of *metabolic equivalents* (METs) for prescribing specific physical activities (table 13.2). One

Table 13.1.   Functional classification of patients with heart disease (New York Heart Association Criteria Committee, 1964).

Class 1: Heart disease with no limitation on ordinary physical activity

Class 2: Slight limitation: ordinary physical activity (e.g. walking) produces symptoms

Class 3: Marked limitation: unable to walk on the level without disability, less than ordinary activity produces symptoms

Class 4: Dyspnoea at rest: inability to carry out any physical activity

Table 13.2.   Approximate energy requirements for selected activities.

Category	METs	Examples
Very light	< 3	Washing, dressing, driving car, working at desk, washing up dishes, walking at 2 mph
Light	3–5	Light shopping, dancing, golf, tennis (doubles), walking at 3–4 mph, cycling on flat (7 mph)
Moderate	5–7	Stairs, digging soft soil, tennis (singles), walking 4–5 mph, cycling (10 mph), swimming
Heavy	7–9	Jogging (5 mph), non-competitive squash, cycling (12 mph)
Very heavy	> 9	Shovelling snow, running > 6 mph, cycling > 13 mph (or steep hills), competitive sport

MET is defined as the oxygen consumption by the patient at rest, and is roughly equivalent to 3.5 ml of oxygen per minute (1.4 calories per minute).

Three months or more after an uncomplicated myocardial infarction, the average post-infarction patient is capable of performing at a level of up to 9 METs. This is equivalent to running at about 5 miles per hour, cycling at 12 miles per hour or playing 'non-competitive' squash. If less than ordinary activity produces symptoms, it may be necessary for a more suitable activity level to be planned. Patients who have had congestive heart failure, for example, are often limited to 3 to 5 METs at three months.

Physical activity on the coronary care unit

Early ambulation in the uncomplicated myocardial infarction is essential to avert or minimise the deleterious effects of prolonged bed rest, including decreased physical work capacity. It also reduces the anxiety and depression that often follow acute myocardial infarction.

In some coronary care units, patients are encouraged to sit out of bed on the day of admission provided they are free from pain and significant dysrhythmias. If there has been a prolonged period of bed rest, resumption of activity often results in a moderate tachycardia and orthostatic hypotension. Physical activities should there-fore be at a low level of intensity (1 to 2 METs), such as eating, dressing and undressing, washing of the hands and face, use of a bedside commode, simple arm and leg exercises or sitting in a bedside chair. Observation of the patient as he performs these activities is useful to ensure that he can cope, and that an inappropriate tachycardia is not provoked. Early rehabilitation should not be associated with chest pain, dyspnoea, sweating, palpitations or excessive fatigue. Dysrhythmias and ST-segment displacement on the cardiac monitor should not occur, and systolic blood pressure should not fall more than 10 to 15 mmHg.

The patient is usually the best judge of how much he can do, but he should be warned of the feelings of weakness that may accompany increases in activity.

Table 13.3.   In-hospital exercise plan.

Day	METs	Examples
1	1	Self-feeding, washing with help, passive movement of limbs, commode
1–2	2	Active movement of limbs, sitting out of bed for 20 minutes twice daily
2–3	3	Sitting out for an hour twice daily, walking to bathroom
4–5	4	Walking up to 50 yards, short flight of stairs

Physical activity on the ward

Once the patient leaves the coronary care unit, the aim is for him to attain a level of activity that permits personal care and independence (or at least semi-independence) by the time of discharge from hospital. In these days of early discharge following uncomplicated myocardial infarction, patients usually return home after five to seven days.

The ward activity plan should consist of 'warm-up' isotonic (dynamic) exercises which allow the heart rate to increase proportionally to the intensity of the activity. The systolic blood pressure increases slowly and the diastolic blood pressure remains unchanged or decreases slightly. Isometric exercises should be avoided. These result in a minimal increase in heart rate, but a significant and steep increase in the systolic blood pressure. This causes a sudden increase in cardiac afterload which may be poorly tolerated by an ischaemic left ventricle, resulting in angina or malignant tachydysrhythmias (Nutter et al, 1972).

Walking with a gradual and progressive increase in speed and distance should be the major component of the activity plan (table 13.3). It is advisable for most patients who will have to climb stairs at home to try stairs in hospital under supervision. This results in increased confidence and reduced worry for the patient and family. At the time of discharge from hospital, patients should be able to perform activities at peak levels of 3.5 to 4 METs for short periods to simulate usual activities at home.

Exercise stress testing

The current practice of early ambulation and exercise training soon after myocardial infarction has resulted in the more widespread use of exercise testing earlier in the course of the illness, and often before discharge home. A normal response to an early exercise test reliably identifies the patients at low risk of future cardiac events (see

Table 13.4.   Exercise targets following acute myocardial infarction.

Weeks	METs
1–3	2–4
4–12	5–7
> 12	7 and over

chapter 5). It is beneficial for spouses to observe and even participate during stress testing so as to gain more confidence in their husbands' physical and cardiac capability (Taylor et al, 1985).

Physical activity during convalescence

When the patient returns home, progressive increases in physical activity are used to achieve a level of activity that allows normal daily activities and will later permit a return to work. The activity plan within hospital will usually have helped allay the patient's and family's fears of a further heart attack or sudden death resulting from physical exertion. Patients should be encouraged to exercise daily, and it should be stressed that a lack of exercise may be harmful rather than beneficial. The best form of exercise is walking, but golf, swimming, jogging and cycling can be encouraged when the patient feels well enough. Exercises that use less than half of the patient's working capacity will not help to increase fitness.

The benefits of exercise should be stressed, including weight control, improvement of respiratory function and a general feeling of well-being. Practical advice is helpful too: for example, only exercising in warm environments, and not after heavy meals by the fire-side in winter, or in the midday sun in summer. Competitive sports are not advisable in the early months following infarction for obvious reasons.

The levels of activity performed at the end of the hospital stay should be maintained, and gradually increased (table 13.4). Walking speed and distance should be increased, so that by the end of four to six weeks the patient may walk up to five miles per day (Oberman, 1984). The patient and family will usually gain confidence and the patient more independence when he accomplishes each objective.

Formal exercise programmes for outpatients

Although there is some debate about the benefits derived from formal exercise programmes, there are some indications that they may be of value (Shephard, 1986). Most studies claim that patients who have participated in these programmes show increased physical fitness, a better understanding of their illness and treatment, and fewer psychological problems, with an earlier and larger number returning to work (Prosser et al, 1978; Mayou et al, 1981). In particular, fewer fatal re-infarctions have been found to occur in those who have been involved in such programmes (Shephard, 1983).

During exercise sessions, direct observation, including ECG monitoring by telemetry, is recommended. A warm-up period of five minutes is needed to gradually increase the pulse rate and blood pressure and help joint flexibility. Maintaining a target heart rate is a useful guide for achieving the correct intensity of exertion. The level of activity is altered until the desired heart rate is achieved, and the exercise is maintained for the duration of the session (continuous training) or interspersed with brief rest periods (intermittent training). The exercise devices used include the treadmill, arm/leg ergometer, rowing machine and wall pulleys. The ECG is observed for dysrhythmias or ST-segment displacement. Heart rate and adverse signs or symptoms need to be recorded. At the conclusion of the exercise session, it is important to taper the activity down gradually (a 'cool down') rather than to stop it abruptly.

Home-based exercise programmes are probably as effective as group training (Miller et al, 1984), although a rehabilitation programme that is community based may be more beneficial in terms of social contact and support (Bethell et al, 1983).

INFORMATION FOR CONVALESCENCE

Exercise sessions may usefully be combined with education and counselling of the patient and family, and providing information for convalescence.

It is not uncommon for the patient and family to be left to cope by themselves with only vague instructions about discharge and rehabilitation, which results in uncertainty, distress and failure to adjust. A well planned programme is desirable, to anticipate the patient's homecoming and return to work. Patients and spouses often have specific questions about convalescence, medication, diet, drinking, driving and smoking, as well as resumption of leisure and sexual and work activities (Cay, 1982).

Group discussions after the exercise session provide a means of asking questions, sharing feelings and concerns, and learning from others who have similar problems. Patients and spouses who participate in group counselling seem to suffer less anxiety, depression and anger, as well as having improved compliance with advice about treatment (Dracup, 1985). There is good evidence that beneficial effects occur where patients provide each other with information, advice and support (Ibrahim et al, 1974; Rahe et al, 1979). Counselling also reduces depression and promotes independence and sociability (Stern et al, 1983).

General health recommendations to all coronary patients and their families should include:

- A varied diet with appropriate caloric intake to achieve or maintain an ideal body weight
- The cessation of smoking
- A programme of regular and vigorous physical activity
- A regular health examination including testing of the urine for sugar and protein, measurement of blood pressure and assessment of plasma lipids

Psychological aspects

Many patients are confronted by fear and uncertainty when they arrive back home, which, when combined with minor physical symptoms, result in increased anxiety and depression. Considerable psychological distress and a low level of understanding have been found to occur in many post-coronary patients and their spouses (Mayou et al, 1976, 1978). Such reactions may impair the recovery of a group of patients in whom psychological factors are stronger determinants of re-adjustment to normal life than is their physical status (Wiklund et al, 1984).

Predischarge counselling is useful in improving morale and aiding a successful return to home and work. Preparation should include discussions of potential problems that may occur on return home, such as anxiety, depression, poor concentration, irritability, sleeplessness and fear of complications (especially death). The spouse often experiences a greater degree of anxiety than the patient, and may need careful and supportive counselling (Hentinen, 1983; Thompson and Cordle, 1988). The family particularly needs to be cautioned against overprotectiveness towards the patient.

Only a few well controlled studies of in-hospital psychological interventions have been reported in patients following acute myocardial infarction. These have varied from individual daily supportive psychotherapy (Gruen, 1975) to stress management and relaxation techniques (Langosch et al, 1982), or combinations of these (Oldenburg et al, 1985). Such interventions have generally shown significant improvements in psychosocial and physical functioning for at least a year after the infarct. Whether these improvements can be sustained over a longer period remains to be seen.

Because the transition from hospital to home is frequently a traumatic and neglected aspect of post-myocardial infarction management, it may be appropriate to make arrangements that will ensure continuity of care. Periodic checks (e.g. telephoning the patient and spouse, home visits) may be useful in some instances to bridge this gap, and this is probably best achieved by close liaison between hospital and community nurses. The district nurse can play an important role in teaching, counselling and evaluating the care that has been initiated within the hospital. She is also ideally placed for informing the patient and spouse about community resources, including counselling services, home helps and rehabilitation facilities. She may also liaise with the patient's family doctor.

The multidisciplinary health team approach is advantageous as it combines the skills of different professionals, provides continuity between hospital and community care, and thus maximises the resources available to the patient and family. Nevertheless, it is important to avoid encouraging patient and family dependence; ultimately each individual is responsible for his or her own health, and must be encouraged to assume overall responsibility and control.

Sexual counselling

If the patient is to be properly rehabilitated, his sexual needs cannot be ignored. Although discussion of this intimate aspect of the patient's life is a difficult process for both the patient and the medical staff, sexual counselling should be viewed as an integral part of the cardiac rehabilitation programme (Thompson, 1983). It is recommended that the subject of sex should be approached as a matter of routine in the rehabilitation of all coronary patients and their partners.

The energy expenditure during intercourse is not as great as popularly believed, being equivalent to that of climbing about two flights of stairs (4 METs). Experimental data have demonstrated that peak heart rates occur during orgasm, and adequate foreplay will allow the pulse rate to increase gradually from resting levels to a transient peak of about 180 beats per minute. Blood pressure also rises gradually to peak just before or during orgasm, with increases of 20 to 100 mmHg systolic and 20 to 40 mmHg diastolic. Hyperventilation occurs, with respiratory rates recorded of up to 60 per minute. These physiological variables rapidly return to precoital levels after orgasm.

Extramarital and other illicit encounters may, however, expend much more energy, and are often associated with faster heart rates, higher blood pressures, and an increased risk of sudden death.

Sexual problems

Patients recovering from acute myocardial infarction often suffer from a depressed libido which may result in sexual disharmony. Interestingly, impotence is rarely a problem. The spouse is often more concerned than the patient, and may be frightened of resuming sexual activity because of precipitating a heart attack or sudden death (Thompson, 1983). The severity of the infarct and the extent of cardiac decompensation are much less important causes of sexual debility than the psychological condition of the patient.

The PLISSIT model (Annon, 1976) provides a useful framework for those involved in dealing with sexual counselling of coronary patients and their partners. This model provides four levels of approach (Thompson and Cordle, 1986).

Permission

This is permission to discuss and ask questions about sex. For instance, the counsellor can introduce the topic by saying, 'Many people are worried about when they can resume normal sexual relations. I wonder whether there are any questions or concerns that either of you may have regarding your sex life?'

Limited information

This means providing the couple with factual information directly relevant to their particular situation or sexual concern. Many patients lack sufficient information which results in unnecessary worry. For instance, the commonest fear is that of re-infarction or death occurring during intercourse. This is in fact a rare occurrence, accounting for about 0.6 per cent of cases of cardiac deaths (Ueno, 1963). Most of these fatalities occur during extramarital sex. Fear of resuming sexual activity is more harmful than the actual activity, and sexual frustration should be avoided at all costs. In general, most patients can resume sexual intercourse about two to four weeks after discharge home. Typical advice may be: 'If you can make it up the stairs to the bedroom in one go, you can resume sexual activity'. Good sex need not be an athletic feat.

If these two stages are insufficient to resolve sexual concerns, two options are available.

Specific suggestions

This stage involves careful and detailed assessment of the couple's specific problems. There may be a need to advise patients on how to minimise symptoms that may accompany intercourse. A warm bedroom and warm sheets are desirable. If chest pain, breathlessness or palpitations occur during or after sexual activity, they should stop and seek medical advice. Often, all that is required is for GTN to be taken immediately before coitus prophylactically, as the patient might do before any form of physical activity. Beta-blockers are also very useful for limiting heart rate and myocardial work. It should be noted that patients using cutaneous nitrates may deposit some of their medication on their partner, imparting typical nitrate side-effects on them ('Not now, I've got a headache!').

If psychological problems remain unresolved, it may be necessary to refer the patient on for intensive counselling.

Intensive therapy

Specialised sexual counselling by a trained psychologist, often within a sexual dysfunction clinic, may be indicated for intensive therapy in resistant cases.

Medication

Compliance with drug therapy varies from patient to patient, but often remains unacceptably poor. Difficulty in understanding and complying with drug therapy may occur for a variety of reasons, including fear of dependency or of side-effects. The more complex the drug regimen, the less likely compliance seems to be, and careful review of the patient's medication is necessary before discharge. Many patients will not have taken tablets before their heart attack, and the habit of taking regular medication may be unfamiliar.

Information should include correct identification of the drug, what it is for, the dosage and other special instructions (for example, the storage and limited life of GTN). Reissue of prescriptions needs to be covered: patients often stop what is intended to be continuous therapy when they have finished 'the course'. In addition, they should be warned that they should not allow themselves to run out of tablets, or go away on holiday with insufficient supplies. Sudden withdrawal of certain drugs (e.g. beta-blockers) may be associated with sudden cardiac events, including unstable angina, myocardial infarction and sudden death. Patients should enquire about whether or not it would be cheaper to obtain an annual prescription 'season ticket' rather than paying for individual medications.

It may be useful to issue a small record card listing the patient's medications, with dose, time to be taken, action and possible side-effects written on the card. This may be kept with the medication at home, thus serving as a reminder and providing important information about the drugs. The cards are also useful to summarise therapy when prescriptions are being re-issued by the patient's family doctor, and can be taken to hospital appointments so that all concerned know what medication is actually being taken.

Family participation in teaching about drugs may exert a strong influence on the patient's understanding and thus improve compliance with therapy.

Driving

Patients can usually resume driving about four to six weeks after an uncomplicated myocardial infarction. However, they should initially avoid rush-hour traffic and long journeys, as well as aggressive or competitive driving. Patients are precluded from holding licences to drive heavy goods (HGV) or public services vehicles (PSV) after they have had a myocardial infarction. There is a statutory requirement for the patient to inform both the licensing authority (the DVLC at Swansea) and their motor insurance companies about changes in their health circumstances.

Flying

Patients are usually safe to travel by air as soon as the period of convalescence is over, although long flights are probably inadvisable initially.

Return to work

The return to work usually gives the patient increased self-satisfaction, restored self-respect and relief from financial worries. Many consider return to work to be the goal of cardiac rehabilitation, although in the current gloomy employment climate it is increasingly difficult to use the return to work as a valid outcome of post-infarction rehabilitation.

At about six weeks after acute myocardial infarction, the greater part of the affected heart muscle should be healed by the formation of a firm scar, and any collateral circulation should also be well developed. As a consequence, most patients should be ready to resume work, provided it is not physically or mentally too demanding. It is important that the myocardial infarction is not seen as an absolute deterrent to returning to work.

In general the rates of return to work for post-infarction patients are not as good as might be anticipated (Mayberry et al, 1983). Only about one-half to three-quarters of patients return to their former employment. By one month most of these are back at work, although only about half work as well as they had done before their coronary (Cay, 1982). About 25 million working days are lost annually from coronary heart disease in the UK, equivalent to lost production of £1100 million. Several factors influence the return to work, including:

- The severity of myocardial infarction
- Post-coronary complications and symptoms (especially breathlessness and angina)
- Advanced working age
- Stressful work environment
- A sporadic pre-coronary work record
- Family instability

It can be seen from these factors that non-cardiac causes of invalidity are just as important as cardiac causes in failure to return to work (Cay et al, 1973).

Discouragement by the family is a major cause of the patient not returning to work (Mayou, 1979). This may be because of shared fear of further cardiac problems, although possible early retirement and Social Security payments may sometimes create a disincentive to return. Inconsidered advice from the patient's medical advisor to 'lay off work and take things easy for a few months' will not help, and some employers seem to believe that coronary patients cannot or should not work at all.

Those patients likely to do best are those given encouragement from the start of the illness, particularly from their family. It is likely that the better the patient perceives his health to be, the more likely he is to return to work. A multidisciplinary approach is often required, involving the social worker, disablement resettlement officer and the employer (World Health Organisation, 1980). Initially the patient may be advised to return to work on a part-time basis, and occasionally with lighter work. A few patients involved in heavy manual work may need to change their occupation, although this is not always acceptable or practical. When the patient does return to work, his level of activity may need to be closely monitored. Many manual workers continue to try to carry out heavy duties which may be harmful. The patient may dispute this and feel fully capable or not wish to show weakness.

The daily workload of the female patient who is a housewife also needs careful consideration. She has often played a central role in home life, and feels a tremendous responsibility, both while she is in hospital and on her return home. Such patients often feel that the house has been neglected, shopping for essential items has been forgotten and the house has not been cleaned adequately. They worry about being unable to look after their family, including cleaning, shopping and cooking. The family will need careful counselling about the psychological stresses on such women, and must provide both moral and physical support. They should not be left at home alone initially, and will need help in performing the household chores, particularly physically taxing jobs such as making the beds and hanging out the washing.

Sickness benefit

Many patients and spouses are anxious about how and when to claim sickness benefit. It is helpful to provide them with brief details.

In the UK, sickness benefit (factory sickness pay) is paid by the employer provided sufficient NI contributions were paid during the relevant tax year. Sickness benefit will be paid for up to 28 weeks, and thereafter an invalidity benefit may be paid. Supplementary benefit (for items such as the mortgage) may additionally be payable from the DHSS. The old age pension is payable at the age of 65 years for men and 60 for women, the amount being dependent on the length of working life and the contributions paid.

Useful literature for patients

The following are useful sources of information for the post-infarction patient.

1. *British Heart Foundation – Heart Research Series pamphlets* (1980)
Published as a series of eleven pamphlets, these are written for cardiac patients and their families. They cover most aspects of coronary heart disease, and are obtainable from the British Heart Foundation, London. The address is shown in the appendix.

2. *Coronary Heart Disease: The Facts* (1981), Oxford University Press, by J P Shillingford
Written by a distinguished cardiologist, this book is ideal for answering the concerns of most coronary patients and their families.

3. *Look After Your Heart publications (DHSS)*
● *Campaign Strategy Document*
● *A Guide to Healthy Lifestyles*

- *Beating Heart Disease*
- *Exercise. Why bother?*
- *A Guide to Healthy Eating*
- *New Smoking Leaflet*

4. *The Big Kill: Smoking Epidemic in England and Wales* (1985), eds. Roberts J L and Graveling A. Health Education Council/British Medical Association, London

References

Annon J S (1976) *The Behavioural Treatment of Sexual Problems: Brief Therapy.* New York: Harper and Row.

Bethell H J N, Larvan A and Turner S C (1983) Coronary rehabilitation in the community. *Journal of the Royal College of General Practitioners,* **33:** 285-291.

Casey E, O'Conell J K and Price J H (1984) Perceptions of educational needs for patients after myocardial infarction. *Patient Education and Counselling,* **6:** 77-82.

Cay E L (1982) Psychological problems in patients after a myocardial infarction. *Advances in Cardiology,* **29:** 108-112.

Cay E L, Vetter N J, Philip A E and Dugard P (1973) Return to work after a heart attack. *Journal of Psychosomatic Research,* **17:** 231-243.

Deberry P, Jefferies L P and Light M R (1975) Teaching cardiac patients to manage medications. *American Journal of Nursing,* **75:** 2191-2193.

Dorossiev D (1983) *Rehabilitation and Comprehensive Secondary Prevention after Acute Myocardial Infarction: Report on a Study.* EURO Reports and Studies No. 84. Copenhagen: WHO Regional Office for Europe.

Dracup K (1985) A controlled trial of couples group counselling in cardiac rehabilitation. *Journal of Cardiopulmonary Rehabilitation,* **5:** 436-442.

Dracup K, Meleis A I, Clark S, Clyburn A, Shields L and Stanley M (1984) Group counselling in cardiac rehabilitation: effect on patient compliance. *Patient Education and Counselling,* **6:** 169-177.

Gaglione K M (1984) Assessing and intervening with families of coronary care patients. *Nursing Clinics of North America,* **19:** 427-432.

Geissler W, Cay E and Dorossiev D (1985) Educational programmes after myocardial infarction. In: *Rehabilitation after Myocardial Infarction. The European Experience,* eds. Kallio V and Cay E, pp. 89-102. Copenhagen: World Health Organisation.

Gregor F M (1981) Teaching the patient with ischaemic heart disease: a systematic approach to instructional design. *Patient Counselling and Health Education,* **3:** 57-62.

Gruen W (1975) Effects of brief psychotherapy during the hospitalization period on the recovery process in heart attacks. *Journal of Consulting and Clinical Psychology,* **43:** 223-232.

Halhuber M J (1978) Health education in cardiac rehabilitation. *Advances in Cardiology,* **24:** 146-152.

Hentinen M (1983) Need for instruction and support of the wives of patients with myocardial infarction. *Journal of Advanced Nursing,* **8:** 519-524.

Hogan C A and Neill W A (1982) Effects of a teaching program on knowledge, physical activity, and socialization in patients disabled by stable angina pectoris. *Journal of Cardiac Rehabilitation,* **2:** 379-385.

Ibrahim M A, Feldman J G, Sultz H A, Staiman M G, Young L J and Dean D (1974) Management after myocardial infarction: a controlled trial of the effect of group psychotherapy. *International Journal of Psychiatry in Medicine,* **5:** 253-268.

Johnson J E (1980) Preparing patients to cope with stress while hospitalized. In: *Patient Teaching,* ed. Wilson-Barnett J, pp. 19-33. Edinburgh: Churchill Livingstone.

Langosch W, Seer P, Brodner G, Kallinke D, Kulick B and Heim F (1982) Behaviour therapy with coronary heart disease patients: results of a comparative study. *Journal of Psychosomatic Research,* **26:** 475-484.

Linde B J and Janz N M (1979) Effect of a teaching program on knowledge and compliance of cardiac patients. *Nursing Research,* **28:** 282–286.

Mayberry J F, Kent S V, Jenkins B and Colbourne G (1983) Employment of men after myocardial infarction. *British Medical Journal,* **287:** 1262–1263.

Mayou R (1979) The course and determinants of reactions to myocardial infarction. *British Journal of Psychiatry,* **134:** 588–594.

Mayou R, Williamson B and Foster A (1976) Attitudes and advice after myocardial infarction. *British Medical Journal,* **i:** 1577–1579.

Mayou R, Foster A and Williamson B (1978) The psychological and social effects of myocardial infarction on wives. *British Medical Journal,* **i:** 699–701.

Mayou R, McMahon D, Sleight P and Florencio M J (1981) Early rehabilitation after myocardial infarction. *Lancet,* **ii:** 1399–1401.

Miller N H, Haskell W L, Berra K and DeBusk R F (1984) Home versus group exercise training for increasing functional capacity after myocardial infarction. *Circulation,* **70:** 645–649.

Morris J N, Everitt M G, Pollard R, Chave S P W and Semmence A M (1980) Vigorous exercise in leisure time: protection against coronary heart disease. *Lancet,* **ii:** 1207–1210.

Moynihan M (1984) Assessing the educational needs of post myocardial infarction patients. *Nursing Clinics of North America,* **19(3):** 441–447.

New York Heart Association Criteria Committee (1964) *Diseases of the Heart and Blood Vessels; Nomenclature and Criteria for Diagnosis,* 6th edn. Boston: Little, Brown.

Nichols K A (1985) Psychological care by nurses, paramedical and medical staff: essential developments for general hospitals. *British Journal of Medical Psychology,* **58:** 231–240.

Nutter D O, Schlant R S and Hurst J W (1972) Isometric exercises and the cardiovascular system. *Modern Concepts in Cardiovascular Disease,* **41:** 11–15.

Oberman A (1984) Rehabilitation of patients with coronary artery disease. In: *Heart Disease,* ed. Braunwald E, pp. 1384–1398. Philadelphia: W B Saunders.

Oldenburg B, Perkins R J and Andrews G (1985) Controlled trial of psychological intervention in myocardial infarction. *Journal of Consulting and Clinical Psychology,* **53:** 852–859.

Owens J F, McCann C S and Hutelmyer M (1978) Cardiac rehabilitation: a patient education program. *Nursing Research,* **27:** 148–150.

Paffenbarger R S and Hyde R T (1980) Exercise as protection against heart attack. *New England Journal of Medicine,* **302:** 1026–1027.

Prosser G, Carson P, Gelson A, Tucker H, Neophytou M, Philips R and Simpson T (1978) Assessing the psychological effects of an exercise training programme for patients following myocardial infarction: a pilot study. *British Journal of Medical Psychology,* **51:** 95–102.

Rahe R H, Scalzi C and Shine K (1975) A teaching evaluation questionnaire for post-myocardial infarction patients. *Heart and Lung,* **4:** 759–766.

Rahe R H, Ward H W and Hayes V (1979) Brief group therapy in myocardial infarction rehabilitation: three to four year follow-up of a controlled trial. *Psychosomatic Medicine,* **41:** 229–242.

Redman B K (1984) *The Process of Patient Education.* St Louis: C V Mosby.

Runions J (1985) A program for psychological and social enhancement during rehabilitation after myocardial infarction. *Heart and Lung,* **14:** 117–125.

Scheuermann W, Scheidt R, Nussel E and Deckert E (1985) Multicentre study on heart groups. In: *Proceedings of the International Conference on Preventive Cardiology,* Moscow, June 1985. Abstract 123.

Shephard R J (1983) The value of exercise in ischaemic heart disease – a cummulative analysis. *Journal of Cardiac Rehabilitation,* **3:** 294–298.

Shephard R J (1986) Cardiac rehabilitation in prospect. In: *Heart Disease and Rehabilitation,* eds. Pollock M L and Schmidt D, pp. 713–740. New York: Wiley.

Sivarajan E S, Newton K M, Almes M J, Kempf T M, Mansfield L W and Bruce R A (1983) Limited effects of outpatient teaching and counseling after myocardial infarction: a controlled study. *Heart and Lung,* **12:** 65–73.

Stern M J, Gorman P A and Kaslow L (1983) The group counselling versus exercise therapy study: a controlled intervention with subjects following myocardial infarction. *Archives of Internal Medicine,* **143:** 1719–1725.

Taylor C B, Bandura A, Ewart C K, Miller N H and DeBusk R F (1985) Exercise testing to enhance wives' confidence in their husbands' cardiac capability soon after clinically uncomplicated acute myocardial infarction. *American Journal of Cardiology*, **55**: 635–638.

Thompson D R (1983) Sexual counselling and cardiac patients. *British Journal of Sexual Medicine*, **10**: 16–18.

Thompson D R and Cordle C J (1986) Sexual counselling following myocardial infarction. *British Journal of Sexual Medicine*, **13**: 16–17.

Thompson D R and Cordle C J (1988) Support of wives of myocardial infarction patients. *Journal of Advanced Nursing*, **13**: 223–228.

Ueno M (1963) The so-called coition death. *Japanese Journal of Legal Medicine*, **17**: 330–340.

Wenger N K (1975) Patient and family education after myocardial infarction. *Postgraduate Medicine*, **57**: 129–134.

Wiklund I, Sanne H, Vedin A and Wilhelmsson C (1984) Psychosocial outcome one year after a first myocardial infarction. *Journal of Psychosomatic Research*, **28**: 309–321.

Wilson-Barnett J (1979) *Stress in hospital. Patients' Psychological Reactions to Illness and Health Care*. Edinburgh: Churchill Livingstone.

Wilson-Barnett J and Oborne J (1983) Studies evaluating patient teaching: implications for practice. *International Journal of Nursing Studies*, **20**: 33–44.

World Health Organisation (1980) *International Classification of Impairments, Disabilities and Handicaps*. Geneva: World Health Organisation.

14

Treating the Risk Factors of Coronary Heart Disease

Mortality from coronary heart disease has changed appreciably in many countries over the past two decades. Some countries such as Australia, Finland, Israel and the USA have shown fairly dramatic reductions. For example, there have been declines in the mortality from coronary heart disease (down 39 per cent), stroke (down 54 per cent) and other cardiovascular diseases (down 19 per cent) in the 20-year period from 1964 to 1984 in the USA, compared with a reduction of only 12 per cent in non-cardiovascular disorders (National Center for Health Statistics, 1982, 1984). A number of factors have been responsible for this decline, including cardiovascular risk factor modification. Certain major risk factors, of course, cannot be modified, including age, sex, race and heredity. However, hypertension, smoking, hyperlipidaemia and diabetes may often be easily modified.

The early approaches towards the prevention of coronary heart disease concentrated on modifying one risk factor, so that an effect could be defined for each factor. However, these trials did not provide consistent answers, mainly because the atheromatous process is multifactorial, and attacking only one risk factor had (as might have been expected) little or no effect. Nevertheless, these early trials were useful in demonstrating and confirming aetiological factors. More recently, a multifactorial approach has been taken, and many interventions have been recommended in the prevention of coronary heart disease and the rehabilitation of the patient following myocardial infarction. These involve some modification or major changes in the patient's life-style (European Atherosclerosis Society, 1987; Health Education Council, 1984).

The rehabilitation programme should include changes relevant to the patient, particularly those that may result in a reduced risk of myocardial infarction. It is, however, important when talking to patients to explain that changing any life-long habit (whether it be exercise, smoking or diet) will never guarantee that they will be free from heart disease, or any other ailment for that matter. What is being considered are relative risks, and it is important that this is appreciated by all concerned.

Counselling patients on risk factors presumes that the person will change them on being informed about the relative risks involved in ischaemic heart disease. However, life-style modification is not easy; denial frequently has to be overcome and belief that change is necessary has to replace it. Time to consider and reappraise the situation is essential for the patient so that change may be introduced gradually with his cooperation. Modifying behaviour is a difficult and long-term process. Although the hospital setting provides an ideal environment for discussing and motivating the patient to a healthier way of life, educational opportunities are often constrained by the acute illness and associated anxiety. Nevertheless, counselling during the latter part of the patient's stay in hospital provides an ideal foundation for patient and family education.

DIETARY ADVICE

Many health professionals seem to forget that, apart from providing the essential nutrients to the body, eating and drinking are pleasurable experiences. Many misconceptions regarding diet litter the popular press and bookstalls, and the problem is compounded by conflicting and unsubstantiated information given by friends, relatives and even some health professionals.

If the nurse is to be successful in achieving compliance, it is important that she presents factual information objectively, consistently and in a way that can be easily and readily understood by the patient and his family. Dietary modifications often require a major change in the patient's normal eating habits, and gradual changes are more likely to be successful. Involvement of the patient's family is also helpful; eating is usually a family or communal activity, and the women of the household are the ones who are normally responsible for the shopping and preparation of the meals. It is therefore important to both educate them and enlist their help and cooperation in any dietary manipulation.

Modifying the diet is probably helpful in the treatment of hyperlipidaemia, hypertension and congestive cardiac failure, and in the prevention of hypertension and atherosclerosis. However, it is clear that some of these are contentious issues (Thompson, 1983; Oliver, 1986). Many dietary recommendations have been advanced on the basis that they will prevent or minimise the risk of heart disease, and detailed and complicated dietary modification are to be found in abundance in the medical literature and popular press. Nevertheless, it should be appreciated that dietary modification alone has not been shown to prevent heart disease. Many patients become distressed when they make alterations to their diet and life-style only to find that they have heart disease.

Weight control

The single most important dietary measure is the prevention or reduction of obesity. Obesity is often associated with elevated plasma lipids, glucose intolerance and hypertension. It is therefore desirable for obese patients to lose weight by decreasing caloric intake and increasing energy expenditure. Body weight is essentially controlled by food intake, and it is always possible to lose weight by eating less food than the body requires. Long-established Western dietary habits are hard to break, and we are generally encouraged to eat and drink more than is good for us, particularly saturated fats, simple sugars and alcohol.

Acceptable ranges for body weight have been defined by the Royal College of Physicians of London (1983) and the Fogarty Consensus Conference on Obesity (Bray, 1979), although distinction should be made between 'average' weights and 'ideal' weights. The former are always higher in the West, where we all over-eat. Ideal

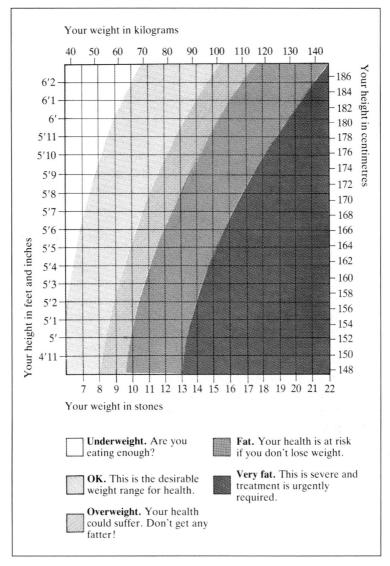

Fig. 14.1 Desirable body weight (From Garrow, 1981. Reproduced by kind permission of Churchill Livingstone, with acknowledgement to the Health Education Council and E Fullard, Oxford)

weights are based on the pooled experience of life assurance companies, who have calculated desirable weight based on excess mortality figures. On average, life expectancy is decreased by 15 per cent for every 10 per cent excess of ideal body weight. Another index of obesity is the *body mass index* (BMI), which is obtained by dividing the height^2 (in metres) into the weight (in kilograms). Obesity begins at a BMI of over 28.

There are many causes of obesity, but alas virtually all are environmental. Affluence, familial obesity (due to role modelling and eating habits) and the Western sedentary life-style all contribute. The instant food market has led to instant obesity. The increasing consumption of alcohol is also a major contributory factor. Hormonal imbalance, although a popular excuse, is not an underlying cause. Such disorders (e.g. myxoedema and Cushing's disease) invariably present with other symptoms.

The nurse needs to ascertain the major cause of obesity when counselling the patient, and needs to establish a mutually agreed goal for weight reduction. A regular record needs to be kept (e.g. with a graph) which gives a quick visual indication of how the patient is progressing. The hospital is an ideal place for launching such a plan, which must be relevant to the patient's life-style, culture and socioeconomic status. Practical advice should include explanation of calorific intake versus expenditure, the regular and slow eating of smaller amounts of food and the participation in regular physical activity. The goal is to achieve a body weight appropriate for age, height and sex (figure 14.1). Attending 'Weight Watchers' or other slimming clubs may be helpful.

It must be noted that it will be more difficult to influence the patient if family members and those counselling the patient are overweight.

Specific advice on diet

There is no doubt that the Western diet is generally appalling, and the recent DHSS recommendations (Committee on Medical Aspects of Food Policy, 1984) are welcomed as a policy for prevention of cardiovascular disease in the future. This general advice is summarised below, but referral to the dietitian may be beneficial when expert advice is required regarding more complex changes.

Dietary restrictions, if necessary, must be realistic and thoroughly understood by the patient and family if they are going to be adhered to. This should be supplemented by leaflets which can be referred to at home. In all cases it is advisable to talk to whoever does the shopping and cooking, and if there are cultural differences, advice from somebody of the same background is desirable as this will aid understanding and acceptability. For most patients it is better to emphasise an alteration in general eating habits rather than the necessity to adhere to a specific dietary plan; patients are not going to change the habits of a lifetime based on a 10-minute chat with a doctor, nurse or dietitian. An infinite variety of foods are now widely available and in most cases it is possible to advise a nutritious, balanced and varied diet. Alternative diets (vegetarian and vegan) are increasingly popular and their possibilities may need to be discussed.

Dietary fats

There are two main categories of fat in the diet, saturated (animal) fats which tend to raise serum cholesterol levels, and unsaturated (vegetable) fats which tend to lower blood cholesterol. The major dietary sources of fats are the spreading fats (butter and margarine), cooking fats, meat and dairy produce. In addition, much of our fat intake is hidden in foods such as cakes and biscuits. Offal (liver, kidney and pate), shellfish and eggs all contain large amounts of cholesterol.

Overall reduction of saturated fat intake with substitution of vegetable fats where possible is desirable, and the World Health Organisation (WHO Expert Committee,

1982) recommends a reduction to 30 per cent of the total food energy intake, with two-thirds of this as vegetable fat. This has been endorsed by the British Hyperlipidaemia Association (Shepherd et al, 1987).

Dietary fibre

An increased fibre intake is recommended. Viscous fibre (e.g. guar or pectin) will help lower plasma cholesterol levels. Fresh vegetables and fruit provide excellent sources of pectin, vitamins and minerals.

Salt intake

Dietary salt is a controversial issue, but a suitable reduction can be made by not adding it to food after cooking. Obviously salty foods should be avoided (e.g. crisps, peanuts or Marmite), especially by those with high blood pressure.

Sugar

Countries with a high per capita intake of sugar have high rates of coronary heart disease (Keys, 1980). However, there is a close link between sugar and fat intake in the poorer countries, and it is unlikely that sugar is an independent risk factor. A reduction in simple sugars and other refined carbohydrates is however helpful in preventing obesity, treating glucose intolerance and reducing the incidence of dental caries.

Alcohol

The evidence relating to alcohol and coronary heart disease is complex, mainly due to concomitant abuses which often accompany alcohol intake (e.g. smoking or overeating). Alcohol may directly damage the myocardium, as well as causing hypertension and hyperlipidaemia. Moderate intake of alcohol (25 to 30 g/day) probably does not increase cardiovascular risk.

Electrolytes and trace elements

The myocardium is more susceptible to damage, dysrhythmias and digoxin in the presence of hypokalaemia. Most chronic hypokalaemia is due to diuretics, and an increased intake of potassium in the diet is desirable. Magnesium depletion (due to thiazide diuretics, diabetes or diarrhoea) usually accompanies hypokalaemia and hypocalcaemia.

Potential benefits from a 'healthy' diet

Diets that are fat-modified, high in fibre and low in salt may help reduce serum cholesterol and blood pressure. Thrombogenicity may also decrease, via the reduced effect of fatty acids on platelet function. In addition, there is improved large bowel function, and a reduced risk of bowel cancer. High-fibre diets are associated with less constipation, diverticular disease, appendicitis, gall-stones and haemorrhoids. Glucose tolerance may be improved, and high-carbohydrate, high-fibre, low refined sugar diets are recommended for patients with diabetes mellitus.

MANAGEMENT OF HYPERLIPIDAEMIA
(see Jowett and Galton, 1987)

Patient screening

The most commonly employed screening test is the measurement of total cholesterol and triglyceride levels in a sample of venous blood taken, preferably without stasis, after an overnight (12-hour) fast. It should be noted that acute illness such as infection, trauma (including surgery) and myocardial infarction may alter serum lipoprotein concentrations. For example, for about three months after acute myocardial infarction, plasma triglycerides may be higher and total cholesterol lower than in the pre-infarction state, although samples taken in the first 24 to 48 hours reflect the pre-infarction levels (Ryder et al, 1984). In the UK, the Coronary Prevention Group (1987) recommends that estimation of serum cholesterol should be available on request by patients, since knowledge of their own blood cholesterol may help them modify future risk. At the same time risk factor counselling can take place, along with blood pressure measurement.

The upper limits of normality of lipid concentrations will vary between laboratories, and take into account both differing analytical methodology and the population that is being assessed. It has become clear that a standard method for lipid measurement needs to be agreed and adopted by hospital laboratories both nationally and, probably, internationally.

There is persuasive evidence that cholesterol is causally related to atherosclerosis and its complications, particularly coronary heart disease. Plasma cholesterol continues to be a risk factor for recurrent myocardial infarction, although less strongly related than for the first attack (International Society and Federation of Cardiology, 1981). It should be noted that the relationship between serum cholesterol concentrations and mortality is not linear, but J-shaped (figure 14.2), with more cases of cancer of the colon and strokes occurring in those at the lower end of cholesterol distribution. Whilst the cause of this is not clear, it may be disadvantageous to lower the cholesterol level too far.

Although the upper level of 6.5 mmol/l for normality continues to be shown on many pathology reports, the threshold for medical intervention should be lowered to 5.2 mmol/l (*Lancet*, 1987). At this plasma cholesterol level, the risk of coronary heart disease is comparatively small (Martin et al, 1986) and this level is therefore considered optimal.

If abnormal values are discovered, fasting levels are re-measured on three occasions at weekly intervals, before a diagnosis of hyperlipidaemia is established. Then:

1. Patients with concentrations less than 5.2 mmol/l should be screened every five years.

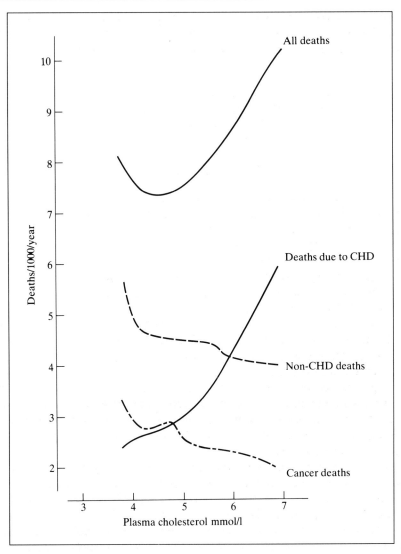

Fig. 14.2   Relationship between plasma cholesterol concentrations, total mortality, cardiac and non-cardiac mortality (data from Rose and Shipley, 1980)

2. Those with plasma cholesterol levels between 5.2 and 6.3 mmol/l should be treated by diet (see below).

If the total cholesterol level is above 6.3 mmol/l, the HDL–cholesterol (HDL–C) level should be obtained, because it is the HDL/LDL–cholesterol ratio and not the total cholesterol concentration which is important. Low HDL–C levels (less than 1.0 mmol/l) and high LDL–C levels (more than 5.0 mmol/l) are associated with atherosclerotic disease, and a ratio of these two lipoprotein subfractions of less than 0.2 appears to be an important predictor of coronary heart disease.

The LDL–cholesterol concentration may be estimated by the formula:

$$\text{LDL-C (mmol/l)} = \text{Total cholesterol} - \left(\text{HDL-C} + \frac{\text{Triglycerides}}{2.19} \right)$$

Family screening

Many of the primary hyperlipidaemias are familial, and lipoprotein abnormalities may be found in the patient's relations. Measurement of serum lipids should therefore always be offered to first-degree relatives, particularly the younger males where early therapy will be of most value. This is especially important in monogenic familial hypercholesterolaemia, a dominantly inherited disorder which carries a high risk of very early coronary death. Early diagnosis and therapy is the only hope of improving the prognosis.

Exercise

Exercise increases HDL levels and HDL/LDL ratios and may decrease the incidence of atherosclerotic heart disease.

Dietary advice

Few constituents in the blood vary between populations as much as cholesterol. Mean levels of total cholesterol in New Guinea are only 2.5 mmol/l as opposed to, for example, East Finland where the level is 7.5 mmol/l. Of course these differences may reflect differing genetic make-up, but dietary factors are probably of equal importance. The mean serum cholesterol concentration in the UK population is 5.7 mmol/l, and more than two-thirds have serum cholesterol levels above the recommended level of 5.2 mmol/l.

Dietary modification must be the first line of treatment for all types of hyperlipidaemia, although the response will depend both on the underlying lipoprotein abnormality and its severity. Fat intake should be reduced to below one-third of total energy requirements, and the proportion of these ingested as polyunsaturated (as opposed to saturated) fats should be increased from the typical 25 per cent found in Western diets to about 75 per cent of the total fat intake. This action alone will reduce cholesterol levels and increase the HDL/LDL ratio, as well as making the fat-depleted diet more tolerable. The calorific deficit can be replaced by unrefined, high-fibre carbohydrates, although replacement should not be complete in the overweight. This applies particularly to those patients with predominantly raised triglyceride levels, as attainment of correct body weight will often be the only therapy required. Alcohol excess may also produce hypertriglyceridaemia, but unfortunately 'excess' will vary from patient to patient, and abstention may sometimes be the only way of reducing triglyceride levels.

Drug therapy

Drug therapy should be used only after a careful trial of diet (employing the most rigorous diet suitable for the individual) and control of other risk factors. Treatment with drugs is rarely justified at cholesterol levels below 6.5 mmol/l, and comparatively few with levels between 6.5 and 7.8 mmol/l (Shepherd et al, 1987). Most cases with cholesterol concentrations above 7.8 mmol/l will need medication, especially if there is associated hypertriglyceridaemia (*Lancet*, 1987). The aim is to reduce the total cholesterol below 5.2 mmol/l. This is most important in young, male patients (under 30 years of age), for those with familial hypercholesterolaemia and for those with strong family histories of coronary heart disease.

Patients will be found to have either hypercholesterolaemia, hypertriglyceridaemia or a mixed picture. Those with hypercholesterolaemia should initially be treated with bile acid sequestrants (e.g. cholestyramine, colestipol). Those with mixed hyperlipidaemias are usually treated with fibric acid derivatives (e.g. bezafibrate), especially if the triglyceride levels are markedly elevated. Treatment of hyper-triglyceridaemia remains controversial. Mild elevations (3 to 6 mmol/l) are usually due to obesity or excess alcohol, but if fasting concentrations persist above 3 mmol/l, associated with depression of HDL-C levels (to less than 1.0 mmol/l), treatment should be considered. Nicotinic acid is sometimes very effective, and has been shown to be safe in long-term usage.

Recent studies have shown the value of combined therapy with drugs and diet in the secondary prevention of coronary heart disease (Blankenhorn et al, 1987; Nikkila et al, 1984), and special consideration should therefore be given to patients with coronary heart disease, especially if they have undergone coronary artery bypass surgery or coronary angioplasty.

SMOKING

Every health worker needs to have a thorough knowledge of the facts concerning smoking and health, and in particular its effects on the cardiovascular system. About 1000 men and women in the UK die each week from diseases of the heart and circulatory system because of smoking.

The main effects of smoking (Klein, 1987) are:

- Decreased oxygen carriage by the blood
- Increased platelet aggregability and adhesiveness
- Increased coronary vasomotor tone
- Coronary and renal arteriolar thickening
- Elevation of serum cholesterol, with decreased HDL-cholesterol levels
- Increased sympathetic stimulation (increasing heart rate and blood pressure and hence myocardial work)

The risk of a further heart attack declines on cessation of smoking, and the risk is halved within five years (Doll and Peto, 1976). Additionally, stopping smoking reduces the excess risk of chronic bronchitis and cancer. It has been estimated that a 20 per cent reduction in cigarette smoking could result in 8000 fewer deaths in the UK every year.

Table 14.1.   Smoking – cardiovascular facts.

● Smoking is responsible for 31 per cent of deaths from coronary heart disease
● Smokers run 2–3 times the risk of myocardial infarction than non-smokers; young smokers are even more at risk; a 45-year-old smoker (25/day) runs a 10–15 times higher risk
● Smoking increases the 'strength' of other risk factors, particularly hypertension and hypercholesterolaemia
● Cigarette smokers are at increased risk of sudden death
● Women smokers taking the pill are at a ten-fold increased risk of myocardial infarction
● The risk of stroke is three-fold; 37 per cent of cerebrovascular accidents are due to smoking
● Subarachnoid haemorrhage is more common in smokers
● Nearly all patients with peripheral vascular disease smoke heavily; over 90 per cent of patients with intermittent claudication smoke

Sources: Doll and Peto, 1976; Royal College of Physicians of London, 1977; Gyntelberg et al, 1981; United States Office of Smoking and Health, 1983; Bonita et al, 1986; Cook et al, 1986.

Advice on smoking

Advice on smoking should involve:

● Educating the patient and the family about the facts (table 14.1)
● Initiating effective intervention
● Enlisting the support of friends, workmates and other organisations (e.g. ASH)

Non-smoking policies are widespread in hospitals these days, and cigarette sales from ward trolleys and hospital shops should become obsolete.

The habit of smoking is a complex addiction with a high level of dependence. It appears to serve multiple functions, and exerts its addictive influence by satisfying a physical need, providing stimulation and pleasure, and relieving anxiety and tension. It is important for counsellors to try to ascertain what particular function smoking serves in each individual case.

Advice on smoking should start on the coronary care unit, and a nurse who is a non-smoker will be a more credible role model. Patients usually know if their nurse smokes, and every nurse should read the leaflet *A guide for hospital nurses – helping people to stop smoking*, available from the Health Education Authority (address in the appendix).

The recent concept of 'passive smoking' should also be kept in mind. There is evidence of deleterious effects of maternal smoking on foetuses, and infants in smoking families are also hospitalised more frequently. Additionally, non-smoking spouses may be at increased risk of developing cigarette-associated diseases, including cancer. All these observations should prompt aggressive anti-smoking approaches. The argument that individual freedom is being infringed is sometimes advanced, but it can be seen that smokers do not just harm themselves. They additionally put financial strain on the limited health resources available to all.

Like all rehabilitation advice, its value depends heavily upon the attending medical and nursing staff adopting an informed, committed and uniform approach. Similar education of the patient's family is equally important and giving such information at the bedside when the patient is suffering from obvious smoking-related symptoms often reinforces the importance of such advice.

A realistic plan can be drawn up with the aim of complete cessation of smoking. Cutting down is not the answer, neither is switching to a low-tar cigarette. This is because the smoking pattern will change to extract the same amount of nicotine from weaker or fewer cigarettes. Although it is widely held that switching to cigars or a pipe will reduce the cardiovascular risk, this is not the case (Kaufman et al, 1987). Anyone who has tried a pipe (without inhaling) will already realise this from the immediate symptoms of tachycardia and tremor.

The benefits should be stressed (Rigotti and Tesar, 1985), including improved health and finances, improvement of the senses of taste and smell, and a greater physical attraction when freed from the smell of smoke and nicotine stains on the skin and teeth. The risk of a further myocardial infarction decreases by about one-half (Mulcahy, 1983), and the onset of angina is delayed (Daly et al, 1985). Shock tactics have been employed in the past, by getting the patient to watch videos of those with lung cancer, respiratory failure or amputations. Others may gain benefit from hypnosis and acupuncture, with a success rate of about 20 per cent at one year.

During the initial period of withdrawal, the patients (and their relatives) should be warned that they may become irritable and unable to concentrate. There may be mood swings, gastrointestinal upsets or even an initial worsening of their 'smokers' cough'. Reassurance that these effects are temporary is required. It is important to ensure that the patient does not succumb to the common temptation of 'just one more'. Distraction is useful when craving is present. Nicotine chewing gum may help by maintaining blood nicotine levels, and easing withdrawal symptoms in the early stages.

Although the hospital setting is ideal for smoking cessation, it is necessary for checks to be made on compliance with advice periodically after discharge. General practitioners can very effectively influence their patients by advice, coercion and support (Russell et al, 1979). The use of a carbon monoxide monitor may be very useful in checking compliance, by measuring the levels of carbon monoxide in the blood when the patient attends for rehabilitation or medical follow-up.

HYPERTENSION

Patients are generally unaware of the risks of hypertension, and many of those admitted to the coronary care unit report never having had their blood pressure taken. The expression of the 'rule of halves' expresses the current state of underdiagnosis.

● Only 50 per cent of hypertensive patients have been diagnosed; of these
● Only 50 per cent are receiving treatment; of these
● Only 50 per cent have their blood pressure controlled

In 1972, 50 per cent of patients with hypertension in the USA were unaware of the fact, but now the figure is less than 25 per cent. What is more, the number taking effective antihypertensive treatment has risen from 4 million to 12 million. This kind of increased awareness and intervention has contributed to the recent fall in cardiovascular mortality in the USA.

It is widely accepted that control of hypertension will reduce the incidence of cerebrovascular disease and renal failure, but the benefits for coronary heart disease (CHD) are uncertain. Nevertheless, the commonest cause of death in patients with hypertension is myocardial infarction, which occurs two or three times more commonly than stroke (Medical Research Council Working Party, 1985). The Medical Research Council's trial on the treatment of mild hypertension (1985) looked at 17 354 patients aged 34 to 64 years with phase 5 blood pressures of 90–109 mmHg. Active treatment with propranolol or bendrofluazide reduced the rates of all cardiovascular events (particularly in smokers), but made no difference to the incidence of coronary events alone. In patients over 60 years, however, cardiac mortality was reduced.

Although there is no convincing evidence that secondary intervention improves outcome, treatment is usually given since the risk of heart failure, angina and stroke is reduced (International Society and Federation of Cardiology, 1981).

Treatment of hypertension should be along traditional lines (WHO/International Society of Hypertension, 1983), with initial advice on exercise, weight reduction and dietary restriction of salt and alcohol. It is probably more important to stop smoking than to treat mildly raised blood pressure.

If drug therapy is required, it must be made clear that it is usually permanent, and patients should not just complete the course of tablets. Special attention must be paid to the related contraindications of any antihypertensive agent employed. For example, beta-blockers are not advisable in patients with cardiac conduction defects or heart failure, and diuretics may adversely affect plasma lipid, urate and potassium levels. Care is also required when treating those with poor left ventricular function. Some of these patients will become hypotensive during exercise, and an excessive fall of the blood pressure may precipitate further cardiovascular events.

Hypertensive emergencies can occur either in patients with a previous history of hypertension or in previously normotensive individuals. Rapid reduction of blood pressure is seldom required, except for perhaps for the following emergencies.

1. *Hypertensive encephalopathy*   This is an acute neurological syndrome associated with a rapid rise in blood pressure. The elevated blood pressure causes excessive vasoconstriction and/or vasospasm causing marked changes in cerebral blood flow which results in cerebral micro-infarcts. Clinically, there is a diastolic blood pressure greater than 130 mmHg, hypertensive retinopathy and proteinuria. Headache is the initial symptom, usually in the occipital region, but later becoming generalised and associated with nausea and vomiting. Signs of cerebral irritation with confusion, restlessness, fitting and coma, and focal neurological signs may develop.

2. *Hypertensive heart failure*   Pulmonary oedema and hypertension often coexist, and one may precipitate the other. Often the blood pressure falls with effective treatment of left ventricular failure.

3. *Hypertension complicating myocardial infarction*   Many patients with acute myocardial infarction will be hypertensive on admission to hospital. Hypertension will often respond to pain relief and sedation, but resistant cases will need the addition of a vasodilator such as sodium nitroprusside (Chiarello et al, 1976). When hypertension represents sympathetic overactivity, treatment with beta-blockers is indicated. However, caution is needed: tachycardia and hypertension may be a compensatory

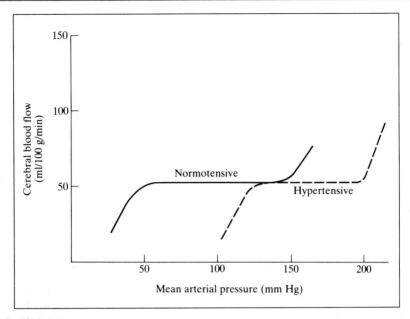

Fig. 14.3 Cerebral autoregulation of blood flow. Note that the control mechanism is set at a higher level in patients with hypertension

mechanism in response to left ventricular dysfunction. This is usually not the case if there is a loud first heart sound, wide pulse pressure and no dyspnoea.

The aim of treatment in hypertension is to lower the blood pressure as safely as possible, rather than as quickly as possible. In patients with chronic hypertension, sudden reduction of the blood pressure may cause a stroke. This is because cerebral autoregulation is set at higher levels (figure 14.3) and 'normal' blood pressures will be insufficient to perfuse the brain, resulting in cerebral ischaemia and infarction.

In hypertensive emergencies, bed rest and oral medication may be all that is required to reduce an elevated blood pressure. The aim should be to reduce the diastolic pressure to around 100 mmHg over 24 to 48 hours using this or standard drug therapy (e.g. beta-blockers or nifedipine). Patients with accelerated hypertension need investigation to look for underlying causes.

STRESS

The role of stress and the stress response in the aetiology of ischaemic heart disease needs to be discussed. Type A characteristics include abrupt gestures, hurried speech, impatience, tenseness, hostility and rapid, illegible handwriting. These behavioural characteristics should be discussed to enable the patient to recognise them. In some patients they may represent outward signs of underlying emotional reactions, such as anger or anxiety, and will need recognising as such.

A marked reduction in the intensity of type A behaviour has been seen in patients undergoing regular counselling (Gill et al, 1985), suggesting that it can be modified in the short term at least. Intervention by counselling after acute myocardial infarction leads to a dramatic and sustained fall in cardiovascular mortality (Friedman et al, 1986).

Methods of relaxation are numerous and varied, and one that is suitable to the individual should be chosen, e.g. progressive relaxation, meditation, biofeedback, yoga, self-hypnosis, group therapy or listening to music. Polyphasic activities must be avoided (e.g. watching television, eating and reading simultaneously). The role of frequent moderate exercise is often underplayed. Jogging, for example, is ideal for reducing muscular tension and giving the patient an opportunity for privacy and self-appraisal as he runs.

Planned periods of rest and relaxation may be beneficial for the majority of patients, and are more productive if the spouse participates. Most methods involve the person selecting a comfortable sitting or reclining position. A quiet, peaceful environment, often with the light subdued, is ideal; otherwise the patient may become distracted or have difficulty in concentrating or relaxing. This particular type of relaxation therapy is assuming increasing importance in the rehabilitation of patients following myocardial infarction, and such techniques have been shown to reduce anxiety and depression (Bohachick, 1984) as well as reducing heart rate, blood pressure and arrhythmias (Benson et al, 1975; Patel, 1975). Relaxation on a regular basis should be encouraged, otherwise many patients cease the practice once they feel better.

ASSESSING PROGNOSIS FOLLOWING MYOCARDIAL INFARCTION

It is often of great importance to be able to assess prognosis following acute myocardial infarction, so that therapy may be optimised and new treatments may be evaluated. Long- and short-term prognosis is dependent on many factors (table 14.2), the most important of which are the extent of coronary arterial disease (which may place the surviving myocardium in jeopardy) and the level of residual left ventricular function (Glover and Littler, 1987). All the prognostic factors are interrelated, and are largely dependent on the modified functional anatomy of the damaged heart. There is an array of different variables which may be identified, but most lack specificity (i.e. may be associated with a large proportion of false positive results (Murray et al, 1987). The Norris prognostic index may be computed from a weighted score for age, history of ischaemia, radiological heart size and evidence of cardiac failure on the first day of admission (Norris et al, 1970). Other prognostic indicators may be apparent from their in-hospital course or may be defined following further investigations. Additionally, prognosis may change because of medical intervention. Stratification of patients according to risk is a continuous process, and should not be based upon one assessment only.

Most patients who are going to die from heart attack do so within the first few weeks, and the majority of these from ventricular fibrillation before reaching

Table 14.2. Factors associated with a poor prognosis following acute myocardial infarction.

Age > 60 years
Male sex
Poor left ventricular function (heart failure, hypotension)
Post-infarction angina
Cardiomegaly on the chest radiograph
Previous evidence of coronary heart disease
ECG:
● Persistent ST/T wave changes
● Ventricular ectopic activity
● Atrial fibrillation
● Conduction defects
● Left ventricular hypertrophy
Other coexisting diseases:
● Hypertension
● Diabetes

hospital. Later, in-hospital deaths are mainly due to 'pump failure' or re-infarction. The overall mortality of patients surviving to be discharged from hospital is 10 to 15 per cent in the first year. Deaths are often sudden, presumably due to dysrhythmias or re-infarction. Most of these will have shown problems within the first three months following the acute myocardial infarction (Theroux et al, 1979). For those who survive 12 months, the annual death rate is about 5 per cent.

Prognostic factors include the following.

Age

Mortality rises steadily with age. Hospital mortality is twice as great in the over-65 age group as in those under 65 years of age.

Myocardial damage

The degree of myocardial damage may be shown by clinical, electrocardiographic or radiological methods, often aided by monitoring enzyme concentrations in the blood. Most poor prognostic signs are due to increased myocardial damage, for example shock, anterior myocardial infarction, previous myocardial infarction and left ventricular failure. Myocardial damage may be assessed by estimating the size of the infarct, its location, and the extent of coexistent coronary vascular disease.

Infarct size

It is the size of the infarct that influences the outcome, and loss of more than 40 per cent of left ventricular myocardium is usually associated with cardiogenic shock. There is a strong correlation between the peak creatine kinase (CK) levels and four-year mortality (Thompson et al, 1979). Enzymatic markers of myocardial infarction are closely linked to other prognostic indices, including site and thickness of the infarct, the degree of ventricular dysfunction and the frequency of ventricular dysrhythmias. More accurate information may be obtained by echocardiography or radionuclide assessment of left ventricular function.

Infarct location

A more favourable prognosis is associated with inferior as opposed to anterior infarction, even when estimates of infarct size are identical. Extension of the infarct, acute dilatation with aneurysm formation, thrombus formation or rupture are also more common with anterior infarcts (Bulkley, 1981). As might be expected, the short-term prognosis is better with non-transmural than full thickness infarcts, although this does not apply in later years; the underlying lesion may progress and cause further events (De Wood et al, 1986).

The extent of coexisting coronary arterial disease

It is the blood supply to surviving myocardium which influences prognosis (Betriu et al, 1982). Most patients presenting with acute myocardial infarction have two or more diseased coronary vessels, a clue to which may be reciprocal changes on the admission electrocardiogram. Persistent and recurrent ischaemic pain following acute myocardial infarction is a poor prognostic sign. ECG evidence of transient ischaemia in the early phase following acute myocardial infarction is common (particularly in those with non-Q-wave infarction), and correlates with residual ischaemia and the extent of the myocardium 'at risk'. Early ST monitoring may therefore be useful for selecting these at-risk patients in whom aggressive investigation and treatment may be indicated (Bosch et al, 1987). This may be carried out using Holter monitors or low-level exercise stress testing.

Dysrhythmias and conduction defects

For those patients who survive myocardial infarction complicated by bundle branch block (particularly left bundle branch block), the prognosis is poor. In general, bundle branch block occurs in those with extensive infarction and mechanical problems.

Atrial fibrillation in the first 72 hours following acute myocardial infarction is associated with a high mortality, usually reflecting post-infarction complications such as heart failure and raised atrial pressures (Cristal et al, 1976). Ventricular dysrhythmias (including ventricular fibrillation) are very common in the first 24 to 48 hours following infarction, and are usually a transient complication. However, after 48 hours, their presence is of poor prognostic implication, and associated with a high in-hospital mortality. Ventricular dysrhythmias are usually associated with poor left ventricular function. Those patients who show frequent ventricular ectopic beats (10 or more per hour) on 24-hour Holter recording in the first four weeks following myocardial infarction delineate a subset of patients who are at risk of sudden death. This also applies to those who demonstrate frequent ventricular ectopics during exercise stress testing (Pratt et al, 1984).

With the exception of beta-adrenergic blocking agents, treatment with anti-dysrhythmic agents has not yet been shown to reduce mortality.

Exercise tolerance

It may be very difficult clinically to distinguish patients with extensive coronary artery disease (poor prognosis) and those with single coronary artery disease (better prognosis). Limited exercise testing prior to discharge from hospital is a simple, non-invasive investigation, and may be useful to assess prognosis. Provided there is no heart failure, ventricular dysrhythmias, hypotension or post-infarction angina, the test can safely be performed even in the first week following infarction (Crean and Fox, 1987). Those who show evidence of myocardial ischaemia or poor blood pressure responses during exertion have a poorer prognosis. The outlook in this group of patients may be improved by further investigation, including coronary angiography and cardiac surgery (see chapter 15).

Other prognostic factors

Mortality is higher in those who continue to smoke tobacco. Persuading a post-infarction patient to stop smoking is the most useful advice that may be given to improve prognosis. Diabetes and hypertension have been related to early (less than 30 days) mortality (Henning et al, 1979) although the main reason for controlling blood pressure is to prevent non-cardiac mortality (i.e. stroke). A high admission blood glucose is indicative of a poor prognosis. This may be because it denotes pre-existing diabetes, or because it reflects the severity of the attack. Obesity and hyperlipidaemia are minor risk factors associated with a poor prognosis. The routine use of beta-blockers following infarction may be prevented by conduction defects or heart failure. As such, the inability to tolerate beta-blockade following acute myocardial infarction delineates a group of patients at high risk. Whether it is because this group have more myocardial damage or because they are denied the 'protective' value of beta-blockade is not known.

Conclusions

Combining information from clinical assessment, investigations and exercise stress testing can be used to assess post-infarction prognosis, and seems to be of greater value than considering individual risks since these lack specificity. Important variables include reciprocal changes on the ECG at the time of infarction, severe myocardial damage, inability or a poor result in a post-infarction stress test, and an inability to tolerate post-infarction treatment with beta-adrenergic blocking agents. These patients might benefit from more rigorous medical treatment or surgical intervention.

References

Benson H, Alexander S and Feldman C L (1975) Decreased premature ventricular complexes through the use of relaxation response in patients with stable angina. *Lancet,* **ii**: 380–382.
Betriu A, Castaner A, Sanz G A, Pare J C, Roig E, Coll S, Margrina J and Navarro-Lopez F (1982) Angiographic findings one month after myocardial infarction: a prospective study of 259 survivors. *Circulation,* **65**: 1099–1105.

Blankenhorn D M, Nessim S A, Johnson R L, Sanmarco M E, Azen S P and Cashin-Hemphill L (1987) Beneficial effects of combined colestipol–niacin therapy on coronary atherosclerosis and coronary venous bypass grafts. *Journal of the American Medical Association,* **257**: 3233–3240.

Bohachick P (1984) Progressive relaxation training in cardiac rehabilitation: effect on psychologic variables. *Nursing Research,* **33**: 283–287.

Bonita R, Scragg R, Stewart A, Jackson R and Beaglehole R (1986) Cigarette smoking and the premature risk of stroke in men and women. *British Medical Journal,* **293**: 6–8.

Bosch X, Theroux P, Waters D D, Pelletier G B and Roy D (1987) Early post-infarction ischaemia: clinical, angiographic and prognostic significance. *Circulation,* **75**: 988–995.

Bray G A (1979) Obesity in America. An overview of the Second Fogerty International Center conference on obesity. *International Journal of Obesity,* **3**: 363–375.

Bulkley B H (1981) Size and sequelae of myocardial infarction. *New England Journal of Medicine,* **305**: 337–338.

Chiarello M, Gold H K, Leinbach R C, Davis M A and Maroko P R (1976) Comparison between the effects of nitroprusside and nitroglycerine on ischaemic injury during acute myocardial infarction. *Circulation,* **54**: 766–773.

Cook D G, Shaper A G, Pocock S J and Kussick S J (1986) Giving up smoking and the risk of heart attacks. *Lancet,* **ii**: 1376–1379.

Committee on Medical Aspects of Food Policy (1984) *Panel on Diet in Relation to Cardiovascular Disease.* London: Department of Health and Social Security.

Coronary Prevention Group (1987) Risk assessment: its role in the prevention of coronary heart disease. *British Medical Journal,* **295**: 1246.

Crean P A and Fox K M (1987) Exercise electrocardiography in coronary artery disease. *Quarterly Journal of Medicine,* **62**: 7–13.

Cristal N, Peterburg I and Schwarcberg J (1976) Atrial fibrillation developing in the acute phase of myocardial infarction: prognostic implications. *Chest,* **70**: 8–11.

Daly L E, Graham I M, Hickey N and Mulcahy R (1985) Does stopping smoking delay onset of angina after infarction? *British Medical Journal,* **291**: 935–937.

De Wood M, Stifter W F, Simpson C S et al (1986) Coronary angiographic findings soon after non-Q-wave myocardial infarction. *New England Journal of Medicine,* **315**: 412–422.

Doll R and Peto R (1976) Mortality in relation to smoking: 20 years' observations on male British doctors. *British Medical Journal,* **ii**: 1525–1536.

European Atherosclerosis Society (1987) Strategies for the prevention of coronary heart disease: a policy statement of the European Atherosclerosis Society. *European Heart Journal,* **8**: 77–88.

Friedman M, Thorensen C E and Gill J J (1986) Alteration of Type A behaviour and its effect on cardiac recurrences in post-myocardial infarct patients: summary results in the Recurrent Coronary Prevention Project. *American Heart Journal,* **112**: 653–665.

Gill J J, Price V A, Friedman M, Thoreson C E, Powell L H, Ulmer D, Brown B and Drews F R (1985) Reduction in type A behaviour in healthy middle-aged American military officers. *American Heart Journal,* **110**: 503–514.

Glover D R and Littler W A (1987) Factors influencing the survival and mode of death in severe ischaemic heart disease. *British Heart Journal,* **57**: 125–132.

Gyntelberg F, Pedersen P B, Lauridsen L and Schubell K (1981) Smoking and risk of myocardial infarction in Copenhagen men aged 40–59 with special reference to cheroot smoking. *Lancet,* **i**: 987–989.

Health Education Council (1984) *Coronary Heart Disease Prevention: Plans for Action.* London: Pitman.

Henning H, Gilpin E A, Covell J W, Swan E A, O'Rourke R A and Ross J (1979) Prognosis after acute myocardial infarction: a multivariate analysis of mortality and survival. *Circulation,* **59**: 1124.

International Society and Federation of Cardiology (1981) Secondary prevention in survivors of myocardial infarction. *British Medical Journal,* **282**: 894–896.

Jowett N I and Galton D J (1987) The management of the hyperlipidaemias. In: *Drugs for Heart Disease,* ed. Hamer J, 2nd edn. London: Chapman and Hall.

Kaufman D W, Palmer J R, Rosenberg L and Shapiro S (1987) Cigar and pipe smoking and myocardial infarction in young men. *British Medical Journal*, **294:** 1315-1316.

Keys A (1980) *Seven Countries*. London: Harvard University Press.

Klein L W (1987) Cigarette smoking and coronary artery disease: recent findings and implications for patient management. *Heart and Lung*, **16:** 74-78.

Lancet (1987) Prevention of coronary heart disease. *Lancet*, **i:** 601-602.

Martin M J, Hulley S B, Browner W S, Kuller L H and Wentworth D (1986) Serum cholesterol, blood pressure and mortality: implications from a cohort of 361 662 men. *Lancet*, **ii:** 933-936.

Medical Research Council Working Party (1985) MRC trial of treatment of mild hypertension: principal results. *British Medical Journal*, **291:** 97-105.

Mulcahy R (1983) Influence of cigarette smoking on morbidity and mortality after smoking. *British Heart Journal*, **49:** 410-415.

Murray D P, Salih M, Tan L B, Murray R G and Littler W A (1987) Prognostic stratification of patients after myocardial infarction. *British Heart Journal*, **57:** 313-318.

National Center for Health Statistics 1982 (1984) Advance report of final mortality statistics. *Monthly Vital Statistics Report*, 33 (Suppl.): 1-43.

Nikkila E A, Viikiukoski P, Valle M and Frick M H (1984) Prevention of progression of coronary atherosclerosis by treatment of hyperlipidaemia: a seven year prospective angiographic study. *British Medical Journal*, **289:** 220-223.

Norris R M, Caughey D E, Mercer C J, Deeming L W and Scott P J (1970) Coronary prognostic index for predicting survival after recovery from acute myocardial infarction. *Lancet*, **ii:** 485-488.

Oliver M F (1986) Prevention of coronary heart disease; propaganda, promises, problems and prospects. *Circulation*, **73:** 1-9.

Patel C (1975) 12 month follow-up of yoga and bio-feedback in the management of hypertension. *Lancet*, **i:** 62-64.

Pratt C M, Seals A A and Luck J C (1984) The clinical significance of ventricular arrhythmias after myocardial infarction. *Cardiology Clinics*, **2**(1): 3-11.

Rose G and Shipley M J (1980) Plasma lipids and mortality: a source of error. *Lancet*, **i:** 523-526.

Royal College of Physicians of London (1977) *Smoking or Health: A Report*. London: Pitman Medical.

Royal College of Physicians of London (1983) Report on obesity. *Journal of the Royal College of Physicians of London*, **17:** 3-58.

Rigotti N A and Tesar G E (1985) Smoking cessation in the prevention of cardiovascular disease. *Cardiology Clinics*, **3:** 245-257.

Russell M A, Wilson C, Taylor C and Baker C D (1979) Effect of general practitioners' advice against smoking. *British Medical Journal*, **ii:** 231-235.

Ryder R E, Hayes T M, Mulligan I P, Kingswood J C, Williams S and Owens D R (1984) How soon after myocardial infarction should plasma lipid values be assessed? *British Medical Journal*, **289:** 1651-1653.

Shepherd J, Betteridge D J, Durrington P, Laker M, Lewis B, Mann J, Miller J P, Reckless J P D and Thompson G R (1987) Strategies for reducing coronary heart disease and desirable limits for blood lipid concentrations: guidelines of the British Hyperlipidaemia Association. *British Medical Journal*, **295:** 1245-1246.

Theroux P, Waters D D, Halphen C, Debaisieux J C and Mizgala H F (1979) Prognostic value of exercise testing soon after myocardial infarction. *New England Journal of Medicine*, **301:** 341-345.

Thompson D R (1983) Dietary advice and heart disease: a nursing dilemma? *International Journal of Nursing Studies*, **20:** 245-253.

Thompson P L, Fletcher E E and Katavatis V (1979) Enzymatic indices of myocardial necrosis: influence on short and long term prognosis after myocardial infarction. *Circulation*, **59:** 113.

United States Office of Smoking and Health (1983) *Cardiovascular Disease: The Health Consequences of Smoking - A Report of the Surgeon-General*. Department of Health, Education and Welfare Publication No. DHHS (PHS) 84-50204.

WHO Expert Committee (1982) *Prevention of Coronary Heart Disease.* WHO Technical
   Reports Series No. 678. Geneva: World Health Organisation.
WHO/International Society of Hypertension (1983) Guidelines for the treatment of mild
   hypertension. *WHO Bulletin,* **61:** 53–56.

15

The Role of Surgery in Coronary Heart Disease

The risks of cardiac surgery have been greatly reduced over the last decade as operative techniques and peri-operative management have been improved. The two main factors that probably constitute the major risks for mortality and morbidity are the general condition of the patient undergoing surgery and the state of the functional myocardium. When considering patients for surgical management of coronary heart disease, the first point to take into account is whether the operation will involve fewer risks for the patient than continuing with medical therapy. Surgical intervention must also improve the quality of the patient's life, and not just the quantity.

The main role of surgery in coronary heart disease is to improve blood supply to the ischaemic myocardium. However, operations may be required for mechanical defects that have arisen as a consequence of a myocardial infarction (e.g. mitral incompetence or ruptured interventricular septum). It is most often (and most safely) performed electively, but is sometimes required urgently when these complications occur suddenly (table 15.1).

Although many operations have been described in the past for improving myocardial blood supply, coronary artery surgery has only been practised since the late 1960s (Favaloro, 1969). Since that time, the numbers of operations performed have increased exponentially (there were 7403 operations in the UK in 1982), placing an ever-increasing demand on the limited existing facilities of the National Health Service (English, 1984). The most frequently performed operation for ischaemic heart disease is coronary artery bypass grafting (CABG). This has become an important adjunct to current medical therapy, and is highly effective in the treatment of angina. As experience of this operation has improved, there has been a major fall in operative mortality and morbidity which is attributed to better patient selection and

Table 15.1. Indications for surgery in coronary heart disease.

Elective surgery
Stable angina uncontrolled by medical therapy
Left ventricular aneurysms producing complications
Advanced coronary artery disease

Urgent surgery
Mechanical defects following acute myocardial infarction:
● Mitral incompetence
● Ventriculoseptal defect
Crescendo angina which does not settle with medical therapy
Cardiogenic shock

---

preoperative assessment. Attention is now being directed to evaluation of the long-term results of bypass surgery, the development of new techniques (including per-cutaneous transluminal coronary angioplasty) and the effect of surgical intervention in the acute phase of myocardial infarction.

CORONARY ARTERY BYPASS SURGERY

Indications

The main indication for bypass surgery is relief of symptoms, although the following indications are usually considered.

- Symptoms despite maximal medical therapy
- Three-vessel disease
- Left main stem stenosis
- Unstable angina

Left main stem coronary artery disease is associated with serious coronary events (Mock et al, 1982), including myocardial infarction and sudden death. Although disease of this artery is usually symptomatic, it may only be revealed at coronary angiography. The European Coronary Surgery Study Group (1980) showed that the five-year survival rate for three-vessel and left main stem disease was greater in those treated surgically rather than medically (table 15.2). Single and two-vessel disease (with the exception of the left main stem) are better treated either medically or by coronary angioplasty. Some centres consider a 50 per cent occlusion of the left main stem ('the widow maker') sufficient for urgent surgery, regardless of symptoms.

The prognosis for patients with severe symptoms or strongly positive exercise stress tests will improve with surgery, especially if there is impaired left ventricular function. Patients with asymptomatic left main stem or triple artery disease will also benefit. Those with moderate angina or single or double arterial disease (excluding left main stem) are probably managed better by medical therapy or coronary angioplasty (see below) if the lesions are accessible.

Britain's first Consensus Development Conference for coronary artery bypass grafting met in November 1984, and considered the implications for bypass surgery in the UK. The approach for the patient with stable angina and for asymptomatic patients following myocardial infarction is shown in figures 15.1 and 15.2.

Table 15.2. Results of the European Coronary Surgery Study Group (1980).

Group	5-year survival (%)	
	Medical	Surgical
Left main stem	62	93
Three vessels	85	95
Two vessels	88	92

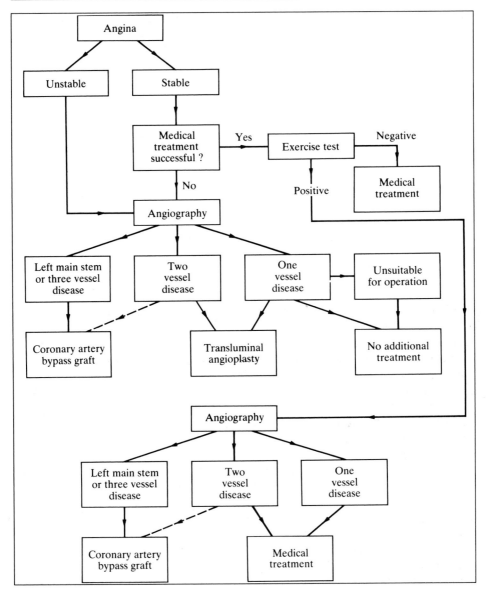

Fig. 15.1 Suggested assessment and treatment for patients with angina (Reproduced by kind permission of the *British Medical Journal*)

About 60 to 80 per cent of patients undergoing coronary artery bypass surgery are free from angina at one year, and the various trial reports indicate that results have improved as the skill of the surgeons has increased (European Coronary Surgery Study Group, 1982; CASS Principal Investigators and their Associates, 1983; Hampton, 1984). Greater care at operation has led to improved graft patency acutely, which has also been helped by the use of aspirin and persantin as antiplatelet agents in the first year (Loop, 1983). Cardiac surgeons are now attempting to attain a

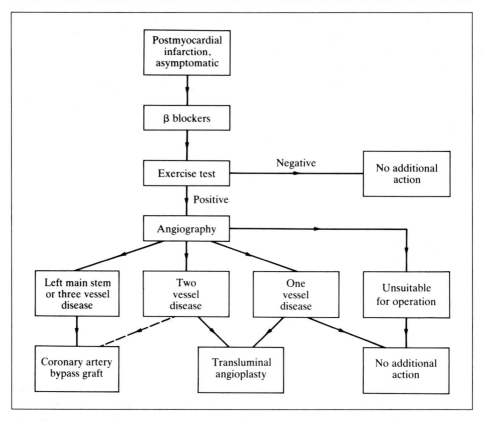

Fig. 15.2 Suggested assessment and treatment for asymptomatic patients who survive myocardial infarction (Reproduced by kind permission of the *British Medical Journal*)

greater degree of revascularisation by bypassing more of the diseased vessels, so that what was originally known as a 'triple bypass' now often involves up to five or six vein grafts. Nevertheless, it must be remembered that these costly and time-consuming operations are palliative, and do not arrest the progression of the underlying atherosclerotic process. The role of primary and secondary prevention of myocardial infarction is of major importance. Most surgeons will not consider patients who have not stopped smoking or reduced their body weight to acceptable levels.

Operative procedures

The object is to revascularise the myocardium by grafting all significantly diseased arteries more than 1 mm in diameter. The decision regarding the number of arteries bypassed is taken after inspection of the coronary angiogram, because many stenotic lesions cannot be appreciated at operation. A lesion leading to greater than 50 per cent occlusion is considered a significant obstruction.

The heart is exposed through a median sternotomy, and cardiopulmonary bypass established via cannulae in the atria and ascending aorta. The body temperature is lowered to 32 °C and cardiac arrest induced with potassium.

Whilst this is going on, a second group of surgeons is stripping the long saphenous vein from the leg, which is then flushed with heparinised blood and checked for leaks.

Endarterectomy of the major coronary arteries is sometimes carried out first if there is diffuse disease or complete stenosis. The distal ends of the bypass vein grafts are then sutured to as many vessels as require it. The aorta is then unclamped, the patient rewarmed and normal cardiac rhythm established by defibrillation. Using special side-biting clamps, the proximal end of the grafts are sutured to the ascending aorta, cardiopulmonary bypass is stopped, cannulae removed and the chest closed.

Postoperative management

Patients are normally ventilated until haemodynamically stable and awake. Arterial lines and Swan–Ganz catheters monitor cardiac pressures for the first 24 hours, after which time the majority of patients can usually leave the intensive care unit. Patients are mobilised quickly, and are often fit for discharge from hospital within 7 to 10 days.

Problems following surgery

Early effects

The morbidity and mortality rates following coronary arterial surgery have fallen with increased expertise; in most centres overall mortality is less than 3 per cent (Treasure, 1983). The main determinant of operative risk is left ventricular function, although several other factors have been implicated:

- Poor left ventricular function
- Emergency surgery
- Previous myocardial infarction (especially if very recent)
- Left main stem disease
- Number of diseased vessels
- Mitral regurgitation
- Hypertension

The commonest problem is perioperative myocardial infarction, although the majority of these do not have significant sequelae. Pain from the median sternotomy and cracked ribs can cause discomfort for a few weeks, as can pain around the long incision used for removing the saphenous vein. Cerebral embolisation is rare, since the operation is essentially closed apart from the cardiopulmonary bypass cannulae. A small number of patients have a temporary impairment of concentration or memory attributable to small atheromatous emboli from the aorta at the time of the operation (Smith et al, 1986). Although embolic events have been considered to be the major cause of stroke during heart surgery, hypoperfusion of the brain may be contributory. Current evidence seems to suggest that these complications are due to cardiopulmonary bypass rather than the operation itself.

Immediate and complete relief from angina is reported by about 80 per cent of patients, and most of the remainder have a marked improvement in their symptoms. The majority of patients are able to return to work between two and six months after the operation.

Long-term effects

The long-term effects of coronary artery bypass surgery are determined by changes in left ventricular function, progression of atherosclerosis and patency of the grafts. Many grafts become occluded in the first month, especially if endarterectomy has been required. Operative technique is obviously important to minimise the risk of thrombosis, including the meticulous preparation of the saphenous vein graft before anastomosis. At one year, about one-quarter of the grafts have become occluded, after which the rate falls to about 2 per cent per year. Anticoagulants and antiplatelet agents are usually prescribed for the first year to minimise this complication. Angina returns in about one-quarter of patients within five years, although it will not necessarily be so severe.

Re-operation will produce nearly as good results (60 per cent angina-free at one year) although operative mortality may be a little higher, probably because of technical difficulties which need to be considered preoperatively.

Left ventricular function may improve postoperatively if poor function has been due to myocardial ischaemia rather than infarction, and provided any left ventricular aneurysm has been removed. The only operative treatment for severe left ventricular dysfunction following infarction is cardiac transplantation.

Coronary bypass using the internal mammary artery

Although technically more difficult, arterial grafts will fare much better than traditional saphenous vein grafts (*Lancet*, 1984) because the graft has its own blood supply left intact, and thus forms a 'living' graft with potential for growth. The left internal mammary artery is usually selected for bypass grafting, mostly for cases of proximal occlusion of the left coronary artery (left main stem disease). The internal mammary artery is mobilised from its origin at the subclavian artery, and its branches tied. It is then anastomosed directly to the left coronary vessel distal to the occlusion.

This operation seems likely to play an increasing role in coronary arterial surgery. It is best suited to the younger patient in whom a longer surviving graft is required. At 10 years, when on average 50 per cent of saphenous vein grafts will have stenosed, about 90 per cent of artery grafts are still functioning.

Bypass surgery for unstable angina

Patients with crescendo angina do badly unless stabilised preoperatively. Fewer than 25 per cent will deteriorate despite medical intervention. For the majority of patients who stabilise, exercise testing should be performed and coronary angiography carried out in those with strongly positive tests.

Peri-infarction bypass surgery

The role of immediate coronary artery bypass surgery is at present being investigated, and results are awaited from trials using early revascularisation within six hours of the infarct. Peri-infarction mortality is about 5 per cent, but long-term results are not yet known. Surgery in the first six weeks is also being carried out in those considered to have a poor 12-month survival, based on exercise stress testing. Those with angina, ST depression and poor haemodynamic responses (tachycardia and hypotension) will be selected for operation. Again, the results of trials are awaited.

OPERATIONS FOR COMPLICATIONS OF MYOCARDIAL INFARCTION

There are three commonly performed operations in patients who have developed mechanical post-infarction complications. These are resection of left ventricular aneurysms, replacement of the mitral valve and repair of the interventricular septum.

Resection of left ventricular aneurysms

After myocardial infarction, the damaged left ventricle may be *akinetic* (i.e. does not move) or *dyskinetic* (i.e. moves paradoxically). This will improve as the infarct heals. Left ventricular aneurysms usually present several weeks or months after acute myocardial infarction, and may be associated with angina, heart failure, dysrhythmias and thromboembolic events. Surgery will usually help overall left ventricular function, but the prognosis following surgery will depend on how the ventricle performs postoperatively, and the overall perfusion of the remaining myocardium. Coronary artery bypass grafting is often carried out at the same time as excision of the aneurysm.

Mitral valve replacement

This is often required for acquired mitral regurgitation due to papillary muscle rupture or dysfunction. The degree of valvular incompetence is variable from slight to massive. Mild cases may respond to diuretic therapy, but uncontrolled heart failure requires mitral valve replacement. Acute rupture is usually fatal within one or two days and, although operation carries a high mortality, mitral valve function may be restored by replacement with a prosthetic valve.

Repair of a ruptured ventricular septum

Rupture of the interventricular septum occurs in about 1 per cent of all infarcts, and untreated will kill 90 per cent of patients, most within a few days. The clinical picture varies considerably, but it usually presents in the first four days after myocardial infarction with severe heart failure in the presence of a loud pansystolic murmur, often with a palpable thrill at the left sternal edge.

Initial therapy is with diuretics and offloading with peripheral vasodilators such as sodium nitroprusside. Insertion of an intra-aortic balloon pump (see below) may augment coronary, cerebral and renal blood flow. Early surgical repair is the best option, although perioperative mortality is high (20 to 30 per cent).

BALLOON PUMPING IN CARDIOGENIC SHOCK

Pathological studies show that fatal cardiogenic shock occurs when over 40 per cent of the left ventricular myocardium has been damaged. This may be due to an acute massive infarction (usually due to left main stem occlusion) or a further infarct in an already damaged heart (acute-on-chronic infarction). Alternatively, it may be due to a mechanical defect resulting from the infarct, such as rupture of the intraventricular septum or acute mitral incompetence. Cardiogenic shock following myocardial infarction is associated with:

● Arterial systolic blood pressure < 90 mmHg
● Oliguria (< 20 ml/h of urine)
● Peripheral hypoperfusion

When these three features are present, mortality approaches 100 per cent whatever medical therapy is instituted. Use of the intra-aortic balloon pump has been advocated for these patients (Mundth et al, 1973).

An inflatable balloon is inserted into the upper part of the descending aorta via the femoral artery. Inflation takes place during diastole, thus raising mean arterial diastolic pressure, allowing improvement of coronary blood flow and perfusion of other vital organs. Deflation is triggered by the R wave on the electrocardiogram, so that the heart never contracts against an occluded aorta.

Haemodynamic improvements include an increased arterial blood pressure of about 10 mmHg, a rise in the cardiac index of about 50 per cent, and a reduction in pulmonary arterial wedge pressure (PAWP) of about 25 per cent. As a consequence, cardiogenic shock is reversed in the majority of patients and is associated with relief of pain and limitation of infarct size.

Unfortunately, the main problem is that it is very difficult to withdraw treatment with the pump without serious haemodynamic decompensation. However, it does give time for the patient to be assessed with a view to emergency surgery. A small proportion of those with cardiogenic shock will have potentially remediable causes (e.g. ruptured interventricular septum), and may benefit from emergency open heart surgery (Resnekov, 1978).

SURGERY FOR TACHYDYSRHYTHMIAS

Surgery has been shown to be effective in the treatment of tachydysrhythmias in patients with and without accessory atrioventricular connections. Electrophysiological investigation is normally carried out first to determine the site and mechanism of the dysrhythmia. Operative therapy is then carried out to destroy or remove the abnormal focus or interrupt the accessory pathway.

1. Areas of irritable myocardium can be excised or destroyed by catheter ablation. An electrical shock is delivered via a pacemaker catheter to the irritable myocardium, which may destroy its ability to conduct or generate impulses. Cryodestruction can also be used.

2. Destruction (by cryotherapy or electricity) or surgical incision of the AV node or other atrioventricular pathways will prevent transmission of supraventricular tachycardias. A permanent ventricular pacemaker will then need to be inserted.

3. Implantable defibrillators with an output of 2 to 30 J have been used to sense tachydysrhythmias and deliver a d.c. shock to restore sinus rhythm (Mirowski et al, 1980). If the discharge is ineffective, they can typically recycle up to three further times, with the energy delivered being increased for the third and fourth shocks. They are not a definitive treatment for recurrent serious dysrhythmias, and are not a substitute for traditional antidysrhythmic therapy.

PERCUTANEOUS TRANSLUMINAL CORONARY ANGIOPLASTY (PTCA)

Following original work on lower limb arterial dilatation by a balloon catheter described by Dotter and Judkins in 1964, a modified procedure for dilatation of the coronary arteries was first described by Gruentzig in September 1977 (Gruentzig et al, 1979). It has since become an established and effective way of treating many serious arterial stenoses (Gruentzig, 1984). In 1984, it was estimated that 40 000 coronary angioplasties had been carried out in the USA: in the UK experience is still limited, and only 500 cases had been undertaken in the same year. Angioplasty has obvious clinical and financial advantages since it is performed under local anaesthesia, and the patient is fully mobile 24 hours after the procedure, with discharge from hospital within two days. Considerable benefit may be obtained in these individuals without recourse to open heart surgery. The main limitation at present is that only about 10 to 15 per cent of patients have lesions suitable for this sort of therapy (Cumberland, 1985; table 15.2). The procedure involves introducing a thin double lumen balloon catheter through a guiding catheter into the affected coronary artery. Steerable wire guiding systems have recently been introduced, which has helped with access to the more difficult arteries, such as the circumflex branch and the distal arterial tree. The balloon is advanced to lie within the stenosis, and then inflated to a pressure of 5 to 10 atmospheres for about 30 to 60 seconds. This is repeated several times until there is angiographic evidence of improved patency. This can be confirmed by measurement of the pressure gradient across the stenosis. On average, a 50 per cent improvement in patency is obtained, and is thought to be due to a combination of atheroma splitting and compression, stretching of the arterial media and endothelial desquamation. Chest pain is frequently experienced during dilatation, so the procedure is usually covered with drugs that minimise coronary arterial spasm. Nifedipine (10 mg

Table 15.3.   Selection criteria for PTCA.

Ideal criteria
Single, short, non-calcified lesions
Proximal lesions
Stable angina

Possible criteria
Multiple lesions in one vessel
Multiple lesions in two or more vessels
Distal lesions
Unstable angina
Acute myocardial infarction
Occluded saphenous vein grafts

sublingually) is given at the start of the procedure, and intracoronary nifedipine or nitrates can be given if there is peroperative spasm. Heparin is usually given until the patient leaves hospital, but aspirin, nifedipine and nitrates are given for six months. About 1 per cent of patients sustain a myocardial infarction, and a further 2 per cent need emergency coronary artery bypass surgery. Overall mortality is less than 1 per cent. The problem in assessing the value of coronary angioplasty is that the definition of success will differ from centre to centre. Early reports claimed success rates of 50 to 60 per cent (where the lumen was increased by more than 20 per cent) and, with improved equipment and technique, the rates have substantially improved (around 90 per cent success). The best operative results are obtained in single- as opposed to multivessel disease. Additionally, patients with single-vessel disease have a much lower mortality and morbidity rate. Acute coronary events (including myocardial infarction, perforation, embolism or death) occur in about 13.6 per cent of patients. Of these, nearly two-thirds are of a major nature (Cowley et al, 1984). Not surprisingly, the best results are obtained in young patients with a recent history, when the atheromatous plaques are short, concentric and uncalcified.

Although the patency improves in the early weeks following operation due to healing and remodelling, re-stenosis occurs in about a quarter of patients within four months; recurrence seldom occurs after nine months (Gruentzig, 1984). Second operations are usually easier to perform, with lower risk and with a larger degree of patency obtained (Dorros et al, 1983). At one year, 95 per cent of patients are symptomatically improved and 80 per cent have normal exercise stress tests.

The technique has also been used to recanalise the saphenous vein grafts used for coronary artery bypass, with varying results.

Percutaneous laser-assisted coronary angioplasty

The potential for laser energy to clear the lumen during angioplasty was first described during coronary artery bypass surgery in 1982, but has been held back by the major problem of vessel perforation (Choy et al, 1982). However, reports have started to emerge of successful use during percutaneous coronary angioplasty (Cumberland et al, 1986), although further problems of thrombosis and arterial spasm have been encountered. Certainly the technique is feasible, if only to clear a path through completely occluded vessels for passage of a traditional balloon. Clearly, this field is going to prove very interesting in the future.

Indications for angioplasty

About 10 per cent of patients awaiting coronary artery bypass surgery are suitable for this method of therapy, the procedure being limited by accessible lesions. Eccentricity and calcification of the lesions do not limit the chances of success. The prime indication for angioplasty is isolated discrete stenoses in the three major coronary arteries (left anterior descending, right and circumflex arteries). The procedure is appropriate in multivessel disease where there is one major stenosis and borderline stenoses elsewhere.

Angioplasty is not indicated for severe stenoses of the left main stem, as acute occlusion is often met with disastrous results. Long (more than 3 cm) and old stenoses are usually not treatable by this method.

TRANSPLANT SURGERY

The usual patients considered for cardiac transplantation are those with ischaemic and non-ischaemic cardiomyopathy. This is usually due to advanced ischaemic myocardial damage leading to dyskinetic or akinetic left ventricular contraction. However, primary cardiomyopathies are probably more deserving cases, and are less likely to be affected by those factors that lead to myocardial ischaemia in secondary cases. Less commonly, the operation has been performed for certain forms of congenital heart disease, or following difficult valvular replacement. The first human heart transplant was carried out in December 1967, and it has now become sufficiently commonplace not to attract public notice. Of those patients selected for transplantation, only 5 per cent will live for six months unless a donor heart can be found. Following transplantation, two-thirds of patients will survive for one year, and over one-third for five years.

Heart/lung transplantation has more recently stolen the headlines, and is carried out on patients with pulmonary hypertension. The first heart/lung transplant was performed in 1968, just a year after the first heart transplant, but it was not until 1981 that this operation began to be successful. Anatomically, it would seem much easier to transplant the heart and lungs together, since there are fewer great blood vessels to anastomose. However, the trachea needs to be connected, and since this is a relatively avascular structure healing is poor. Furthermore, the trachea is in direct contact with the air and airborne pathogens.

Heart/lung patients have other problems too. Because the nerve fibres to the lungs are divided, the cough reflex is abolished and vigorous physiotherapy is therefore required, both perioperatively and for the rest of the patient's life. The lung is also much more susceptible to ischaemic and immunological damage.

Undoubtedly, the major postoperative problem has been rejection, but the introduction of cyclosporin has revolutionised transplant surgery. The pioneering

Stanford group used this agent for the first time in March 1981 following a heart/lung transplant, with instant success (Jamieson et al, 1983). The recipient, a 45-year-old woman, is still alive. The use of cyclosporin has enabled the reduction of high-dose steroids previously required to suppress rejection, thus helping healing. The major drawback is that it is associated with progressive renal impairment in those taking it long term. Regular monitoring of the body's immune system and endomyocardial biopsies (obtained at cardiac catheterisation) must be maintained for the rest of the patient's life to detect rejection in its early stages.

The Stanford group has recently reported a summary of their work (Burke et al, 1986). Between March 1981 and August 1985, 28 heart/lung transplants had been carried out in 28 patients. Eight died in the perioperative period; ten later developed obliterative bronchiolitis, resulting in four deaths; the remaining ten patients returned to a normal life. The survival at present in these patients ranges from 3 to 53 months. So far, 34 heart/lung transplants have been carried out in Britain, the first in 1983; 23 are presently still alive.

The technical, ethical and financial problems of the heart and heart/lung transplants have made each subsequent operation a public issue. There is no doubt about the value of such an operation in terms of prolonging and increasing the quality of life. Medical research and progress needs such transplantation programmes to continue, and must be supported despite financial implications.

References

British Medical Journal (1984) Consensus Development Conference: coronary artery bypass grafting. *British Medical Journal,* **289:** 1527-1529.

Burke C M, Theodore J, Baldwin J C, Tazelaar H D, Morris A J, McGregor C, Shumway N E, Robin E D and Jamieson S W (1986) Twenty-eight cases of human heart–lung transplants. *Lancet,* **i:** 517-518.

CASS Principal Investigators and their Associates (1983) A randomised trial of coronary artery bypass surgery: survival data. *Circulation,* **68:** 939-950.

Consensus Development Conference (1984) Coronary artery bypass grafting. *British Medical Journal,* **289:** 1527-1529.

Choy D S J, Stertzer S, Rotterdam H Z, Sharock N and Kaminow I P (1982) Transluminal laser catheter angioplasty. *American Journal of Cardiology,* **50:** 1206-1211.

Cowley M J, Dorros G and Kelsey S F (1984) Acute coronary events associated with percutaneous coronary angioplasty. *American Journal of Cardiology,* **53:** 12c-16c.

Cumberland D C (1985) The current status of percutaneous coronary angioplasty. *Acta Radiologica,* **26:** 497-505.

Cumberland D C, Starkey I R, Oakley G D, Fleming J S, Smith G H, Goiti J J, Tayler D I and Davis J (1986) Percutaneous laser-assisted coronary angioplasty. *Lancet,* **ii:** 214-215.

Dorros G, Cowley M J, Simpson J, Bentivoglio L G, Block P C, Bourassa M, Detre K, Grosselin A J, Gruentzig A R, Kelsey S F, Kent K M, Mock M B, Mullin S M, Myler R K, Passamani E R, Stertzer A M and Williams D O (1983) Report of complications from the National Heart, Lung and Blood Institute PTCA register. *Circulation,* **67:** 723-730.

Dotter C T and Judkins M P (1965) Transluminal treatment of arteriosclerotic obstruction. Description of a new technique and a preliminary report of its application. *Circulation,* **30:** 654-670.

English T A H (1984) The UK cardiac surgical register (1977-1982). *British Medical Journal,* **289:** 1205-1208.

European Coronary Surgery Study Group (1980). Second interim report. *Lancet,* **ii:** 491-495.

European Coronary Surgery Study Group (1982) Longterm results of a prospective randomised study of coronary artery bypass surgery in stable angina pectoris. *Lancet,* **ii:** 1173–1180.

Favaloro R G (1969) Saphenous vein grafts in the surgical treatment of coronary artery disease. *Journal of Thoracic and Cardiovascular Surgery,* **58:** 178–185.

Gruentzig A R (1984) Percutaneous transluminal angioplasty: six years' experience. *American Heart Journal,* **107:** 818–819.

Gruentzig A R, Senning A and Siegenthaler W E (1979) Non-operative dilatation of coronary artery stenosis. *New England Journal of Medicine,* **301:** 61–68.

Hampton J R (1984) Coronary artery bypass grafting for the reduction of mortality: analysis of the trials. *British Medical Journal,* **289:** 1166–1170.

Jamieson S W, Reitz B A, Stinson E B, Oyer P E, Hunt S, Billingham M, Theodore J, Modry D, Bieber C P and Shumway N E (1983) Combined heart and lung transplantation. *Lancet,* **i:** 1130–1132.

Lancet (1984) Coronary bypass with the internal mammary. *Lancet,* **ii:** 1253–1254.

Loop F (1983) Progress in surgical treatment of coronary atherosclerosis. Parts 1 & 2. *Chest,* **84:** 611–624, 740–755.

Mirowski M, Reid P R, Mower M M, Watkins L, Gott V L, Schayble J F, Langer A, Heilman M S, Kolenik S A, Fischell R E and Weisfeldt M L (1980) Termination of malignant ventricular arrhythmias with an implanted automatic defibrillator in human beings. *New England Journal of Medicine,* **303:** 322–324.

Mock, M, Ringqvist I, Fisher L, Davis K, Chaitman B R, Kouchoukos N, Kaiser G, Alderman E, Ryan T, Russell R, Mullen S, Fray D and Killip T (1982) The survival of medically treated patients in the Coronary Artery Surgery Study (CASS) registry. *Circulation,* **66:** 562–568.

Mundth E D, Buckley M J, Leinbach R C, Gold H K, Daggett W M and Austen W G (1973) Surgical intervention for the complications of myocardial infarction. *Annals of Surgery,* **178:** 379–390.

Resnekov L (1978) Cardiogenic shock. *British Journal of Hospital Medicine,* **20:** 232–241.

Smith P L, Treasure T, Newman S P, Joseph P, Ell P J, Schneidau A and Harrison M J (1986) Cerebral consequences of cardiopulmonary bypass. *Lancet,* **i:** 823–825.

Treasure T (1983) Coronary artery bypass surgery. *British Journal of Hospital Medicine,* **30:** 259–263.

16

Therapeutics

The following is a list of some of the drugs frequently used on the coronary care unit, with doses and common side-effects. Trade names are shown in brackets. It is not fully comprehensive or complete, and serves only as a guide. Further information should always be sought from the hospital pharmacy department, manufacturers' data sheets, the *Monthly Index of Medical Specialities* (MIMS) or the *British National Formulary* (BNF), particularly if the drug is unfamiliar. The BNF is published jointly by the British Medical Association and the Pharmaceutical Society of Great Britain, and additionally contains useful sections on drug interactions, intravenous additives and advisory labelling.

ADRENALINE

Adrenaline acts on both alpha- and beta-adrenergic receptors and increases heart rate and contractility. A 1 : 10 000 solution is recommended during cardiopulmonary resuscitation (see chapter 11).
Doses 0.5–1.0 mg (5–10 ml of a 1:10 000 solution).

AMILORIDE

Amiloride (Midamor) is a potassium-conserving diuretic which acts by direct action on the distal renal tubules. Diuresis occurs over 24 hours, but full activity may be delayed for two to three days. It should not be used in renal failure or with potassium supplements or ACE inhibitors unless serum potassium is closely monitored.
Doses 5–10 mg orally.

AMIODARONE

Amiodarone (Cordarone X) is really the only potent Class III antidysrhythmic agent. It prolongs the duration of the action potential, and increases the effective refractory period of both the atria and the ventricles. Intravenously it may also have quinidine-like effects and some beta-blocking properties. It is of value in many different atrial and ventricular dysrhythmias, including re-entry tachycardias.
Doses The dose is usually 150–300 mg intravenously (5 mg/kg over 20 to 120 minutes) followed by intravenous infusion of 1 g over 24 hours. It should be given

by a centrally placed cannula, or thrombophlebitis may result. Oral therapy is usually started at the same time, since this will only be maximal after four to six days. This is because the half-life of the drug is very long (30 to 45 days). The dose is 200 mg three times daily for one week, 200 mg twice daily for one week, then 200 mg per day. Some patients require a faster loading rate and higher maintenance doses.

Side-effects Chronic use is limited by side-effects (McGovern et al, 1983), which are virtually all extracardiac.

1. Corneal deposits are universal, but usually not a problem. Periodic slit lamp examination is recommended.

2. Photosensitivity is very common, as is a bluish discoloration of the skin.

3. Thyroid dysfunction occurs in 2 to 3 per cent of patients, and there may also be problems with biochemical analysis of serum thyroid hormone levels. Thyroid function tests should be carried out before treatment, and then every six months during therapy.

4. Interstitial pulmonary fibrosis or pulmonary alveolitis may occur.

5. Abnormal liver function tests may develop.

6. Peripheral neuropathy.

ANALGESICS

Narcotic analgesics (opiates) are used to relieve moderate to severe pain. Drugs in the group all have similar effects and side-effects, but differ in their duration of action. Although primarily analgesics, they are also sedative in high doses, particularly when used in combination with other centrally acting drugs (e.g. tranquillisers). They suppress cough, cause euphoria, stimulate the vomiting centres in the brain and remove the sensation of pain. They are usually given with an anti-emetic drug.

Narcotic analgesics are usually given by slow intravenous injection or infusion following acute myocardial infarction, since intramuscular absorption may be unpredictable if there is peripheral hypoperfusion of the patient. Diamorphine is probably the best choice of analgesic, since it produces a smaller fall in blood pressure. It also produces vasodilatation, thereby reducing myocardial work and oxygen consumption. It is also much more soluble, and allows injection of smaller volumes of fluid.

Doses
- Diamorphine (heroin): 5–10 mg i.v. or i.m. repeated as required
- Morphine and cyclomorphine: 10 mg i.v. or i.m., repeated as required
- Papaveretum (Omnopon) is a mixture of the alkaloids of opium (20 mg is roughly equivalent to 12.5 mg of morphine).

Side-effects Nausea, vomiting, constipation, urinary retention, bradycardia and respiratory depression.

ANGIOTENSIN CONVERTING ENZYME INHIBITORS

Angiotensin converting enzyme (ACE) inhibitors inhibit the conversion of angiotensin-I to the potent vasoconstrictor angiotensin-II, thereby causing vasodilatation of arteries and veins. Aldosterone levels and sodium retention are also reduced. Captopril was first introduced in 1981, and enalapril followed. Both are now extensively used in the treatment of hypertension and heart failure, and both are equally effective. The once daily dosage of enalapril is, however, an advantage. In severe heart failure, peripheral arterial vasoconstriction may adversely affect the performance of the failing myocardium by increasing afterload. More importantly, vasoconstriction is responsible for symptoms such as fatigue and dyspnoea. Both captopril and enalapril have been shown to relieve symptoms and increase exercise capability in patients with heart failure. They may also reduce mortality in patients with heart failure (Consensus Trial Study Group, 1987).

ACE inhibitors lower systemic arteriolar resistance through vasodilatation without provoking an increase in heart rate. Stroke volume and cardiac output increase without a significant increase in stroke work. Renal blood flow is promoted because renovascular resistance is reduced, and naturesis is increased. Venodilatation also occurs, which reduces preload.

Doses
- Captopril (Capoten, Acepril): 6.25–150 mg daily in divided doses
- Enalapril (Innovace): 2.5–40 mg daily

Side-effects   Headache, fatigue and taste dysfunction. The first dose can produce a large and rapid fall in blood pressure, particularly in patients on diuretics. This effect is not so rapid with enalapril. The first dose should therefore be small (captopril 6.25 mg; enalapril 2.5 mg) and given with the patient in bed. Renal function and potassium levels need monitoring since the levels of creatinine, urea and potassium all rise.

ASPIRIN

Aspirin inhibits cyclo-oxygenase, an enzyme found in all cell membranes. In platelets this reduces the production of thromboxane A2 which is involved in platelet aggregation and precedes thrombosis. A single dose of aspirin (325 mg) reduces the activity of cyclo-oxygenase by 90 per cent for at least two days, thus reducing platelet aggregation.

The most beneficial use of aspirin for coronary heart disease is in unstable angina, where risk of death or progression to myocardial infarction is approximately halved (Petch, 1986). Aspirin prophylaxis after myocardial infarction probably reduces the risk of death or re-infarction by about 20 per cent.

Doses   325–1300 mg daily.

Side-effects   Upper gastrointestinal side-effects (heartburn, abdominal pain, vomiting) are common, especially at high doses.

ATROPINE

Atropine is an acetylcholine agonist at muscarinic sites, and gives rise to parasympathetic blockade. Within the heart, this means that the vagus is blocked. It is used for bradycardia causing hypotension following acute myocardial infarction.

Doses 0.3–1 mg intravenously.

Side-effects Dry mouth, confusion, tachycardia.

BETA-ADRENERGIC BLOCKING AGENTS

Since beta-adrenergic blocking agents first became clinically available in the early 1960s, they have been increasingly used in the treatment of ischaemic heart disease, dysrhythmias and hypertension (Vedin and Wilhelmsson, 1985).

Beta-blockers antagonise the effects of catecholamines by occupying their receptors, and competitively reducing occupancy. They will therefore reduce heart rate (particularly exercise-related tachycardias), myocardial contractility and systemic blood pressure. The overall effect is to reduce myocardial work and oxygen consumption. Unfortunately, the effects are sometimes offset by an increased oxygen requirement due to an increase in left ventricular end-diastolic pressure (LVEDP) and left ventricular ejection time. This may, to a certain extent, be balanced by the concomitant use of nitrates. Although there is only one type of adrenergic transmitter, there are two types of adrenergic receptor. These have been termed alpha and beta. Alpha-receptors seem to be associated with most of the usual adrenergic excitatory function such as vasoconstriction and dilatation of the pupils. Beta-functions, such as inhibition of vasoconstriction (resulting in vasodilatation) and inhibition of bronchial constriction (resulting in bronchial dilatation), are usually inhibitory. In tissues with both receptors, functions are balanced, but in tissues with only one type of receptor adrenergic activity is either excitatory or inhibitory. The heart and the bronchi have only beta-receptors; stimulation is excitatory in the heart (causing positive inotropic and chronotropic effects) but inhibitory in the bronchi (causing bronchial relaxation). To explain these opposing actions, beta-receptors have been divided into two types, termed beta-1 (cardiac) and beta-2 (bronchial). Beta-blocking agents differ in their affinity for beta-1 and beta-2 receptors (see below).

The choice of agent is usually influenced by the following properties (see table 16.1).

Half-life

Unlike the plasma half-life, the pharmacological half-life depends on the dose. Most beta-blockers can be prescribed twice daily, provided a big enough dose is given. Hydrophilic agents, however, are better suited to once daily dosage, because they have longer plasma half-lives.

Table 16.1 Properties of beta-adrenoceptor blocking drugs.

Generic name	Cardio-selectivity	Intrinsic sympathomimetic activity	Membrane-stabilising activity	Potency (propranolol = 1)	Elimination half-life (h)	Predominant route of elimination	Lipophilicity
Acebutolol	+	+	+	0.3	3–4	Renal	Low
Atenolol	+	0	0	1.0	6–9	Renal	Low
Labetalol	0	0	0	0.3	3–4	Hepatic	Low
Metoprolol	+	0	0	1.0	3–4	Hepatic	Moderate
Nadolol	0	0	0	1.0	14–24	Renal	Low
Oxprenolol	0	+ +	+	0.5–1.0	2–3	Hepatic	Moderate
Pindolol	0	+ + +	+	6.0	3–4	Renal (40%) Hepatic	Moderate
Practolol	+	+ +	0	0.3	6–8	Renal	Low
Propranolol	0	0	+ +	1.0	3–4	Hepatic	High
Sotalol	0	0	0	0.3	8–10	Renal	Low
Timolol	0	0	0	6.0–8.0	4–5	Renal (20%) Hepatic	Low

0   no effect
+   small effect
+ +   moderate effect
+ + + strong effect

Cardioselectivity

Beta-blockers differ in their relative affinity for beta-1 or beta-2 sites. Timolol, propranolol and nadolol act on both sites, and are termed 'non-specific'. However, atenolol and metoprolol act predominantly on the beta-1 cardiac sites, and are therefore termed 'cardioselective'. These drugs (e.g. metoprolol, atenolol) may therefore be safer in patients with peripheral vascular disease, or those prone to bronchospasm.

Cardioselectivity is relative, and is lost at high doses. No beta-blocker is completely safe in the presence of bronchospasm.

Intrinsic sympathomimetic activity

Intrinsic sympathomimetic activity (ISA) is the property of coexistent partial agonist activity, i.e. the drug partially stimulates the beta-sites. This property is believed to reduce the degree of cardiodepression. It is doubtful whether ISA confers any real advantages in the treatment of angina, but such drugs may have smaller effects on peripheral circulation, in congestive cardiac failure and in depression of the conducting tissue. These potentially useful properties are not useful in those patients with angina at rest, although they are of value in patients with marked resting bradycardia. Patients with asthma or diabetes are less likely to develop problems with cardioselective agents, although beta-blockers are probably not first-line therapy in these cases. Catecholamines increase glycogenolysis and lipolysis, and mobilise free fatty acids to raise blood sugar levels. As a result, not only are catecholamine-induced symptoms of insulin-induced hypoglycaemia masked, but recovery from hypoglycaemia is delayed.

Lipid solubility

Pharmacokinetics of beta-blockers vary widely depending upon whether they are soluble in fat (lipophilic) or water (hydrophilic). Lipophilic agents (e.g. propranolol) are well absorbed orally and have a short half-life. They can cross the blood–brain barrier, and may be responsible for central nervous system side-effects (e.g. nightmares) as a consequence. They are metabolised by the liver. Hydrophilic agents (e.g. atenolol), however, are poorly absorbed orally, and excreted unchanged by the kidneys. They have a long plasma half-life, and do not easily cross the blood–brain barrier.

Variation in oral bio-availability is largely influenced by 'first-pass' metabolism of lipid-soluble compounds by the liver. A reduction of dose is therefore required in liver disease. Lipid-insoluble agents (atenolol, nadolol, sotolol) are excreted only by the kidneys.

Side-effects

Common side-effects include bradycardia, heart failure, bronchospasm, nightmares, insomnia, depression and peripheral coldness. There is no good evidence that beta-blockers induce coronary artery spasm (Sleight, 1986). A small number of patients will develop Raynaud's phenomenon, partly due to unopposed alpha-adrenergic action, and partly due to a fall in cardiac output. Central nervous system side-effects are common with beta-blockers that cross the blood–brain barrier (lipid-soluble agents), especially propranolol. These may produce sedation, depression and nightmares.

Beta-blockers adversely affect serum lipid profiles (Jowett and Galton, 1987), although this may not be so severe with agents having strong ISA.

Sudden withdrawal of beta-blockade

Following sudden withdrawal of beta-blockade, there may be an increase in the number of beta-receptor sites. This manifests as an increased sensitivity to catecholamines, with an increase in myocardial work, heart rate and oxygen consumption. Angina, hypertension or even myocardial infarction may result. Patients should be warned of the dangers of suddenly stopping medication, and, if this is required, the dose should be tapered.

Therapeutic uses

There are major benefits on the oxygen supply/demand balance with the use of beta-blockers. Ninety per cent of patients with stable angina pectoris due to coronary atheroma demonstrate improved exercise tolerance and reduced chest pain (Frishman, 1981). With increased exercise capability, there is a secondary benefit in allowing patients to join training programmes. Beta-blockers also have Class II antidysrhythmic activity, and are also of particular value in supraventricular dysrhythmias. Beta-blockers reduce catecholamine concentrations in ischaemic myocardium, decrease platelet stickiness, and have been shown to modify type A behaviour (Sleight, 1986).

Beta-blockers and acute myocardial infarction

In an acute myocardial infarction, the amount of myocardial tissue that remains viable is the major determinant of patient survival. The extent of damage appears to depend upon the ratio between oxygen supply and demand. Increased demand is placed on the heart by increased sympathetic drive, producing increased chronotropic and inotropic effects. Since beta-blockers reduce myocardial work, their administration in the early phase of acute myocardial infarction might limit infarction size, as well as preventing oxygen-consuming tachydysrhythmias. Any benefits in the long term, however, would have to work by a different mechanism.

Over 65 trials (involving 50 000 patients) have so far been carried out to determine whether beta-blockers are of use in acute myocardial infarction (Yusuf et al, 1985). Despite the findings of such trials, there is still much confusion and conjecture over the use of beta blockers in acute myocardial infarction. Certainly, there is no debate where the patient has heart failure, bronchospasm or heart block, where beta-blockade is clearly contraindicated. Patients with normal left ventricular function and no rhythm disturbances form a low-risk group, and treatment is probably not justified. Those forming a high-risk group have suffered larger infarcts, often resulting in poor left ventricular function and dysrhythmias. Treatment with beta-blockers will reduce the rate of re-infarction and sudden death if they can be tolerated. Those in the intermediate group will probably gain some benefit from beta-blockade.

The evidence that early commencement of beta-blockade improves outcome is difficult to interpret. It is necessary to treat 100 to 150 patients at average risk with an intravenous beta-blocker before one life is saved, so the benefit is not large (*Lancet*, 1986). This is probably not surprising since over 50 per cent of myocardial damage takes place in the first six hours, and institution of any therapy often takes longer. However, acute intravenous beta-blockers may have a role in infarct limitation, so for selected patients therapy is often moderately and safe. For other patients who are haemodynamically stable, treatment started within the first two weeks and continued for many months seems to reduce the re-infarction rate by about 25 per cent, with a similar reduction in the occurrence of sudden deaths. This effect is most noticeable with agents without intrinsic sympathomimetic activity. Prime candidates are those patients with post-infarction angina and hypertension. Therapy should be continued for at least 18 months, and the agents at present recommended are metoprolol, timolol and propranolol.

BRETYLIUM TOSYLATE

Bretylium (Bretylate) is an adrenergic neurone-blocking agent which suppresses noradrenaline release. It has Class II antidysrhythmic properties, and is useful in ventricular dysrhythmias, especially resistant ventricular fibrillation. It is not commonly used in the UK, but is in the USA, where the choice of antidysrhythmic agents is limited.

Doses 5–10 mg/kg infused intravenously over 10 to 30 minutes. This may be repeated after one to two hours, to a total dose of 30 mg/kg.

Side-effects Postural hypotension is common, and dopamine support may be required if there are severe hypotensive episodes. Bretylium is excreted by the kidneys, and reduced doses are required in renal impairment.

BUMETANIDE

Bumetanide (Burinex) is a loop diuretic similar to frusemide. Following an intravenous injection, a diuresis starts within a few minutes to a maximum within 15 to 30 minutes. Orally, the onset is usually after 30 to 60 minutes, and the diuresis continues for about three to four hours. One milligram is about equivalent to 40–60 mg of frusemide, but at high doses direct comparison of doses is not possible, and dosage requires titration. Bumetanide may increase urine output in patients with renal failure who are unresponsive to frusemide.

Doses 1–2 mg orally or intravenously, but in renal failure doses over 5 mg are required.

Side-effects Potassium depletion, myalgia and skin rashes.

CALCIUM CHLORIDE

Although the mechanism is not fully understood, calcium ions can cause a heart in asystole to resume beating, and can increase the force of contraction. Calcium chloride is also of use in counteracting hyperkalaemia. However, its routine use during cardiac resuscitation is no longer recommended (Vincent, 1987).

Doses   It is always given intravenously, since it can cause tissue necrosis if given intramuscularly or subcutaneously. The usual dose is 2 ml of a 10 per cent calcium chloride solution (1.36 mEq/ml) repeated every five minutes.

Side-effects   If the patient is digitalised, it may cause sudden death, and should be avoided.

CALCIUM-CHANNEL BLOCKING AGENTS

Calcium-channel blocking agents are an important group of therapeutic agents with a widening range of indications (Kenny, 1985; Braunwald et al, 1985). They are remarkably safe, considering the importance of transmembrane calcium flux in many biological systems. Calcium is needed in the formation of the cardiac action potential, the regulation of cardiac contractility and the contraction of arterial smooth muscle. By preventing calcium uptake by cells, these effects are reduced, resulting in an antidysrhythmic activity, a reduction in myocardial work and vasodilatation. The calcium-channel blocking agents are able to modify the transmembrane transport of calcium ions in various tissues, although their mechanism of action and pharmacological effects differ. The main agents are nifedipine, nicardipine, verapamil and diltiazem. Verapamil has marked effects on the cardiac conduction system whereas nifedipine and nicardipine produce peripheral vasodilatation, as well as preventing coronary vasospasm. Diltiazem acts preferentially on coronary vessels producing vasodilatation, with little effect on systemic vessels.

Diltiazem (Tildiem)

Diltiazem inhibits transmission in cardiac conducting tissue, and gives rise to a mild resting bradycardia. It vasodilates the coronary arteries, whilst having little effect on peripheral vasculature. It is therefore of use in angina, but not in hypertension. It is not so negatively inotropic as other calcium-channel blockers.

Doses   60–120 mg eight hourly.

Nicardipine (Cardene)

This agent is similar to nifedipine, although cardiodepression is not so marked. It is used in the treatment of angina and hypertension.

Doses   20–30 mg eight hourly.

Nifedipine (Adalat)

Nifedipine reduces peripheral and coronary vascular resistance. It has a mild negative inotropic effect which is usually offset by increasing sympathetic activity secondary to its vasodilator effect. The dose is 15–60 mg/day in divided doses, although a sustained release form is available (Adalat SR) which is of particular value in the treatment of hypertension (up to 320 mg/day).

Verapamil (Cordilox, Berkatens, Securon)

The most striking effect of verapamil is on AV nodal conduction, making it very useful for treatment of supraventricular tachycardias. Verapamil is a Class IV antidysrhythmic agent which inhibits calcium influx through slow channels into the myocardial cells. Electrical activity in the sino-atrial and atrioventricular nodes is largely dependent on calcium ions, so verapamil is of major value in supraventricular tachycardias. As re-entry is responsible for 70 per cent of cases of supraventricular tachycardias, verapamil is the drug of choice. Following an intravenous injection (5–10 mg), AV conduction is quickly reduced, and re-entry tachycardias at the AV node are terminated (Talano and Tommaso, 1982). Orally it is not so effective because much is metabolised by the liver. If given to a patient on beta-blockers, profound hypotension or bradycardias may be produced, and care is needed. Although it is useful with digoxin in controlling the ventricular rate in atrial fibrillation and atrial flutter, it is contraindicated in atrial fibrillation complicating the Wolff–Parkinson–White syndrome, as it gives rise to preferentially accessory conduction which may result in ventricular fibrillation.

Doses The recommended dose is 5–10 mg intravenously over two to three minutes, which may be repeated after 30 minutes. Care is needed if the patient is taking other agents that act on the sino-atrial and atrioventricular nodes (especially beta-blockers), to prevent heart block and heart failure developing. Oral therapy is 40–120 mg three times a day. Higher doses are required for the treatment of angina (40–120 mg three times daily) and hypertension (120–240 mg twice daily).

Uses of the calcium-channel blocking agents

Angina

The calcium blocking agents have been used most extensively in the treatment of myocardial ischaemia. The main indication for these drugs is stable angina, and all are effective. They probably work by reducing myocardial work. Nifedipine used alone may produce a tachycardia, thus worsening stable angina, and is often better combined with a beta-blocker. The well documented anti-anginal effects of beta blockers may be augmented by the addition of a calcium-channel blocker. Verapamil usually slows the heart, and is probably superior to nifedipine when used alone (Subramanian et al, 1982). However, the combination of verapamil and a beta-blocker may depress myocardial function and conduction to produce heart block and heart failure (Winniford et al, 1985).

Calcium-channel blockers are effective in coronary artery spasm, and are useful in variant angina. Spasm also plays an important role in the genesis of crescendo angina, and the calcium-channel blockers are effective, providing symptomatic relief and reducing the rate of myocardial infarction or the need for coronary arterial surgery. Diltiazem is probably the drug of choice in these cases.

Hypertension

Nifedipine and nicardipine are powerful peripheral vasodilators, and do not have much effect on cardiac conduction. Nifedipine has emerged as a potent antihypertensive agent, and is often prescribed as a first-line agent. It is also useful in hypertensive crises. Verapamil and diltiazem are also useful, but their place in the routine treatment of hypertension is unclear (Breckenridge, 1984). This specific peripheral vasodilator effect makes them good agents for treating Raynaud's disease, and perhaps in the prevention of migraine attacks.

Cardiac dysrhythmias

Intravenous verapamil is the drug of choice in supraventricular tachycardia, with a success rate of 85 per cent (Talano and Tommaso, 1982). It may be given as a prophylactic drug for paroxysmal supraventricular dysrhythmias, and is also sometimes successful in ventricular tachycardia.

Diltiazem similarly impairs atrioventricular and sino-atrial conduction, and may also be useful in the management of supraventricular dysrhythmias.

Side-effects

The calcium-channel blocking agents are remarkably safe drugs. The most serious side-effects are those on cardiac conduction. Varying degrees of heart block and asystole can occur, especially in those with nodal disease or in patients taking beta-blockers. The drugs should not be given intravenously to those taking beta-blockers. Myocardial depression can also produce heart failure. Vasodilator effects (flushing, headache and dizziness) sometimes occur at the start of therapy, and these are most pronounced with nifedipine. Fluid retention is common, often resulting in ankle oedema. Verapamil can produce constipation, and also reduces digoxin excretion. If these two drugs are given together, the dose of digoxin should be halved. Diltiazem appears to produce fewer side-effects than the other calcium blockers as it has less effect on the heart than verapamil, and less effect on the peripheral vessels than nifedipine.

Like beta-blockers, sudden withdrawal of calcium blockers may be associated with symptoms of myocardial ischaemia or even myocardial infarction.

CORTICOSTEROIDS

Very large doses of intravenous steroids cause vasodilatation in patients with shock and peripheral vasoconstriction. This enables fluids to be given and tissue perfusion to be re-established.

Doses Variable. Single doses of methylprednisolone (30 mg/kg) have been used, with vasodilatation occurring after two to four hours.

Side-effects Many and usual. Gastrointestinal haemorrhage and hypokalaemia are often a problem.

DIAZOXIDE

Diazoxide (Eudemine) is useful in lowering systemic vascular resistance, and is most effective when given with a loop diuretic. It has a very rapid action intravenously and should thus be given with care.

Doses 300 mg in 20 ml as an intravenous bolus. For oral treatment: 400–1000 mg in two or three daily doses.

Side-effects Hyperglycaemia is inevitable and often needs concomitant treatment with tolbutamide. Fluid retention may require diuretic therapy.

DIGOXIN

Digoxin (Lanoxin) increases the force of myocardial contraction and, via the vagus, exerts a slowing of conduction at the sino-atrial and atrioventricular nodes. Therapeutic doses cause shortening of the QT interval and flattening (or inversion) of the T waves with ST segment sag. False positive ST changes may develop during exercise stress testing.

Digoxin is rapidly and almost entirely absorbed, but the effects are not directly correlated with blood levels of the drug. This is because of variable protein binding, penetration and uptake by the myocardium, and other factors. It is primarily metabolised by the kidneys within two to three days, but may accumulate in renal impairment. In some patients, digoxin is inactivated by gut flora, necessitating large oral doses to achieve satisfactory blood levels. If these patients are given broad spectrum antibiotics which affect the gut flora, digoxin toxicity may be precipitated.

The principal use of digoxin is for controlling the ventricular rate in atrial fibrillation, especially when it occurs with heart failure. Digoxin has an acute positive inotropic effect, although whether this is maintained chronically is debated (*Lancet*, 1985). It is of little value in cases of high-output failure, cor pulmonale and restrictive cardiomyopathy. Long-term use in congestive cardiac failure without rhythm disturbance is controversial, since many patients in sinus rhythm remain well after therapy with digoxin is discontinued. In patients with paroxysmal atrial fibrillation, digoxin may maintain sinus rhythm, although it is contraindicated in atrial fibrillation complicating the Wolff–Parkinson–White syndrome. Atrial flutter is converted to atrial fibrillation and sinus rhythm may then be reinstated on stopping the drug. In patients with thyrotoxicosis very large doses may be required to slow the ventricular rate, often supplemented with propranolol.

Ventricular ectopics and ventricular tachycardia have been treated with digoxin, although it must be ensured that the dysrhythmia is not actually caused by digoxin.

Digoxin following myocardial infarction

The role of digoxin in acute myocardial infarction is very controversial. In patients with left ventricular failure following acute myocardial infarction digoxin is effective, but concern surrounds increased myocardial work by the positive inotropic effect of the drug which may extend the area of myocardial necrosis. Beneficial haemodynamic effects are greatest in patients with moderate left ventricular failure, and the risk of extending myocardial damage is probably least in these patients. Post-infarction survival in patients with congestive cardiac failure and with multifocal ventricular ectopics may be improved by withholding or discontinuing digoxin.

Doses

Digoxin is very irritant to the tissues and should only be given orally or intravenously. A single intravenous dose of 1 mg by infusion produces an effect in about 10 minutes, with maximal effect at one to two hours. The half-life is 36 to 48 hours. By mouth, the effect is noted within an hour and persists for two to three days. However, some effect may still be present for a week. Digitalisation will take about a week if no loading dose is given (0.125–0.25 mg twice daily). The faster method is by giving 1–1.5 mg over 24 hours in divided doses. The usual amount of digoxin required to produce a therapeutic blood level (in a patient weighing 70 kg) is about 0.75–1.0 mg. Care is needed in the elderly, and if there is coexistent hypokalaemia, hyponatraemia or hypocalcaemia.

Radioimmunoassay techniques are available for determining blood levels of digoxin, which should not be measured within six hours of the last oral dose. Therapeutic levels are quoted at 0.5–2.5 ng/ml, but it must be remembered that the diagnosis of digoxin toxicity is clinical and too much reliance should not be placed upon laboratory results. For example, digoxin toxicity can occur at normal blood levels if there are concomitant electrolyte upsets, thyroid disease, renal impairment or hypoxia. Additionally, patients with levels greater than 2.5 ng/ml may display no signs of toxicity.

Digoxin toxicity

A major drawback to the treatment with digoxin is the narrow margin between therapeutic doses and toxicity. Hence, adverse drug actions are very common, with as many as 20 per cent of patients on the drug manifesting toxicity at some time (Aronson, 1983). There are many factors that may result in toxicity, including electrolyte imbalance and deteriorating renal function, especially in the elderly (who are most likely to be on digoxin). The early symptoms of overdose are nausea, vomiting and diarrhoea. Headache and confusion, often with visual disturbances, are more serious. Classically, *xanthopsia* (yellow vision) is reported, but flickering dots, halos and scotomata can occur.

In severe cases, there may be life-threatening dysrhythmias. Digitalis can produce virtually any sort of dysrhythmia, especially sinus bradycardia and ventricular ectopics (bigemini). Digoxin must not be used in heart block, and preferably not in those undergoing cardioversion.

Management consists of withdrawal of the drug, and restoration of electrolyte imbalance. Dysrhythmias will need therapy. In particular, supraventricular and ventricular tachycardias may respond to potassium supplementation, beta-blockade and Class 1 antidysrhythmic agents. Bradycardia will need treatment by atropine or temporary cardiac pacing.

Until recently there was no specific antidote, but a digoxin-specific antibody (Digibind) is now available, which not only binds and deactivates circulating digoxin, but additionally rapidly unloads digoxin from cardiac tissue. It therefore constitutes an effective and highly specific means of reversing advanced, life-threatening digitalis toxicity.

DISOPYRAMIDE

Disopyramide (Rythmodan, Dirythmin) is a Class I antidysrhythmic agent, with electrophysiological properties similar to quinidine. It decreases automaticity in ectopic pacemaker cells and lengthens the effective refractory period in atrial and ventricular muscle. It thus has both ventricular and supraventricular activity.

Doses The dose is 2 mg/kg by very slow intravenous injection, to a maximum of 150 mg in the first hour. An infusion of 0.4 mg/kg/h may then be employed, or oral therapy (400–800 mg in four doses). If the drug is going to work, it does so in the first 15 to 20 minutes. The usual therapeutic plasma levels are 2–4 μg/ml. Over half the drug is excreted unchanged in the urine, and dose reduction is required in patients with hepatic and renal impairment. The half-life is between 6 and 12 hours.

Side-effects It has a marked negative inotropic effect, related to both serum levels and speed of administration. It should therefore be used cautiously in patients with heart failure. Sinus node depression also sometimes occurs, so care is needed in heart block. Anticholinergic activity may cause glaucoma, retention of urine and constipation.

DOBUTAMINE

Dobutamine (Dobutrex) is a synthetic adrenergic agent, modified from isoprenaline. It stimulates beta-adrenergic cardiac receptors and thereby directly increases the force of myocardial contraction, with only small increases in heart rates. Unlike dopamine, there is little systemic vasoconstriction. This is because dopamine acts indirectly (by causing noradrenaline release) whereas dobutamine acts directly.

It is used short term in the treatment of cardiogenic shock and heart failure, and is best administered when full cardiovascular monitoring techniques are available (including Swan–Ganz catheterisation). The left ventricular filling pressure falls and the cardiac output rises.

Doses It is supplied in ampoules containing 250 mg dobutamine. Following dilution, it is added to 250 or 500 ml of dextrose or saline, giving 1000 μg/ml or 500 μg/ml respectively. It is infused intravenously, and most patients respond to a dose of

2.5–10 µg/kg/min. Some patients may need 40 µg/kg/min. Dobutamine is often given in combination with low-dose dopamine, which is used to promote renal perfusion.

DOPAMINE

Dopamine (Intropin) is the natural precursor of noradrenaline and has similar alpha- and beta-stimulatory actions, particularly at beta-1 sites. Stroke volume is increased with little effect on heart rate. It causes peripheral vasoconstriction which raises blood pressure but, unlike other sympathetic agents, produces selective renal and cerebral arterial vasodilatation. This is therefore of great use in renal hypoperfusion. At low doses, the renal effects are most marked, but as the dose increases, vasoconstriction and positive inotropic and chronotropic effects are more marked (see below). Dopamine is of major value in cardiogenic and other types of shock, and prolonged low-dose infusion is useful in heart failure.

It is given intravenously by continuous infusion, preferably by a central line. This is because of the dangers of extravasation. Profound localised tissue ischaemia may result in gangrene. This can even result in the absence of extravasation when large doses are used for long periods. Should signs of tissue necrosis develop, the area should be infiltrated with phentolamine (10 mg in 10 ml saline).

Doses   Each ampule contains 800 mg dopamine which is diluted in 500 ml of dextrose or saline, yielding 1600 µg/ml.

Calculating the rate of administration

Dopamine exerts it effect (table 16.2) by action on different receptors. The infusion is given by continuous metered infusion.

Administration of the required dose is calculated in drops per minute by the formula: Required dose (µg/kg/min) × Body weight (kg) × Total volume of infusion (ml) × Number of drops/ml dispensed by infusion pump; divided by Amount of dopamine added to infusion (mg) × 1000.

For example, for an infusion of 5 µg/kg/min in an 80 kg man given via a standard drip (20 drops/ml), the infusion rate would be:

$$\frac{5 \times 80 \times 520 \times 20}{800 \times 1000} = \frac{4\,160\,000}{800\,000}$$
$$= 5.2 \text{ drops/min}$$

Table 16.2.   Effects of dopamine at different doses.

Dose (µg/kg/min)	Effect
1–5	Dilates renal and mesenteric arterioles to produce increased renal blood flow and glomerular filtration rate and urine output.
5–20	Direct inotropic effect on the heart with dose-related increase in cardiac output and heart rate.
> 20	Direct alpha-action leads to peripheral vasoconstriction which raises blood pressure. There are further inotropic and chronotropic effects on the heart.

Dopamine is contraindicated in patients with uncontrolled dysrhythmias and those taking monoamine oxidase inhibitors. Hypovolaemia should always be corrected before its use, and therapy should be withdrawn slowly and not stopped abruptly.

FLECAINIDE

Flecainide (Tambocor) is a Class Ic agent which has no effect on the duration of the action potential, but slows conduction through the His–Purkinje system and prevents retrograde conduction through accessory pathways. It is useful in chronic ventricular dysrhythmias and in re-entry tachycardias, especially the Wolff–Parkinson–White syndrome.

Doses It is available for intravenous and oral use, and its long half-life allows a twice daily dosage. Intravenously it should be given by slow injection or infusion (2 mg/kg). Oral maintenance is 100–200 mg twice daily.

Side-effects Pro-arrhythmic side-effects have been described in patients with pacemakers, and caution is therefore required. It is also negatively inotropic. Dizziness and blurred vision may occur.

FRUSEMIDE

Frusemide (Lasix, Dryptal, Aluzine) is a powerful loop diuretic, similar to bumetanide. When given intravenously for left ventricular failure, the relief is almost immediate, and occurs before a diuresis has taken place. This suggests that the prime value in acute heart failure is due to a vascular effect, by causing increased venous capacitance, and the diuretic effect is secondary.

Doses The usual dose is 40–80 mg orally, intramuscularly or intravenously. Patients with refractory oedema or renal impairment may require very large doses (500–1000 mg).

Side-effects Transient or permanent deafness may result if frusemide is injected too rapidly, particularly in those with renal impairment. Large doses must be diluted, and intravenous infusion is then a preferable method of administration.

HEPARIN

Heparin is naturally occurring high molecular weight mucopolysaccharide with marked anticoagulation properties. It is inactive orally, and must therefore be given subcutaneously or intravenously. Intramuscular injection may produce large haematomas. It has been used prophylactically to prevent thromboembolism, and in the treatment of deep vein thrombosis and pulmonary emboli (Goldberg et al, 1984).

It acts by combining with antithrombin III in the coagulation cascade, preventing the formation of factor Xa. It probably also reduces platelet stickiness. Unlike warfarin, it does not block prothrombin formation in the liver.

The activated partial thromboplastin time (APTT) is used as an index of efficacy, and should be maintained at about twice normal. Thrombocytopenia often occurs and platelet counts should be checked on alternate days.

Overdose producing prolonged coagulation times should be corrected by reducing the dose or stopping the drug altogether (the half-life is only 1.5 hours). More urgent cases can be treated with protamine sulphate (1 mg neutralises 100 units heparin within five minutes). However, since protamine is a weak anticoagulant itself, doses exceeding 50 mg should not be given.

Heparin regimens

- *Low dose* (prophylaxis)   5000 units twice daily, subcutaneously. APTTs are not required.
- *Medium dose* (treatment of deep vein thrombosis or disseminated intravascular coagulation)   30 000–45 000 units daily by infusion or four hourly by intravenous injection. After 48 hours the dose is reduced by about 50 per cent and adjusted according to APTTs. Warfarin is usually started at the same time.
- *High dose* (pulmonary embolism, systemic embolisation)   A bolus loading dose of 5000–10 000 units should be given followed by intravenous infusion, but there should be no reduction in dose at 48 hours as above. Warfarin is usually not started acutely.

HYDRALAZINE

Hydralazine (Apresoline) is an arteriolar vasodilator used in the treatment of aortic dissection, heart failure and hypertension. It increases heart rate and cardiac output by reducing afterload, and also increases renal and cerebral perfusion. However, myocardial work and oxygen consumption are also increased, and angina may be precipitated.

Doses   The oral dose is 25–75 mg three to four times daily.

Side-effects   Due to vasodilatation, with postural hypotension, headache and flushing. Long-term therapy may cause a lupus syndrome with positive LE cells (SLE).

INSULIN

Hyperglycaemia in the peri-infarction period is best treated with insulin, since oral hypoglycaemic agents may cause unwanted metabolic side-effects, particularly if there is renal and hepatic hypoperfusion. Soluble insulin of human origin (e.g. Humulin S) is probably the best choice (to prevent formation of insulin antibodies) and should preferentially be given by intravenous infusion. Hypoglycaemia should be avoided, as the induced catecholamine response may lead to tachydysrhythmias.

LIGNOCAINE

In addition to its local anaesthetic properties, lignocaine (Xylocard) is a Class I antidysrhythmic agent of particular value in ventricular dysrhythmias. It has mild negative inotropic and chronotropic activity and may produce marked side-effects in the central nervous system (sedation, respiratory depression or convulsions).

The drug is first choice in the treatment of ventricular dysrhythmias following acute myocardial infarction, although about 20 per cent of patients do not respond.

Doses   The usual dose is a 100 mg bolus injection, followed by an intravenous infusion at 4 mg/min. After 30 minutes this is reduced to 2 mg/min for two hours and then 1 mg/min. However, smaller doses may be as effective, and prevent cardiodepression and central nervous system side-effects. Hence, a 50 mg bolus (0.75–1.0 mg/kg), followed by an infusion of 1–2 mg/min (25–50 µg/kg/min) is probably preferable. Blood levels can be measured, and should not exceed 5 µg/ml. A 100 mg intramuscular injection into the deltoid muscle has been claimed to be useful if there is delay in transport of the patient to the coronary care unit. However, absorption of lignocaine is erratic, and the injection may cause elevation of creatinine phosphokinase levels. The efficacy of lignocaine in preventing primary ventricular fibrillation is still unproven (Kertes and Hunt, 1984).

Side-effects   Fits and respiratory arrest may be provoked by high doses. Bradycardia and cardiac arrest may occur.

METOCLOPRAMIDE

Metoclopramide (Maxolon) is a centrally acting anti-emetic agent, which also promotes gastric emptying. Oesophageal reflux is reduced, and small bowel transit time is increased.

Doses   10 mg orally, i.v. or i.m.

Side-effects   Drowsiness, dizziness and dystonic movements of the head and neck.

MEXILETINE

Mexiletine (Mexitil) is very similar to lignocaine but can be given orally, and sometimes works in lignocaine-resistant dysrhythmias. It is used in the treatment of ventricular dysrhythmias in ischaemic heart disease and following myocardial infarction.

Doses   An intravenous loading dose of 100–250 mg is given over 5–10 minutes, and is followed by a reducing infusion starting at 2 mg/min for one hour, then 1 mg/min for two hours, down to 0.05 mg/min until no longer required or oral therapy is instituted.

Oral loading is with 400 mg, followed by 200–250 mg three or four times daily. A slow release preparation is available.

Side-effects   These are related to blood levels, and reduction in doses may be required for light-headedness, tremor and blurred vision. Gastrointestinal side-effects sometimes limit its value (nausea, vomiting, hiccoughs).

NITRATES

Organic nitrates have been the mainstay in the treatment of angina pectoris for over 100 years, and more recently in the treatment of heart failure. The benefits arise from the combination of coronary and non-coronary actions, and different forms of ischaemic heart disease may respond differently. Nitrates relax vascular smooth muscle, mainly in the venous system, to increase capacitance and thus reduce preload to the heart. Arteriolar relaxation also occurs with a fall in peripheral resistance (afterload). Although not a main action, coronary dilatation probably occurs, which may improve regional myocardial blood flow. These effects are most marked when the coronary arterial stenosis is due to spasm rather than a fixed lesion. Nitrates are, however, less effective when compared with calcium antagonists in the treatment of coronary artery spasm and Prinzmetal angina (Conti, 1985). Sublingual glyceryl trinitrate (GTN) is accepted as standard treatment for acute episodes of angina, and the longer acting variants are used as prophylaxis against attacks. Tolerance may develop rapidly after the initiation of therapy, but disappears quickly after disconti-nuing the drug (Cowan, 1986). Cross-tolerance with different preparations is also thought to occur. Tolerance appears to be a function of constant plasma levels of nitrates and is less likely to occur when nitrate levels fluctuate. Preparations designed to give 24-hour therapeutic plasma levels (e.g. transdermal nitrates) may therefore be associated with tolerance, and should probably only be used at night in cases of nocturnal angina. Long-acting oral nitrates should therefore be given as intermittent therapy, two or three times daily, and allowing a nocturnal nitrate-free period (Parker et al, 1987).

Uses

The commonest indication for nitrate therapy is in the treatment and prophylaxis of angina. Recently nitrates have been used in acute left ventricular failure, hypertension and the early phase of evolving acute myocardial infarction, with the hope of diminishing peri-infarction ischaemic zones, and thus limiting the size of infarction (Conti, 1985; Johansson, 1986).

Choice

The haemodynamic effects of GTN are short lasting, and therefore many different preparations have been developed to prolong their effect and make them useful as prophylactic agents.

Sublingual GTN (0.3, 0.5 or 0.6 mg)

These tablets should be used as early as possible after the onset of angina, or prophylactically before physical activity. If the pain persists, the tablets may be repeated
at five-minute intervals until relief is obtained. It must always be explained that the
drug is neither addictive nor to be reserved for emergencies only. Headache and
hypotension are common, and may be avoided if the pill is swallowed or spat out as
soon as relief is obtained. The tablets are deactivated by heat and light, and must
therefore be kept cool and in a dark bottle. The activity of the drug after opening
is only eight weeks, and old tablets should be discarded. Tablets are also deactivated
if cotton-wool is placed in the bottle: the chemicals are absorbed by it.

Oral nitrates

There is an extensive 'first-pass' effect on nitrates when taken orally. That is, the
amount of drug reaching systemic circulation is very much reduced because of metabolism by the liver (the first major organ encountered after drug absorption from the
gut). As a result, as little as 10 per cent of the drug may reach the circulation, although
prolonged action can be achieved by using higher or more frequent doses. Isosorbide
dinitrate (Isordil, Sorbitrate, Cedocard) is swallowed whole in doses of 10–60 mg four
to six hourly. The onset of action is after about 30 minutes, but faster if the tablet
is chewed. Isosorbide mononitrate (Ismo 20, Elantan) is thought not to be so extensively removed on first pass, and allows smaller doses to be given (20–40 mg eight
hourly).

Buccal nitrates

Sublingual GTN, Sorbichew and Nitrolingual sprays are rapidly acting preparations
which can bypass the hepatic circulation, and consequently may have better effect.
Suscard Buccal is a form of nitrate which has been impregnated into an inert polymer
matrix, allowing slow diffusion of the drug across the buccal mucosa. The pill is
tucked under the top lip without chewing, and a gel-like coating forms around the
drug, allowing it to adhere to the buccal mucosa. Slow absorption can then take place
as long as the pill remains intact (usually three to five hours).

Transdermal nitrates

The use of cutaneous nitrates has been known for 30 years, and GTN ointment and
slow release skin preparations which hold a reservoir of GTN are available.
Cutaneous applications circumvent the first-pass metabolism of swallowed nitrates.
Therapeutic blood levels are achieved within an hour, and last for up to 24 hours.
The patches are applied to any clean, dry, non-hairy part of the skin, although the
extremities should be avoided. Their absorption depends upon site and blood flow,
and large amounts are sometimes required to produce therapeutic blood levels. Skin
irritation and variable absorption limit their use, but there is a high placebo effect,
especially if patches are applied over the heart. GTN ointment (Percutol) is messy to
use, and requires frequent application to produce a sustained effect. Each tube is

provided with a measure so that the required length of cream (1–2 inches) can be applied under waxed paper, applied for four to eight hours. Cutaneous prepacked patches containing 5 or 10 mg of GTN behind a special slow release membrane (Transiderm-Nitro, Deponit 5) prevent the application from being rubbed or washed off, and may last much longer. About 5 mg GTN is released in 24 hours.

Intravenous nitrates

Intravenous GTN (Tridil) and isosorbide dinitrate (Isoket) are useful in the management of unstable angina, prolonged infarction pain and left ventricular failure. The dose required for pain relief varies widely, and the infusion rate (1–10 mg/h) must be titrated against pain and blood pressure.

Side-effects

The major side-effects of nitrates are due to vasodilatation which may give rise to hypotension, tachycardia and headache. Alcohol will potentiate the effects. Side-effects will not be so prominent with continued use, if the patient can be persuaded to persevere. Beta-blockers given at the same time may help slow the heart, and relieve the headache. The nitrate ion reacts with haemoglobin to produce methaemoglobinaemia, but quantities are usually trivial.

Hypotension and reflex tachycardia during intravenous infusion can be treated by slowing or stopping the infusion, since the half-life of intravenous GTN is only one to two minutes.

NORADRENALINE

Noradrenaline stimulates cardiac beta-1 receptors to produce a positive inotropic effect and raise the blood pressure (especially the systolic blood pressure). Baroreceptor stimulation limits a simultaneous tachycardia. Alpha-adrenergic vasoconstriction takes place in vascular beds except in the cerebral and coronary vessels, which dilate.

Noradrenaline may be useful in septic shock, although not following acute myocardial infarction. It augments coronary perfusion and raises the blood pressure, although peripheral vasoconstriction may increase cardiac afterload and myocardial work without increasing cardiac output. It may also constrict renal capillary beds, leading to renal hypoperfusion.

Doses   1–2 µg/min are infused centrally until the blood pressure rises.

Side-effects   Renal hypoperfusion and increased myocardial work. If the drug is allowed to run in too fast, hypertensive crises may occur, leading to stroke and myocardial infarction.

OUABAIN

Ouabain is a potent digitalis glycoside, obtained from the *Strophanthus* seed. It is not active orally, but when given intravenously has a quicker onset of action and shorter effect than intravenous digoxin. Ouabain has been withdrawn in the UK, but may still be available in some places.

PHENYTOIN

Although primarily used as an anticonvulsant, phenytoin (Epanutin) has Class Ib antidysrhythmic action, and is particularly of value in ventricular dysrhythmias, especially if digitalis induced. This is because it shortens prolonged QT intervals, increases AV nodal conduction and suppresses ventricular ectopic activity.

Doses An intravenous dose of 250 mg produces an effect in 5 to 20 minutes. Oral doses are from 200 to 600 mg daily.

Side-effects Ventricular fibrillation, heart block and respiratory depression may result following intravenous administration. Oral therapy may be limited by ataxia, skin rashes and blood dyscrasias.

PROCAINAMIDE

Procainamide (Pronestyl) is derived from the local anaesthetic procaine, and has Class I antidysrhythmic properties, similar to quinidine (see below). It is seldom an agent of first choice, but is of value in the treatment of ventricular ectopics, ventricular tachycardia, and paroxysmal atrial tachycardia.

Doses Oral treatment is preferred: 250 mg four times daily. The usual effective antidysrhythmic plasma concentration is 4–8 µg/ml.

Intravenous administration should be under ECG control, with 100 mg being given over five minutes or by infusion.

Side-effects Toxicity is rare at plasma levels under 12 µg/ml. Gastrointestinal side-effects are common, and a lupus syndrome (SLE) has been described with long-term usage.

PROCHLORPERAZINE

Prochlorperazine (Stemetil) is a phenothiazine derivative often used in the treatment of nausea and vomiting. It may be associated with postural hypotension, and metoclopramide may therefore be a better choice in coronary care units.

Side-effects Dry mouth, drowsiness and extrapyramidal signs.

Doses Can be given orally (5–10 mg), rectally (5 mg) or by deep intramuscular injection (12.5 mg). Intravenous injection is not recommended, as it is an irritant.

QUINIDINE

Quinidine (Kinidin) is the dextro-isomer of quinine and, in addition to antipyretic properties, has Class I antidysrhythmic properties similar to procainamide. It also has anticholinergic activity, thus aiding AV conduction. It is not commonly used now because it is unpleasant to take (nausea, vomiting), and can cause severe side-effects such as ventricular fibrillation and heart block.

Doses   Orally, 500 mg twice daily, adjusted as required.

Side-effects   Gastrointestinal symptoms are common. Cardiodepression and heart block may occur, and the drug should be stopped if the QRS duration increases to longer than 0.14 second.

SODIUM BICARBONATE

Sodium bicarbonate is widely used intravenously for the correction of acidaemia. It may be of value to correct the metabolic acidosis which precedes or follows cardiorespiratory arrest, and can also be used as a temporary measure to correct hyperkalaemia.

Its use during cardiopulmonary resuscitation is no longer recommended, and correction of acidosis should be primarily by alveolar hyperventilation (see chapter 11).

Sodium bicarbonate is irritant to the tissues, particularly the 8.4 per cent solution frequently made available. Additionally, since the drug is very alkaline, many other drugs will precipitate out if mixed (e.g. calcium chloride).

SODIUM NITROPRUSSIDE

Sodium nitroprusside (Nipride) is a well tolerated and potent parenteral vasodilator which may be employed in hypertensive emergencies and severe left ventricular failure. It relaxes both arteriolar and venous smooth muscle. It acts rapidly (within two minutes), and should be given by controlled intravenous infusion. The drug is light sensitive. Solutions are normally red/brown in colour, and deterioration is marked by a colour change to blue.

Doses   The drug should be freshly prepared (in 5 per cent dextrose), and used within four hours. The normal adult dose for heart failure is 10–15 µg/min, adjusted as required. Doses should normally not exceed 400 µg/min. The maximal dose is 700–800 mg in 24 hours, and the drug is best not given for periods exceeding 72 hours because of the build-up of plasma cyanide. If therapy is needed for more than three days, cyanide and thiocyanate levels should be assayed.

Side-effects   Nausea, sweating, dizziness and twitching denote toxicity. These should be treated by stopping the drug and administering sodium thiosulphate if signs persist. Unexplained cyanosis may be due to formation of methaemoglobinaemia. Large doses of hydroxocobalamin (vitamin B12, 1.5 mg/kg) may be used prophylactically to reduce plasma cyanide levels.

TOCAINIDE

This Class Ib agent (Tonocard) is similar to lignocaine and mexiletine, but is virtually completely absorbed following oral administration. It is used in the therapy of severe and recurrent ventricular dysrhythmias, associated with compromised left ventricular function.

Doses 500–750 mg by slow intravenous injection or infusion, followed by 600–800 mg orally. Maintenance therapy is by 1200–2400 mg in divided doses.

Side-effects Gastrointestinal side-effects are very common, and morbilliform skin rashes may be severe.

VERAPAMIL

See Calcium-channel blockers.

WARFARIN

Warfarin (Marevan) inhibits the action of vitamin K in the liver, and thus inhibits synthesis of four plasma procoagulants (II, VII, IX and X). Its effect commences at about 12 hours, and lasts between two and five days. Numerous dosage schedules have been described (e.g. 10 mg daily for three days and then adjusted to keep the prothrombin time at two to three times normal). Over-anticoagulation is treated by reducing the daily dose or stopping the drug altogether. If required, vitamin K1 (phytomenadione) may be given (10 mg over two to three minutes).

Many factors affect the potency of warfarin.

- *Increased potency* Heart failure, liver disease, fever, alcohol, aspirin, cimetidine, diuretics, antibiotics, oral hypoglycaemics.
- *Decreased potency* Diabetes, hypothyroidism, hyperlipidaemia, sedatives, oral contraceptives, cholestyramine, antacids.

The introduction of the World Health Organisation system for international standardisation of prothrombin times has allowed comparison of anticoagulant control regimens based upon common systems of reporting, termed international normalised ratios (INR). (See table 16.3.)

Table 16.3. Proposed therapeutic ranges of warfarin (after Poller, 1985).

INR	Condition
2–2.5	Prophylaxis
2–3	Treatment of deep vein thrombosis, pulmonary emboli and transient ischaemic attacks
3–4.5	Recurrent thromboembolic phenomena, arterial grafts, prosthetic valves, myocardial infarction and heart failure

Anticoagulant therapy in acute myocardial infarction

In theory, anticoagulants should be given in all cases of acute myocardial infarction to prevent or limit the progression of coronary thrombosis. In addition, they may help prevent deep venous thrombosis and subsequent pulmonary embolisation. However, despite many trials, there is no evidence for or against the early usage of anticoagulants (Goldberg et al, 1984). Acute anticoagulation with heparin (subcutaneous or intravenous) is probably the therapy of choice, with long-term warfarin therapy being used in cases of atrial fibrillation, cardiac dilatation and severe heart failure.

References

Aronson J K (1983) Digitalis toxicity. *Clinical Science,* **64:** 253–258.
Braunwald E, Muller J E and Stone P H (1985) Use of calcium channel blocking agents in the management of ischaemic heart disease. *European Heart Journal,* **6:** 31–34.
Breckenridge A (1984) A third drug in hypertension. *British Medical Journal,* **289:** 859–860.
Consensus Trial Study Group (1987) Effects of enalapril on mortality in severe congestive heart failure. *New England Journal of Medicine,* **316:** 1429–1435.
Conti C R (1985) Nitrate therapy in ischaemic heart disease. *European Heart Journal,* **6:** 3–11.
Cowan J C (1986) Nitrate tolerance. *International Journal of Cardiology,* **12:** 1–19.
Frishman W H (1981) Beta-adrenergic antagonists. New drugs and new indications. *New England Journal of Medicine,* **305:** 500–506.
Goldberg R J, Gore J M and Dalen J E (1984) The role of anticoagulant therapy in acute myocardial infarction. *American Heart Journal,* **108:** 1387–1393.
Johansson B W (1986) Nitrate therapy today. *Acta Pharmacologica et Toxicologica,* **59** (Suppl. 6): 7–16.
Jowett N I and Galton D J (1987) The management of the hyperlipidaemias. In: *Drugs for Heart Disease,* ed. Hamer J, 2nd edn., p. 359. London: Chapman and Hall.
Kenny J (1985) Calcium channel blocking drugs and the heart. *British Medical Journal,* **291:** 1150–1152.
Kertes P and Hunt D (1984) Prophylaxis of primary ventricular fibrillation in acute myocardial infarction. *British Heart Journal,* **52:** 241–247.
Lancet (1985) Needless digoxin. *Lancet,* **ii:** 1048.
Lancet (1986) Intravenous beta-blockade during acute myocardial infarction. *Lancet,* **ii:** 79–80.
McGovern B, Garan H, Kelly E and Ruskin J N (1983) Adverse reactions during treatment with amiodarone hydrochloride. *British Medical Journal,* **287:** 175–180.
Parker J O, Farrell B, Lahey K A and Moe G (1987) Effect of intervals between doses on the development of tolerance to isosorbide dinitrate. *New England Journal of Medicine,* **316:** 1440–1444.
Petch M C (1986) Aspirin for unstable angina? *British Medical Journal,* **293:** 1–2.
Poller L (1985) Therapeutic ranges in anticoagulant administration. *British Medical Journal,* **290:** 1683–1686.
Sleight P (1986) Beta-adrenoreceptor blockade in the treatment of coronary heart disease. *European Heart Journal,* **7** (Suppl. C): 79–91.
Subramanian V B, Bowles M J, Khurmi M S, Davies A B and Raftery E B (1982) Randomized double blind comparison of verapamil and nifedipine in chronic stable angina. *American Journal of Cardiology,* **50:** 696–703.
Talano J V and Tommaso C (1982) Slow channel calcium antagonists in the treatment of supraventricular tachycardia. *Progress in Cardiovascular Diseases,* **25:** 141–156.
Vedin A and Wilhelmsson C (1985) Medical treatment of ischaemic heart disease – beta blockers. *European Heart Journal,* **6:** 13–27.

Vincent J L (1987) Should we still administer calcium during cardiopulmonary resuscitation? *Intensive Care Medicine,* **13:** 369–370.

Winniford M D, Fulton K L, Corbett J R, Croft C H and Hillis L D (1985) Propranolol–verapamil versus propranolol–nifedipine in severe angina of effort: a randomised double blind crossover study. *American Journal of Cardiology,* **55:** 281–285.

Yusuf S, Peto R, Lewis J, Collins R and Sleight P (1985) Beta-blockade during and after myocardial infarction: an overview of the randomised trials. *Progress in Cardiovascular Diseases,* **27:** 335–371.

Appendix

Useful addresses

ASH (Action for Smoking on Health), 5-11 Mortimer Street, London W1N 7RH.
Tel: 01-637 9843

British Anti-Smoking Education, 78 Langley Road, Watford, Herts. WD1 3PL.
Tel: (0923) 21348

British Heart Foundation, 102 Gloucester Place, London W1H 4OH.
Tel: 01-935 0185

British Holistic Medical Association, 23 Harley House, Marylebone Road, London NW1 5HE.
Tel: 01-487 4227

Chest, Heart & Stroke Association, Tavistock House North, Tavistock Square, London WC1H 9JE.
Tel: 01-387 3012

Coronary Artery Disease Research Association (CORDA), 47 Wimpole Street, London W1M 7DG.
Tel: 01-834 5000

Familial Hypercholesterolaemia Association, PO Box 116, Kidlington, Oxford OX5 1OT.
Tel: (08675) 79125

Health Education Authority, 78 New Oxford Street, London WC1A 1AH.

International Society for Humanism in Cardiology, 43 Weymouth Street, London W1.
Tel: 01-486 4191

National Society of Non-Smokers, Latimer House, 40-48 Hanson Street, London W1P 7DE.
Tel: 01-636 9103

Resuscitation Council, Department of Anaesthetics, Royal Postgraduate Medical School, Hammersmith Hospital, London W12 0HS.

Index